Ten Key Formula Families
in Chinese Medicine

TEN KEY FORMULA FAMILIES IN CHINESE MEDICINE

....

Huang Huang

....

TRANSLATED BY MICHAEL MAX

EASTLAND PRESS ❧ SEATTLE

Originally published in Chinese in 1994 by
Jiangsu Science and Technology Publishing House.
A revised edition was published in 2007.

English language edition ©2009 Eastland Press, Inc.

Published by Eastland Press, Inc.
P.O. Box 99749
Seattle, WA 98139, USA
www.eastlandpress.com

ISBN: 978-0-939616-68-8
Library of Congress Control Number: 2009900832
Printed in the United States of America

4   6   8   10   9   7   5   3

Cover illustration by Arne Bendik Sjur
Cover design by Patricia O'Connor

Book design by Gary Niemeier

TABLE OF CONTENTS

....

. . . .

THERE IS a defining moment in the study of Chinese language when you realize that the page of text you are looking at is actually right side up. While this seems like a ridiculously simple skill, it is, in fact, one of the cornerstones on which one builds a foundation of understanding. In any endeavor, we must be able to orient ourselves; we need a compass that helps us to navigate.

Doctor Huang's book *Ten Key Formula Families in Chinese Medicine* provides us with a clinical perspective that not only helps us orient and focus our clinical thinking around the prescription of herbal medicines, but also gives us deeper insight into how herbal formulas are related to each other, and how those formula families relate to constitution.

Doctor Huang's perspective is new to many of us in the West, and for that matter in China as well, as his methods of clinical reasoning and treatment are not considered to be mainstream. The methods he shares with us are rooted in streams that stretch back to the early Qing-dynasty writings of Xu Ling-Tai (徐靈胎), and even to passages in *Discussion of Cold Damage* (傷寒論 *Shāng hán lùn*). Additionally, they touch on the Kampō tradition of Japan that has also influenced his thinking. We are fortunate to have practitioners like Dr. Huang who are able to draw deeply from the well of Chinese medicine's knowledge, have the liveliness of mind to synthesize the contributions of doctors from the past, apply it clinically in our modern life, and explain it all in a way that allows it to come alive in the minds of his students.

Ten Key Formula Families in Chinese Medicine was slipped into my hands by Craig Mitchell shortly after I had failed in my studies with a *Discussion of Cold Damage* doctor in Beijing in the winter of 2002. My Chinese was just not up to the task at that time. "Keep working on your Chinese," he said, "it takes time, and plenty of it. In the meantime, read this. It has some interesting perspectives." Indeed it does. Doctor Huang's consideration of constitution and how that relates to formula families helped me see how certain patients are a 'match' for a particular herb, and how that kind of clinical reasoning can provide both a platform and perspective for making sense out of an herbal tradition woven over the course of millenia. No wonder we find Chinese medicine to be so confusing in our day; it is a tapestry of methods and reasoning that spans both time and culture. The book you hold in your hands is not in any way an integrative work, and I suspect it may raise as many questions as it answers. But it does have a particular perspective that can help us focus our clinical eye.

This English edition of *Ten Key Formula Families in Chinese Medicine* differs from the original in that it includes useful insights that have come from conversations I had with Dr. Huang, both in working through the translation itself, and from the time I spent with him in his clinic. These clinical gems are woven into the text, along with the words of Zhang Zhong-Jing and Dr. Huang's own clinical experience.

It has been a great pleasure to know and work with Dr. Huang, and to experience how the knowledge he readily shares has helped the patients I have seen in my own clinic. I am delighted to be able to introduce, through the translation of this book, some methods that will allow you to be of more service to your patients.

It is deceiving, the amount of work and energy required to dig the English out of one little book on Chinese medicine. It is not a task that is accomplished single-handedly. A word of thanks to Eastland Press for their interest in doing this book and to the various friends who have helped with proofreading; their comments and suggestions have added depth and clarity to the book. Gratitude to my editor, Dan Bensky, for his support and challenge in bringing this book into English; his appreciation of Chinese medicine and knowledge of *Discussion of Cold Damage* have added immeasurably to this work.

Finally, a special word of thanks to Xiaozhu who saw me reading *Ten Key Formula Families* on a lazy fall afternoon in Yangshuo, and upon hearing me say that "Someday, I'd like to translate this and share it with English-speaking doctors of Chinese medicine around the world," asked the simple question that has been a guiding star on this journey: "What's stopping you?"

— MICHAEL MAX

TEN KEY FORMULA FAMILIES IN CHINESE MEDICINE was published 15 years ago, and since that time, this little volume has received extensive favorable comments from its readers. Not only has it been reprinted many times in China, it has also been translated into Japanese and Korean, printed with traditional characters in Taiwan, and even published in pirated editions. I am much indebted to Eastland Press for their kindness and support of the English publication of this book. This has been a major joy in my professional career.

Chinese medicine originated here in China, but it is a cultural heritage in which all people can share. It allows the ancient medicine of China to contribute to the health and well-being of people in our times, which is an ideal of many of us who practice Chinese medicine. In my life as a professor of Chinese medicine, whenever I see a group of foreign friends that have come to China to increase their knowledge of Chinese medicine, my heart often feels a complicated mixture of joy and concern. The joy comes from knowing that the influence of Chinese medicine abroad is greatly increasing; the world has begun to use and understand Chinese medicine. The concern is for those from abroad who are unable to engage the medicine in Chinese. Will they be able to learn anything of Chinese medicine in a short amount of time? Will they study the genuine medicine of China?

Chinese medicine is not easy, and the fundamentals are a difficult study. What I have realized from 35 years of involvement with Chinese medicine is that there are different forms of Chinese medicine as a result of its extremely long history, with a multitude of currents of thought and practice, each with its own complexities and techniques. These differences are augmented by the changing conditions across dynasties, across geographical locations, and among the many practitioners who have used this medicine through the ages. There is a danger that those just entering into the study of Chinese medicine, should they take the wrong road, will end up working twice as hard for half the result, or worse yet, have to undo all their previous work. So, the key to studying Chinese medicine well is to choose the right path.

The best approach to Chinese medicine is through a study of the classic formulas. These famous formulas, which mostly come from *Discussion of Cold Damage* (傷寒論 *Shāng hán lùn*) and *Essentials from the Golden Cabinet* (金匱要略 *Jīn guì yào lüè*), have been used over and over again as they have been passed down through the generations over thousands of years to the present day. These classic formulas not only have proven effectiveness, but also contain the classical medical conceptions of the human body along with how illnesses should be treated. They contain the essence and spirit of Chinese medicine that provide the standards and foundation for Chinese traditional medicine.

Sixty-four main formulas were selected for inclusion in this book; it is not a book that discusses the definition of formulas, but one that describes formula presentations. A formula presentation consists of the signs and symptoms that confirm that a formula is appropriate to use. Formula presentations are as easy to grasp as they are objective and practical; they are the keys to studying the classic formulas. To aid the reader's understanding and memory, in this book the classic formulas have been grouped together by their indications.

The cinnamon twig formula family, ephedra formula family, bupleurum formula family, and the others chosen for inclusion in this book are ten influential families in the world of Chinese medicine that will allow the reader to gain a clear understanding of the patient's condition from a single glance. Although these classic formulas are not the entirety of Chinese medicine, it could be said that they embody the essence of this medicine, as they are a summary of the wisdom and knowledge of the ancient Chinese use of naturally occurring medicinals. By learning the fundamentals of the classic formulas, it is easy to reach a high level of proficiency; in this way, it is not difficult to go deeply into the study of Chinese medicine.

This book was written for those beginning their study of Chinese medicine. As much as possible, I have used simple language that is easy to understand. Furthermore, the use of technical explanatory language commonly found in the textbooks used in China has been minimized. I hope that this will not be an obstacle to the translation of this book into other languages. The classic formulas are used to treat illnesses; therefore, the content strives as best it can to be eminently practical. Especially because this book highlights modern uses of the classic formulas, it makes these famous classical formulas quite attractive to the contemporary reader! As a result, young people beginning their study of medicine will be especially fond of this book.

Michael Max is a practitioner from America who has a love for China and Chinese medicine as well as the classic formulas; he is the person responsible for the translation of this book. He has been to China many times in the past and is a close associate who has a good understanding of my thinking and clinical style. In the process of translating this book, Michael and I have had many discussions concerning how to shrink the cultural divide between China and the West so that the beauty of the classic formulas could unfold in the minds of Western readers. I am grateful to Michael for his effort. As Chinese medicine spreads around the world, we will need more people with his enthusiasm for the subject.

It is my heartfelt desire that readers of *Ten Key Formula Families in Chinese Medicine* will gain inspiration and assistance from this book. I hope that this study and use of the classic formulas will be a contribution to the health and well-being of all humanity.

I NEVER STOP hearing the familiar old complaints from those who love Chinese medicine: that there are too many herbal formulas, the combining of herbs is terribly complex, remembering it all is so difficult, and, in general, it is just plain hard to learn.

It is true, too!

Students majoring in Chinese medicine at Chinese medical schools must memorize at least 150 formulas. The Japanese national health insurance also recognizes more than 140 formulas. What is more, when actually using these formulas in the clinic, simply knowing their names just does not cut it. One must have a comprehensive understanding of the herbs that comprise the formulas, the signs and symptoms that constitute the formulas' patterns or presentation, the significance of the way herbs are paired and combined within the formulas, along with knowing the clinically relevant times to use them.

Therefore, for those studying Chinese medicine, not only is the most important thing to be deeply familiar with herbal formulas, but it is the most difficult thing as well.

In response to this challenge, doctors in the past compiled the *Versified Prescriptions* (湯頭歌訣 *Tāng tóu gē jué*). These prescriptions, written in a rhyming format for easy memorization, would be recited daily by heart. This memorization leads to a deep familiarity, which allows doctors to be facile with these formulas when seeing patients. There is also the method of categorizing by prominent indications; this is called 'categorization of formulas' or 'formula families' (類方 *lèi fāng*). Examples include the Qing-dynasty physician Xu Ling-Tai's book *Categorization of Formulas from the Discussion of Cold Damage* (傷寒論類方 *Shāng hán lùn lèi fāng*); Zuo Ji-Yun's *Collection of Categorized Formulas from the Discussion of Cold Damage* (傷寒論類方匯參 *Shāng hán lùn lèi fāng huì cān)*; and the Japanese doctor Yoshimasu Todō's *Categorized Collected Formulas* (類聚方 *Ruijuhō*).

Using these methods of comparing and contrasting formulas, intimately learning how they are different and alike, allows the practitioner of Chinese medicine to relatively quickly grasp each formula's unique presentation. This, indeed, is an excellent method for learning to use herbal formulas.

Figuratively speaking, all the different types of formulas can be regarded as families or clans. This is to say, based on one or a few ingredients that make up the core, they can be sorted into groups of formulas that have similar effects. Let's take, for example, cinnamon twig (*guì zhī*) type formulas. This is the group of formulas of which cinnamon twig is the most important component. Formulas such as Cinnamon Twig Decoction (*guì zhī tāng*), Minor Construct the Middle Decoction (*xiǎo jiàn zhōng tāng*), Cinnamon Twig Decoction plus Dragon Bone and Oyster Shell (*guì zhī jiā lóng gǔ mǔ lì tāng*), Cinnamon Twig Decoction plus Peony (*guì zhī jiā sháo yào tāng*) and all the others that are based on Cinnamomi Ramulus (*guì zhī*) are referred to as the 'cinnamon twig family of formulas.'

In the same way, formulas based on Bupleurum radix (*chái hú*) are those in which bupleurum plays a major role in the overall formula function. These include formulas such as Minor Bupleurum Decoction (*xiǎo chái hú tāng*), Major Bupleurum Decoction (*dà chái hú tāng*), Bupleurum and Cinnamon Twig Decoction (*chái hú guì zhī tāng*), Frigid Extremities Powder (*sì nì sǎn*), Bupleurum plus Dragon Bone and Oyster Shell Decoction (*chái hú jiā lóng gǔ mǔ lì tāng*), and others. These are referred to as 'bupleurum-based formulas.'

It is just like individual members of a family that all share a blood connection. Each one possesses both an individual character while also demonstrating certain family characteristics. Every formula family has its basic actions and symptoms for which it is appropriate. At the same time, each formula, due to its own unique makeup, is especially effective for treating specific illnesses.

Dividing up the complex mass of formulas by taking the main medicinal substances and their actions, separating them into groups of formula categories, and then comparing each formula category with the others, as well as comparing each formula within the same formula category, is a shortcut used by adept practitioners of Chinese medicine.

While there are dozens of formula categories in Chinese medicine, large and small, in this book we will discuss ten key families. Familiarity with these formula categories and their constituent herbs will not enable the reader to have complete mastery over all aspects of Chinese medicine, yet it will enable the practitioner to grasp the general rules for using Chinese herbal formulas, to understand the basic principles of Chinese medicine's differentiation of patterns as a basis of treatment, and to handle these with ease in the clinic, thus laying down a firm foundation for the further study of Chinese medicine.

This book introduces ten major formula families:

1. Cinnamon twig *(guì zhī)*
2. Ephedra *(má huáng)*
3. Bupleurum *(chái hú)*
4. Rhei Radix et Rhizoma *(dà huáng)*
5. Astragalus *(huáng qí)*
6. Gypsum fibrosum *(shí gāo)*
7. Coptis Rhizoma *(huáng lián)*
8. Dry ginger root *(gān jiāng)*
9. Aconite *(zhì fù zǐ)*
10. Pinelliae Rhizoma preparatum *(zhì bàn xià)*

Although Poria *(fú líng)*, Tangkuei *(dāng guī)*, Paeoniae Radix *(sháo yào)*, Rehmannia *(dì huáng)*, White Atractylodes *(bái zhú)*, Gardenia Fructus *(zhī zǐ)*, Kudzu *(gé gēn)*, and Ginseng Radix *(rén shēn)* have not been viewed in terms of formula families, those who are interested in working on these 'branch families' are certainly encouraged to do so.

This book is in no way a comprehensive look at Chinese herbal formulas; it merely shows readers a way to understand and become proficient with Chinese formulas. If readers acquire the ability to utilize the method of comparing and contrasting, master the herbal and formula presentations and pulse and tongue indications, and differentiate clearly which of the commonly used prescriptions should be used in a clinical setting, then the author's purpose in writing this book will have been achieved.

Are there more than ten formula families? Of course! The title of this book, *Ten Key Formula Families*, is simply an attempt to lighten things up while reading the book.

To make things easier for beginners and to facilitate practice, this book does not go into great depth in explaining traditional theories of combining herbs. Furthermore, the key points regarding herb combinations, as well as clinically relevant uses, are found in the discussion of formula presentations.

The clinical scope of the formulas is based primarily on reports in journals. Formula presentations are based on the text of such classics as *Discussion of Cold Damage* (傷寒論 *Shāng hán lùn*) and *Essentials from the Golden Cabinet*

(金匱要略 *Jīn guì yào lüè*). These are combined with references to the experiences of skilled doctors in the past, and, of course, my own clinical experience.

The dosages of herbs used in formulas are those which I use. Dosage in Chinese herbal medicine is actually hard to strictly set. Generally, the practitioner must consider changes in the patient's condition, the environment, the illness, as well as preparation and delivery methods. Through one's practical and personal experience, these subtleties become clear.

To facilitate easy memorization, this book uses some relatively objective signs that are associated with proper herb usage. These are directly referred to as such and such a symptom, this type of tongue, that kind of pulse, or thus and such body type; for example, cinnamon twig presentation, rhubarb tongue, aconite pulse, bupleurum body type, and so on. This type of wording is actually used in *Discussion of Cold Damage* itself. Readers are advised that the book in their hands uses this type of shorthand, which is not consistent with the modern technical terminology of formal Chinese medical language.

In reality, using an herb or formula name to stand for a presentation is more objective, concrete, and reproducible than terms like yin deficiency, Spleen deficiency, or blood deficiency.

There are quite a few schools of thought in Chinese medicine as well as many types of differential diagnostic systems. No matter which system is used, whether it is *zàng fǔ*, eight principle, qi-blood-*jìn-yè*, illness causative factor, *sān jiāo*, four levels, or six stages, in the final analysis, the result is always an herbal formula.

Thus, herbal and formula presentations are the basic building blocks of treatment based on the differentiation of patterns. The matching of herbs and presentations, or formulas and presentations, is the fundamental principle of clinical work in Chinese medicine. From the past to the present, clinicians, without exception, have applied this kind of attentive focus. The explanations in this book also thoroughly follow these principles.

The original title of this book was *Ten Major Kampō Formula Families*, based upon my lecture notes from teaching in Japan. Since returning to China, I have continually added material, talked and written about the formula presentations, tested and verified these ideas in the clinic, and completely revised the text. Be that as it may, there still remain portions of the book that leave much to be desired.

Research into formula presentations remains a huge area in traditional Chinese medicine that is open to further study and discussion. On the one hand, the experience and knowledge that have been passed down through the years must be summarized and put into an accessible format, but on the other hand, we must urgently use the knowledge and research methods of modern medicine and science to further test and verify traditional experience.

In this way, formula presentations will become both more standardized and objective, which in turn will facilitate the use of this method in the clinic. It is my heartfelt desire that more of our Chinese medicine community will see this research as important and participate in its advancement.

CINNAMON TWIG FORMULA FAMILY

....

桂枝類方 *guì zhī lèi fāng*

The clinical applications of the cinnamon twig formula family are quite broad. It is one of the first formula families that practitioners of Chinese medicine should understand and become familiar with. And, to become familiar with Cinnamon Twig Decoction (*guì zhī tāng*), it is first necessary to understand the characteristics of cinnamon twig, Cinnamomi Ramulus (*guì zhī*).

Cinnamomi Ramulus (*guì zhī*) is the dried twig of the cassia tree, which belongs to the camphor family. It is primarily produced in Guangdong and Guangxi provinces and is particularly fragrant and aromatic. It has a slightly sweet taste and acrid and spicy properties.

The clinical application of Cinnamomi Ramulus (*guì zhī*) is indeed broad. It is included in 44 of the 113 formulas in *Discussion of Cold Damage* (傷寒 論 *Shāng hán lùn*). A look at the clinical literature shows that Cinnamomi Ramulus (*guì zhī*) can be used for symptoms of fever, spontaneous sweating, body aches and pain, joint pain, headache, abdominal pain, diarrhea, cold limbs, feeling flushed, seminal emissions, palpitations, irregular heartbeat, wheezing, shortness of breath, superficial edema, stagnant blood, and emotional disturbances.

There is not just one curative function to Cinnamomi Ramulus (*guì zhī*), and it would be extremely difficult to use modern medical disease names to describe the appropriate scope of this medicinal. You could say that Cinnamomi Ramulus (*guì zhī*) is one of the most difficult to use herbs. You could also say, however, that it is one of the most fascinating herbs. This is because it is an herb that confirms and treats a pattern of disharmony, but not one that cures a 'disease.' In this way, it is a quintessentially Chinese medicinal herb. In Chinese medicine, technically speaking, its function can be summarized as having the ability to harmonize the yin, open the yang, benefit water, cause the qi to descend, promote the dissipation of stasis, and tonify the middle.

It is really difficult to explain these technical terms in a clear way. For now, let's just bypass this issue and first take a look at how Cinnamomi Ramulus (*gui zhī*) is used in the clinic.

Cinnamon Twig Presentation (桂枝證 *guì zhī zhèng*)

In Chinese medicine, the symptom pattern or signs that point to the use of a particular herb is referred to as the 'herb presentation' (藥證 *yào zhèng*); thus, the symptom pattern that should be treated with Cinnamomi Ramulus (*gui zhī*) is the 'cinnamon twig presentation' (桂枝證 *guì zhī zhèng*). In essence, this is a summary of the distinctive functions and appropriate uses of Cinnamomi Ramulus (*guì zhī*).

In other words, a cinnamon twig presentation is a situation where, in accordance with the evidence reflected in the signs and symptoms, Cinnamomi Ramulus (*guì zhī*) should be prescribed. Over the course of several thousand years, Chinese doctors have accumulated significant and extremely practical experience understanding on what basis, and for which patterns, Cinnamomi Ramulus (*guì zhī*) is useful.

Let's draw a metaphor here: If Cinnamomi Ramulus (*guì zhī*) is an arrow, then the cinnamon twig presentation is the target. Accurate aim results in a better score. Similarly, if the herb presentation accurately corresponds to the patient's presentation, treatment will of course be effective. The logic of this method is just that simple. Therefore, it is said, Prescribe the herbs in accordance with the presentation or Treat by the corresponding herb presentation.

It can be said that herb presentations are the foundation of clinical practice in Chinese medicine and are a basic tenet of treatment by differential pattern diagnosis. There is not a single genuine Chinese doctor who does not spend a lot of effort working on the determination of herb presentations.

A cinnamon twig presentation is composed of two aspects:

1. Fever or a subjective feeling of fever; sweats easily, even to the point of spontaneous sweating; aversion to wind, sensitivity to cold, joint pain
2. A subjective feeling of upward movement or pulsations in the abdomen; palpitations, being easily startled, feeling flushed, insomnia

The fever in cinnamon twig presentations is a low-grade fever or merely a subjective sense of fever accompanied by sweating, aversion to wind, and fear of cold. While examining the patient, it is common to find the skin of the abdomen and palms to be relatively moist. A feeling in the abdomen of pulsation or a sensation of something moving upward is known in Chinese medicine as 'running piglet' (奔豚 *bēn tún*) or 'struts above the navel' (臍築 *qí zhù*). Normally, it is not easy to be aware of the pulsing of the aorta in one's abdomen; only when there is a certain sensitivity of the nervous system is the pulsation felt. In the same way, being easily startled, insomnia, and palpitations are all considered part of the same response. From this it can be inferred that the cinnamon twig presentation relates to pathological patterns that result from functional imbalances in such processes as thermal regulation, sweat gland secretions, blood vessel tension, and nervous tone.

Cinnamon Twig Constitution (桂枝體質 *gùi zhī tǐ zhì*)

A cinnamon twig constitution refers to the frequently seen constitutional body type that often exhibits signs for which Cinnamomi Ramulus (*gùi zhī*) and the cinnamon twig formula family are indicated.

Distinguishing this type of constitution is accomplished by utilizing the traditional Chinese medicine methods of looking, asking, and palpating to examine the patient's body, skin, pulse, and tongue.

- *External distinguishing characteristics.* The body tends to be thin, the skin is comparatively fair with a fine texture, and the flesh appears moist and firm. The abdomen is usually relatively flat, and the abdominal muscles tend to be tight. The eyes have a spirited look; the lips are pale red or dark. The pulse is often floating and large and can be felt when barely touching the skin. The tongue body is soft and pale red or dark pale in color. The tongue surface is moist with a thin, white coating.
- *Predisposition.* The patient sweats easily or has spontaneous sweating, night sweats, or sweaty palms and soles. In addition, the patient has emotional or physical sensitivity to cold temperatures, frequent colds, tendency toward abdominal pain, palpitations, shallow or dream-filled sleep, or muscle spasms.

From looking at the external distinguishing characteristics, you can see that those with a 'cinnamon twig physique' resemble what people might call 'effeminate bookworms.' They are like the fragile and sentimental characters Lin Mei-Mei and Lin Dai-Yu in the Chinese classic novel *Dream of the Red Mansions*. In modern Western terms, they might be likened to the vulnerable, emotional heroines of gothic romances.

Compare them with those characters from another classic Chinese novel, *Water Margin*, such as the dark complexioned Feng Li-Kui and the renegade monk Lu Zhi-Shen. These are rough, burly, heroic men, with dark, swarthy skin. Like the heroes of many action movies, they can drink like a fish and eat like a horse, and are clearly not cinnamon twig-type people. There is another type of person seen in the clinical setting: their faces are shiny and red, and they are fat with big bellies or fleshy with a loose musculature. They have dull eyes, fear cold, have slow, languid movements, and a yellowish cast to their big bodies. These are also not cinnamon twig-type people.

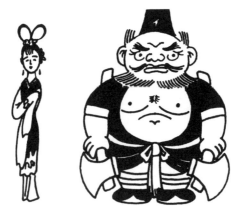

Although practitioners should not decide to write a prescription based simply on a direct correspondence to body type, it can serve to point the prescription in the correct direction. Clearly differentiating body types is extremely important, and is not something that can be neglected.

In my experience, people with a cinnamon twig constitution have a tongue with some rather distinctive characteristics. Namely, the tongue body will be pale red or dark and pale. This is particularly true when they are sick, as most of these patients will have a tongue that is dark and pale, dark and red, or even purple and dark. However, the texture of the tongue body will be tender and moist. This is what I refer to as a 'cinnamon twig tongue' (桂枝舌 *guì zhī shé*).

The pharmacological functions of this herb have been extensively researched in modern times. It has been shown to have antipyretic, anti-inflammatory, anti-allergic, antiviral, stomachic, sedative, analgesic, antitussive, and cutaneous vasodilating effects. When combined with other medicinals, the various functions of Cinnamomi Ramulus (*guì zhī*) can be either modulated or brought out more fully. This leads to an expansion of its use in the clinic.

There are many members of the cinnamon twig family of formulas. Furthermore, the problems for which each and every prescription is appropriate will invariably, to a greater or lesser extent, include some aspects of the cinnamon twig presentation. Similarly, patients with a cinnamon twig constitution will tend toward illnesses that require a cinnamon twig family formula. This is why I started this discussion with an explanation of the cinnamon twig presentation and constitutional body type. Let us now take a look at the cinnamon twig family of formulas.

1.1 **Cinnamon Twig Decoction** (桂枝湯 *guì zhī tāng*)

SOURCE: *Discussion of Cold Damage*

Cinnamomi Ramulus (*guì zhī*) 6-10g
Paeoniae Radix (*sháo yào*) 6-10g
Glycyrrhizae Radix (*gān cǎo*) 3-6g
Zingiberis Rhizoma recens (*shēng jiāng*) 3-6g
Jujubae Fructus (*dà zǎo*) 12g

I recommend that the patient add enough fluid so that the herbs are covered with about one inch of water, soak for 20 minutes, bring to a boil, and simmer for 30 to 40 minutes. Then strain out the dregs and take one-third of the liquid.

While traditionally this was taken with a cup of congee (rice porridge), in today's busy world, patients often do not have the time to do so. In this case, it is fine if the patient has a helping of something warm and easy to digest when they take the strained decoction. Greasy and hard to digest foods, meats, and iced drinks should be avoided. Likewise, most patients are not going to follow the traditional method of covering up to help facilitate a sweat. I usually tell them to try to stay warm and be sure to avoid drafts and getting chilled. If they can, rest for a while. It is best if they take a little nap after ingesting the herbs.

Cinnamon Twig Decoction (*guì zhī tāng*) is the first formula mentioned in *Discussion of Cold Damage*. Legend has it that this ancient prescription was created during the Shang dynasty by the Grand Minister Yi Yin. At that time, the Grand Minister was a highly accomplished chef. He compiled the collective experience of the Chinese people's use of medicinal herbs. Using his skill as a chef, he created all kinds of herbal decoctions. Cinnamon Twig Decoction (*guì zhī tāng*) was composed of the spices and seasonings of that era. There is no telling through how many years this formula has been passed down or how many people have taken it. It is certainly an excellent classic formula that has withstood the test of time and proven to be of great practical use. Chinese doctors call Cinnamon Twig Decoction (*guì zhī tāng*) the crowning glory of all formulas. Everyone who studies Chinese herbal medicine invariably begins their study with Cinnamon Twig Decoction (*guì zhī tāng*).

Just as Cinnamomi Ramulus (*guì zhī*) has the cinnamon twig presentation, Cinnamon Twig Decoction (*guì zhī tāng*) has its scope of appropriate uses. Through the process of fighting disease, the Chinese people have discovered these uses over the course of many years. We are not talking here about a single symptom or just one type of illness; furthermore, there is no way of comparing it to a disease as defined by Western medicine. This concept is a purely Chinese medical perspective on illness.

In his day, Zhang Zhong-Jing, author of *Discussion of Cold Damage*, coined the term 'Cinnamon Twig Decoction presentation' (桂枝湯證 *guì zhī tāng zhèng*). This book continues to use that traditional style of nomenclature. Cinnamon Twig Decoction presentation is a shorthand way of referring to those signs and symptoms that are appropriately treated by Cinnamon Twig Decoction (*guì zhī tāng*).

Chinese doctors often say Use particular herbs for a particular presentation as a turn of phrase to show the relationship between formulas and their presentations. What these doctors focus on is whether or not there is a correspondence between the formula and the presentation.

Formulas address two aspects, the first being the illness itself, the second being a person's constitutional nature. This is because, although disease names are constantly changing through time and vary by location, the presentations that manifest the organism's pathological state are relatively constant. The human organism and its constitutional predilections and responses to disease have not changed. For example, fever, chills, the presence or absence of sweating, and diarrhea or constipation are all examples of how the body responds to a condition of illness.

Using what does not change to respond to the myriad of changes is the standard approach in Chinese traditional medicine. This principle is embodied in the clinical use of Cinnamon Twig Decoction (*guì zhī tāng*).

The Cinnamon Twig Decoction presentation is composed of three aspects:

1. Spontaneous sweating, aversion to wind, and either fever or a sense of feverishness
2. A subjective feeling of upward movement or pulsations (usually in the chest or abdomen), palpitations, and convulsions or stiff and tight muscles
3. A pulse that can be floating, or deficient, or lax, or rapid, or large and without force; a tongue body that is pale and red, or pale and dark, and whose coating is thin and white

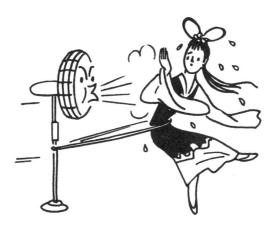

Spontaneous sweating refers to the patient breaking a sweat from simply performing everyday actions. They will sweat even if the weather is not hot, they have not exercised, and have not taken any sweat-inducing medicines. Aversion to wind refers to a sensitivity to wind and cold. They are comfortable only by being in a warm room or wearing extra clothing. Fever could be either an actual measurable fever or a subjective sense of the entire body being feverish. If only one of these three types of symptoms is seen, it cannot be said to be a Cinnamon Twig Decoction presentation. However, if all three appear together, it is significant evidence of a Cinnamon Twig Decoction presentation.

The second group of signs relates to weakened or overactive functions of the nervous system. A sensation of upward-gushing (上衝感 *shàng chòng gǎn*) includes symptoms such as dizziness, feeling flushed, red face, insomnia, excessive dreaming, an upward-surging feeling in the chest and abdomen, or pulsation in the area of the navel. Tight and spasmodic muscles include such problems as spasmodic pain in the stomach and intestines, tight rectus abdominus muscles, and pain from hypertonicity of the muscles of the arms and legs.

A floating pulse means being able to clearly feel the pulse when the fingers just barely touch the skin. This is a finding that is very obvious. In practice, it is common to find that patients whose bodies are on the thin side generally have this type of pulse. The Cinnamon Twig Decoction pulse is not only floating, but also commonly lax and unhurried, or may be simultaneously deficient, which means that there is little or no force when you press on it. Sometimes a deficient and rapid pulse will also be seen.

From the Chinese medicine point of view, a Cinnamon Twig Decoction presentation is the typical expression of exterior deficiency. Exterior and interior are complimentary opposites, as are deficiency and excess. Exterior/interior refers to the location of an illness. An illness located in the outer aspects of the body is considered exterior. Pathology in the sweat glands, skin, and subcutaneous tissues, joints, and upper respiratory tract is, for the most part, a manifestation of an exterior condition. Symptoms include fever, aversion to wind and cold, lack of sweating or abnormal sweating, body aches, a floating pulse, and a thin tongue coating. An illness of the internal organs is regarded as an interior condition. Pathology of the digestive, cardiovascular, endocrine, hematological, or central nervous systems is, for the most part, indicative of an internal condition. Symptoms could include abdominal pain with constipation or diarrhea, listlessness or irritability with an inability to calm down, fever with thirst, or cold limbs with an aversion to cold, a deep pulse, and a red tongue with a thick coating. Clearly, Cinnamon Twig Decoction (*guì zhī tāng*) is indicated for an exterior condition.

Deficiency and excess refer to the patient's condition in terms of analyzing the dynamics and strength of their immune and homeostatic systems. From a systemic perspective, deficiency indicates a lack of normal qi with a decrease in the organism's powers of resistance and a reduction in physiologic functions. Excess indicates an abundance of some strong pathological influence, with a strong toxicity, while the body's resistance to it is not weak. However, just in terms of localized phenomena, deficiency indicates an emptiness, with excessive secretions and insufficient astringency, while excess indicates a condition of congestion, with a surplus of astringency and insufficient secretions.

Figuratively, one can think of it like this: When a door is open, people can come and go through it as they please. This is a good metaphor for deficiency. Now if that same door is closed up so tight that not even a draft can slip through, no one is able to enter or exit; this would represent a condition of excess. Using this concept, it can be said that the human body has many types of doors or gates. For example, the pores of the skin, the cardia of the stomach, the anus and so forth are different types of gates or passageways. During normal biophysiological processes, these gates are sometimes open and at other times are closed. The proper opening and closing of these gates maintains the body's normal biological functions. When there is illness, some of the gates lose their ability to properly open or close. They are either stuck open or locked down and closed. Stuck open is deficiency; locked down and closed is excess.

With exterior deficiency, the pores are stuck open, which results in excessive or spontaneous sweating. Likewise, with exterior excess, the pores are closed down, which results in a lack of sweat, aversion to cold, and dry skin. When the interior is deficient, the anus is 'open,' which results in diarrhea, watery stools, or anal prolapse. When the anus is 'closed,' there is constipation, with many days between bowel movements, and the abdomen is painful and sensitive to pressure. This is a condition of interior excess. The presentation for Cinnamon Twig Decoction (*guì zhī tāng*) is aversion to wind, spontaneous sweating, and fever, which are considered signs of exterior deficiency.

From clinical usage and pharmacological analysis of the individual herbs, it can be inferred that Cinnamon Twig Decoction (*guì zhī tāng*) possesses antipyretic, anti-inflammatory, anti-allergic, analgesic, sedative, and stomachic functions. In particular, it should clearly be stated that it most assuredly has more than a single or localized effect on the body's physiology, and indeed can regulate different parts of the body and various organ systems. The nervous and cardiovascular systems, as well as the body's immune system, are all affected by Cinnamon Twig Decoction's (*guì zhī tāng*) regulatory actions.

This is what Chinese doctors call 'harmonizing the nutritive and protective qi' (調和營衛 *tiáo hé yíng wèi*). Nutritive qi is the subtle yin qi that provides nourishment to the entire body. Protective qi is the yang qi that circulates on the outside and protects the body from attack. When the nutritive and protective qi are in harmony, then the body is in robust health, there is no predisposition toward getting sick, and sweating is normal. Conversely, spontaneous sweating, night sweats, aversion to wind or cold, easily catching colds and falling ill can be seen as a disharmony of the nutritive and protective qi.

It can be seen that these two types of qi, nutritive and protective, are equivalent to the body's homeostatic and immune systems and play extremely important roles in maintaining the health of the body. Therefore, it can readily be seen that Cinnamon Twig Decoction (*guì zhī tāng*), with its function of regulating the nutritive and protective qi, is used for this purpose. Its range of appropriate use is extensive and includes many different branches of medicine:

- Paragraph 13 of *Discussion of Cold Damage* notes: For *tài yáng* illness with headache, fever, sweating, and an aversion to wind, Cinnamon Twig Decoction (*guì zhī tāng*) masters it. In practice, one sees that patients with fevers often present with a Cinnamon Twig Decoction presentation. Regardless of whether it is a fever from an infection, from a noninfectious process, or even a chronic fever of unknown origin, or whether it is a low-grade or a high fever, as long as the signs and symptoms of a Cinnamon Twig Decoction presentation are present, this formula can be used.

- The famous modern physician Yue Mei-Zhong used this method to treat a 14-year-old girl. She had suffered from a fever that reached up to 40°C (104°F) for half a year, with no improvement in spite of taking many kinds of prescriptions. On the basis of her presentation of fever, aversion to wind, sweating from time to time, a floating and lax pulse, lack of thirst, normal bowel movements, and a tongue coating that was pale yellow, Cinnamon Twig Decoction (*guì zhī tāng*) without modifications was prescribed. After three doses she was fine.[1] Lin summarized 68 cases with low-grade fever of unknown origins, five of which had been unsuccessfully treated with antibiotics and other fever-reducing drugs. Using Cinnamon Twig Decoction (*guì zhī tāng*), all recovered.[2]

- Patients with abnormal sweating often show signs and symptoms of a Cinnamon Twig Decoction presentation. As noted in paragraph 54 of *Discussion of Cold Damage*: When a patient has recurrent fevers and sweats that cannot be cured and their yin organs do not have any other disease, ... Cinnamon Twig Decoction (*guì zhī tāng*) is appropriate.

- Cinnamon Twig Decoction (*guì zhī tāng*) can treat spontaneous sweating, night sweats, localized profuse sweating, sweating on the head, and yellow sweat (黃汗 *huáng hàn*). Yellow sweat is a relatively profuse, whole-body sweat that will stain white-colored clothes a yellowish color.

- Cinnamon Twig Decoction (*guì zhī tāng*) can be effective for autonomic dystonia as well as a variety of functional psychological complaints.

- Cinnamon Twig Decoction presentation can occur along with certain cardiovascular diseases such as myocarditis, palpitations from heart disease due to high blood pressure, paroxysmal tachycardia, and Takayasu's arteritis. Because of the large number of treatment options for these types of diseases, those using Cinnamon Twig Decoction (*guì zhī tāng*) must pay special attention to appraising the condition and differentiating properly. Other than the symptom of palpitations, it is common to see spontaneous sweating, aversion to wind, insomnia with vivid dreams, and a tongue that is dark and pale.

• My experience is that Cinnamon Twig Decoction (*guì zhī tāng*) can be used for patients with body types that fall into the cinnamon twig constitution category. Be cautious about using this method for those who are overweight and with red or yellow complexions.

• Cinnamon Twig Decoction presentation also commonly shows up in the course of treating many dermatology cases. Gu has treated many types of erythema, eczema, urticaria, pruritus, winter dermatitis, chilblains, and psoriasis. So long as there is a thin, white tongue coating along with a floating and lax or floating and slippery pulse, using Cinnamon Twig Decoction (*guì zhī tāng*) as a base formula will produce a good result.[3]

I have had similar experiences. However, to confirm that it is suitable, in addition to the tongue and pulse, look for distinguishing characteristics such as a physique that is thin with a pale complexion, susceptibility to catching colds or sweating easily, and an aggravation of symptoms when encountering wind and cold. At the same time, given the number and variety of dermatological disorders and the changes that accompany them, in practice, using Cinnamon Twig Decoction (*guì zhī tāng*) requires the addition of other medicinals or combining it with other formulas.

• In *Discussion of Cold Damage*, it is observed that the Cinnamon Twig Decoction presentation also includes a 'nasal sound' (鼻鳴 *bí míng*). Clinically, what is seen is that patients with aversion to wind and spontaneous sweating usually have an allergic diathesis and therefore not a few of them end up with allergic rhinitis or allergic asthma.

I frequently get good results using Cinnamon Twig Decoction (*guì zhī tāng*) with the addition of Asari Herba (*xì xīn*) or Aconiti Radix lateralis preparata (*zhì fù zǐ*) to treat patients who tend to have allergies and who present with clear and abundant nasal discharge or thin sputum, and have a white, slippery tongue coating. In a study of 20 subjects who were given this formula with the addition of Descurainiae Semen (*tíng lì zǐ*) and Periostracum Cicadae (*chán tuì*) to treat allergic rhinitis, it was reported that two subjects showed no discernable changes, four had relapses, and the other 14 were completely cured.[4]

• Another study reported that 64 subjects were quite satisfied with the use of Cinnamon Twig Decoction (*guì zhī tāng*) in treating morning sickness. Within this group, 54 used Cinnamon Twig Decoction (*guì zhī tāng*) unmodified, while the others took it with the addition of Pinelliae Rhizoma preparatum (*zhì bàn xià*), Ginseng Radix (*rén shēn*), and Zingiberis Rhizoma (*gān jiāng*).[5]

- Another study reported that using Cinnamon Twig Decoction (*guì zhī tāng*) results in quick relief of symptoms for those suffering from morning sickness. Generally speaking, after three doses, the symptoms were reduced, and after seven doses, the patients were cured.[6]

  Often seen with morning sickness is an aversion to wind and dry heaves, similar to this description from paragraph 12 of *Discussion of Cold Damage*: spontaneous sweating, huddling chills, shivering, shuddering fever, nasal resonance, and dry heaves. *Note:* Do not use this formula if the tongue is red with a greasy, yellow coating.

MODIFICATIONS

There are many formulas that are basically Cinnamon Twig Decoction (*guì zhī tāng*) with addition of other ingredients. Among them are the following:

- Add Aconiti Radix lateralis preparata (*zhì fù zǐ*) to get Cinnamon Twig plus Aconite Accessory Root Decoction (*guì zhī jiā fù zǐ tāng*). This treats those with a Cinnamon Twig Decoction presentation who have intense joint pain and cold sweats.

- Add Magnoliae officinalis Cortex (*hòu pò*) and Armeniacae Semen (*xìng rén*) to get Cinnamon Twig Decoction plus Magnolia Bark and Apricot Kernels (*guì zhī jiā hòu pò xìng zǐ tāng*). This formula treats Cinnamon Twig Decoction presentation with fullness in the chest, abdominal distention, cough, panting, and profuse sputum.

- Cinnamon Twig Decoction (*guì zhī tāng*) with double the dosage of Paeoniae Radix alba (*bái sháo*) and Rhei Radix et Rhizoma (*dà huáng*) becomes Cinnamon Twig plus Rhubarb Decoction (*guì zhī jiā dà huáng tāng*). This treats those with a cinnamon twig constitution who suffer from constipation.

- Adding Astragali Radix (*huáng qí*) creates Cinnamon Twig plus Astragalus Decoction (*guì zhī jiā huáng qí tāng*). This formula treats spontaneous, night, and yellow sweating, edema, and urinary difficulty.

- Adding Ginseng Radix (*rén shēn*) and increasing the dosages of Paeoniae Radix alba (*bái sháo*) and Zingiberis Rhizoma (*gān jiāng*) creates Newly Augmented Decoction (*xīn jiā tāng*). Use this to treat excessive sweating, palpitations, dizziness, and poor appetite.

• Adding Puerariae Radix (*gé gēn*) creates Cinnamon Twig Decoction plus Kudzu (*guì zhī jiā gé gēn tāng*). Use this formula to treat Cinnamon Twig Decoction presentation accompanied by a stiff neck and upper back, or diarrhea.

From these examples, it is easy to see that the effective range of use for Cinnamon Twig Decoction (*guì zhī tāng*) is quite extensive.

In accordance with the experience of our predecessors, after administering Cinnamon Twig Decoction (*guì zhī tāng*), porridge or congee should be eaten and the patient should be covered up. Doing so helps to augment the power of the herbs. Cold, raw, greasy, and hard to digest foods should be avoided. Additionally, formulas based on Cinnamon Twig Decoction (*guì zhī tāng*) should be avoided or only used with caution for those who are overweight or have a fever, aversion to cold, and no sweating, or those with a fever, irritability, thirst with a desire to drink, and a red tongue with a coating that is either dry or yellow and greasy.

1.2 Cinnamon Twig plus Aconite Accessory Root Decoction
(桂枝加附子湯 *guì zhī jiā fù zǐ tāng*)

SOURCE: *Discussion of Cold Damage*

Cinnamomi Ramulus (*guì zhī*) 10g
Paeoniae Radix alba (*bái sháo*) 10g
Zingiberis Rhizoma recens (*shēng jiāng*) 6g
Glycyrrhizae Radix (*gān cǎo*) 6g
Jujubae Fructus (*dà zǎo*) 12g
Aconiti Radix lateralis preparata (*zhì fù zǐ*) 10g

Note: Cook Aconiti Radix lateralis preparata (*zhì fù zǐ*) to reduce its toxic nature; it is recommended that this herb be added first and cooked longer. For amounts of 10g or less, cook an additional 20 minutes; up to 20g, cook an additional 40 minutes; up to 30g, cook an additional 60 minutes. For any additional amounts above this, add 20 minutes for every 10g.

A cinnamon twig presentation is categorized as a condition of exterior deficiency. If the degree of deficiency is severe, with ceaseless sweating and cold and clammy skin, or if in fact not only is the exterior deficient, but the interior is also cold from a deficiency of yang qi, leading to an aversion to cold, spasms, and pain of the hands and feet, a pale tongue, and a slow pulse, then simply using Cinnamon Twig Decoction (*guì zhī tāng*) alone will be insufficient. Aconiti Radix lateralis preparata (*zhì fù zǐ*) must be added, which creates the *Discussion of Cold Damage* prescription Cinnamon Twig plus Aconite Accessory Root Decoction (*guì zhī jiā fù zǐ tāng*).

As noted in paragraph 20 of *Discussion of Cold Damage*: When a sweating treatment is given to someone with *tài yáng* disease, but the sweat leaks out continuously and the person has an aversion to wind, urinary difficulty, and a slight tension in the limbs such that they are difficult to flex and extend, Cinnamon Twig plus Aconite Accessory Root Decoction (*guì zhī jiā fù zǐ tāng*) masters it.

Aconiti Radix lateralis preparata (*zhì fù zǐ*) is a commonly used analgesic, tonic, and cardiotonic in Chinese medicine. It has been shown to have many pharmacological effects. It improves cardiovascular function, increases blood circulation, strengthens the heart, raises blood pressure, and regulates micro-circulation, body temperature, and gastrointestinal function, as well as being an analgesic. Chinese medicine considers Aconiti Radix lateralis preparata (*zhì fù zǐ*) to have the ability to warm the yang and dispel cold. It is often used in conditions where there is cold from deficiency (see the aconite family formulas in Chapter 9).

Aconiti Radix lateralis preparata (*zhì fù zǐ*) is a toxic medicinal that is typically prescribed in dosages under 15g. If a large dose is used, Zingiberis Rhizoma recens (*shēng jiāng*) or Zingiberis Rhizoma (*gān jiāng*) must be added. In addition, when decocting, to reduce its toxicity, Aconiti Radix lateralis preparata (*zhì fù zǐ*) should be cooked first, as described above, before adding the other medicinals.

The signs and symptoms for which Cinnamon Twig plus Aconite Accessory Root Decoction (*guì zhī jiā fù zǐ tāng*) is appropriate are as follows:

1. A Cinnamon Twig Decoction presentation with all of the following symptoms: cold sweats, cold and clammy skin, excessive sweating, a pulse that is weak, floating, and large, and a pale tongue body
2. A Cinnamon Twig Decoction presentation accompanied by relatively severe joint pain and cramping in the limbs
3. Cold bulging disorders, abdominal pain, body aches, and cold hands and feet, with a sunken and slow pulse, and a pale tongue

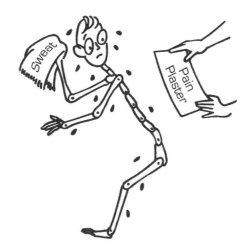

The above signs all belong to the category of exterior deficiency with cold. It is important to emphasize the meaning of deficiency-cold in this context and to clearly explain it. Deficiency is a condition where either the body's ability to function properly has been weakened, or the homeostatic and regulatory capacity of one part or system of the body has been compromised. There can be spontaneous sweating, excessive sweating, or watery diarrhea, incontinence, or other leakage. As previously noted, cold and heat are complimentary opposites; they reflect the nature of the body's ability to react and adapt.

Cold is a sign that the body is lacking warmth, resulting in a decline of physiological and metabolic processes. These patients have signs of cold such as an intense aversion to cold or copious amounts of clear urine. Heat is a sign that the body has an overabundance of warmth such that physiological and metabolic processes are in a state of hyperfunction. These patients present with an aversion to warmth and a preference for cold, red complexion, rough breathing, and yellow or dark urine. Clinically, patterns of cold and deficiency are often seen together, which is called a deficiency-cold pattern. It is the result of insufficient yang qi. This presentation of exterior deficiency-cold is exactly what Cinnamon Twig plus Aconite Accessory Root Decoction (*guì zhī jiā fù zǐ tāng*) is used for.

- Cinnamon Twig plus Aconite Accessory Root Decoction presentation is often seen in the elderly with weak constitutions who catch a cold or those who are constitutionally yang deficient and have excessive sweating and cold limbs when they catch a cold. Guo had an interesting experience treating an in-patient at the hospital for chronic pyelitis. When the patient came down with a cold with symptoms of headache, body aches, sneezing, and a runny nose with clear discharge, he prescribed a single dose of Apricot Kernel and Perilla Drink (*xìng sū yǐn*), thinking to first resolve the exterior before treating the interior. Contrary to his expectations, however, that night the patient was drenched with sweat, was flustered and alarmed, the pulse was faint, and the limbs were frigid with cold. Therefore, Cinnamon Twig plus Aconite Accessory Root Decoction (*guì zhī jiā fù zǐ tāng*) was immediately given to the patient, which not only alleviated the adverse reaction to the previous formula, but cured the cold as well.[7]

• Those patients who have severe spontaneous sweating and autonomic dystonia also often clinically match the Cinnamon Twig plus Aconite Accessory Root Decoction presentation. I have successfully used this formula to treat many patients with recalcitrant severe spontaneous sweating along with aversion to cold, cold limbs, mental and physical fatigue, lusterless complexion, pale and tender tongue, and a thin, deficient, and forceless pulse.

• Based on the experience of using the formula to treat incessant sweating, clinical presentations of allergic rhinitis with constant clear discharge, or women with clear, thin, and profuse vaginal discharge, can also be treated with Cinnamon Twig plus Aconite Accessory Root Decoction (*guì zhī jiā fù zǐ tāng*). It is common in practice to see these types of patients also present with cold limbs, profuse sweating, or a weak constitution with a tendency to sweat easily.

• Cinnamon Twig plus Aconite Accessory Root Decoction (*guì zhī jiā fù zǐ tāng*) can treat all types of joint inflammation that leads to joint pain and sciatica. The famous 18th century Japanese physician Yoshimasu Todō took this formula with the addition of Atractylodis macrocephalae Rhizoma (*bái zhú*) and called it Cinnamon Twig plus Atractylodes and Aconite Accessory Root Decoction (*guì zhī jiā zhú fù tāng*). He used it to treat joints that were both painful and swollen. If in addition to swelling and pain there is floating edema, then Cinnamon Twig, Peony, and Anemarrhena Decoction (*guì zhī sháo yào zhī mǔ tāng*) can be used.

1.3 Minor Construct the Middle Decoction
(小建中湯 *xiǎo jiàn zhōng tāng*)

SOURCE: *Discussion of Cold Damage, Essentials from the Golden Cabinet* (金匱要略 *Jīn guì yào lüè*)

Cinnamomi Ramulus (*guì zhī*) 6-12g

Paeoniae Radix alba (*bái sháo*) 12-30g

Zingiberis Rhizoma recens (*shēng jiāng*) 6g

Glycyrrhizae Radix (*gān cǎo*) 6g

Jujubae Fructus (*dà zǎo*) 12g

Maltosum (*yí táng*) 10g

The secret to Chinese medicine's ability to treat illness is not just in the way that medicinals are combined, but also the way in which the dosage is modified. In this prescription, the basic composition of Cinnamon Twig Decoction (*guì zhī tāng*) has not changed. Simply by adding a single medicinal, Maltosum (*yí táng*), and doubling the amount of Paeoniae Radix alba (*bái sháo*) over that of Cinnamomi Ramulus (*guì zhī*), the function of the modified Cinnamon Twig Decoction (*guì zhī tāng*) changes. This new formula, Minor Construct the Middle Decoction (*xiǎo jiàn zhōng tāng*), has the ability to tonify deficiency and stop pain.

Paragraph 100 of *Discussion of Cold Damage* notes: [When there is] an urgent pain in the abdomen, first give Minor Construct the Middle Decoction (*xiǎo jiàn zhōng tāng*). Another passage in *Essentials from the Golden Cabinet* states: For deficiency due to overwork, chronic intermittent abdominal pain (裡 急 *lǐ jí*), palpitations, nosebleed, abdominal pain, dreaming with seminal emissions, achy limbs, hot hands and feet, dry mouth and throat, Minor Construct the Middle Decoction (*xiǎo jiàn zhōng tāng*) masters it.

What is called 'urgent pain from deficiency overwork' (虛勞 *xū láo*) is, for the most part, in fact an intermittent, spasmodic, and colicky pain. It is not so much that the degree of pain is severe as that it occurs frequently. It is simultaneously accompanied by palpitations, heat irritability, vivid dreams, nosebleed, and other such symptoms of deficiency and weakness. This type of pain is usually accompanied by cinnamon twig constitution type chronic abdominal pain with palpitations and weakness.

The Minor Construct the Middle Decoction presentation is as follows:

1. Chronic abdominal pain accompanied by palpitations, a subjective sense of feverishness possibly accompanied by irritability (煩熱 *fán rè*), weakness, and a flat abdomen with tight muscles
2. Tender tongue body with a sparse coating

Japanese Kampō doctors generally pay considerable attention to the findings of abdominal diagnosis when using Minor Construct the Middle Decoction (*xiǎo jiàn zhōng tāng*). The directions from the Tsumura Pharmaceutical Group state that this formula is for a patient with a weak constitution, easily tired from work, thin abdominal wall, and tight rectus abdominus muscles. In my experience, the above abdominal findings are, for the most part, seen in cinnamon twig constitution patients.

Generally speaking, very few of those with abdominal pain who are obese or whose abdomen protrudes have a Minor Construct the Middle Decoction presentation. A tender tongue—a sign of this presentation—is one that is both soft and shiny. A tongue that is stiff, tough, and has a thick coating usually expresses an excess constitution with internal excess heat and static blood; Minor Construct the Middle Decoction (*xiǎo jiàn zhōng tāng*) is inappropriate in these cases.

- Minor Construct the Middle Decoction (*xiǎo jiàn zhōng tāng*) definitely has an excellent effect on spasmodic abdominal pain. Clinical signs include intermittent abdominal pain with rigid and tight abdominal muscles, or an abdomen that is tight and full, but upon palpation reveals emptiness underneath. The tongue body is generally tender, red, and tending toward dark, and the tongue coating is either thin and white or sparse. This type of abdominal pain can be seen in such diseases as peptic ulcers, allergic colitis, functional gastrointestinal disorders, tubercular peritonitis, stones or biliary ascariasis, and stones in the ureter.

- Some people believe this formula is effective for symptoms such as the epigastric pain seen in early-stage stomach cancer, sloshing water sounds or gurgling in the stomach, acute spasmodic abdominal pain, weak and soft pulse, or vomiting, poor appetite, blood in the stool, and debility from anemia.[8]

- This formula can be used to treat spasmodic constipation. In this condition, there is abdominal pain, and the stools are dry and come out in small pieces about the size of a chestnut. It has been reported that a type of this formula, consisting of Maltosum (*yí táng*) 30g, Paeoniae Radix alba (*bái sháo*) 15g, Cinnamomi Ramulus (*guì zhī*) 6g, Glycyrrhizae Radix preparata (*zhì gān cǎo*) 5g, Zingiberis Rhizoma recens (*shēng jiāng*) 3 slices, Jujubae Fructus (*dà zǎo*) 5 pieces, has been used to treat habitual constipation. The formula was given to 11 subjects for seven days, which was considered one course of treatment. Eventually, all recovered completely. Four required a single course of treatment, and six required two courses of treatment. The final individual, who had been constipated for 16 years, required five courses of treatment.[9]

• This formula can be used to improve the condition of children with weak constitutions. Most of these children are pale with thin physiques, withered hair, are easily startled, sweat profusely, have a depressed appetite, and a floating and deficient pulse. It has been reported that Minor Construct the Middle Decoction *(xiǎo jiàn zhōng tāng)* was prescribed for seven bedwetting children who had weak constitutions, were easily fatigued, and had tight rectus abdominus muscles. On average, within a week, there was obvious improvement.[10] For pale and thin children with abdominal pain and night sweats, this formula is also effective. In Japan, this prescription is used to treat functional gastrointestinal disorders, especially in those with introverted personalities who get stomach pain in the morning because they are anxious about going to school.

RELATED FORMULAS

In discussing the functions of Minor Construct the Middle Decoction *(xiǎo jiàn zhōng tāng)*, one cannot leave out a discussion of Paeoniae Radix alba *(bái sháo)* and Glycyrrhizae Radix *(gān cǎo)*. These two herbs constitute the famous *Discussion of Cold Damage* formula Peony and Licorice Decoction *(sháo yào gān cǎo tāng)*. Zhang Zhong-Jing originally used this formula to treat acute leg spasms resulting from improperly sweating an exterior condition. Later generations of doctors have greatly expanded this formula's scope. It has been reported to be effective in the treatment of spasms of the gastronemius, trigeminal neuralgia, facial ticks, sciatica, gastric spasms, peptic ulcers, recalcitrant hiccup, gallstones, roundworms, urinary tract stones, and thromboangiitis obliterans. The efficacy of this formula has already been proven for spasms of the digestive tract's smooth muscle and for gastronemius muscle pain. This is why it is common for Paeoniae Radix alba *(bái sháo)* and Glycyrrhizae Radix *(gān cǎo)* to be included in formulas that resolve spasms and stop pain. Generally, the amount of Paeoniae Radix alba *(bái sháo)* that is used is 10-20g, but if the pain is particularly severe, 30-45g may be used.

In practice, Minor Construct the Middle Decoction *(xiǎo jiàn zhōng tāng)* is commonly prescribed in a modified form, as follows:

• For a Minor Construct the Middle Decoction presentation with anemia, spontaneous sweating, and vulnerability to catching colds, add Astragali Radix *(huáng qí)* to tonify and benefit the qi and blood. This formula is called Astragalus Decoction to Construct the Middle *(huáng qí jiàn zhōng tāng)*.

• For postpartum women with body aches and abdominal pain, or for painful menses, add Angelicae sinensis Radix *(dāng guī)* to nourish the blood and regulate the menses. This formula is called Tangkuei Construct the Middle Decoction (*dāng guī jiàn zhōng tāng*).

• Removing Maltosum (*yí táng*) from Minor Construct the Middle Decoction (*xiǎo jiàn zhōng tāng*) creates Cinnamon Twig Decoction plus Peony (*guì zhī jiā bái sháo tāng*). This formula is more appropriate for those who do not like sweet foods, those who should not be ingesting sweet foods, or those whose illnesses tend to be relatively acute as well as those patients whose abdominal pain is relatively severe.

1.4 Cinnamon Twig plus Rhubarb Decoction
(桂枝加大黄湯 *guì zhī jiā dà huáng tāng*)

SOURCE: *Discussion of Cold Damage*

Cinnamon Twig (*guì zhī*)	5-10g
White Peony (*bái sháo*)	10-20g
Licorice (*gān cǎo*)	3-6g
Red Dates (*dà zǎo*)	12g
Fresh Ginger (*shēng jiāng*)	6g
Rhei Radix et Rhizoma (*dà huáng*)	3-10g

The differences between deficiency and excess have already been discussed above. Simply stated, they have to do with the 'gates' of the body being either open or closed. Spontaneous or excessive sweating suggests that the pores at the body's exterior open too readily; this is called 'exterior deficiency.' Constipation and abdominal pain occur when the body's interior 'gate' is tightly closed; this is called 'interior excess.' In practice, one sees cinnamon twig constitution patients whose exterior easily becomes deficient while their interior easily becomes excessive. These patients have spontaneous or excessive sweating due to exterior deficiency; simultaneously, they readily develop constipation and abdominal pain. Cinnamon Twig plus Rhubarb Decoction (*guì zhī jiā dà huáng tāng*) was made precisely for this type of exterior deficiency, interior excess condition.

Cinnamon Twig plus Rhubarb Decoction (*guì zhī jiā dà huáng tāng*) is made from Cinnamon Twig Decoction with a double dose of Paeoniae Radix (*sháo yào*) plus the addition of Rhei Radix et Rhizoma (*dà huáng*). Or, it can be seen as a modification of Minor Construct the Middle Decoction (*xiǎo jiàn zhōng tāng*) without the Maltosum (*yí táng*) and with the addition of Rhei Radix et Rhizoma (*dà huáng*). Rhei Radix et Rhizoma (*dà huáng*) is an important medicinal in Chinese medicine used to drain downward and clear heat. It has been called the fierce and invincible general that cuts through barriers to force his way in. It knocks down the door and barges in and thus purges retained stool from the intestines, along with internal accumulation and heat. It is therefore the exemplary herb for excess interior heat conditions.

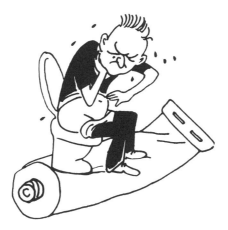

Cinnamon Twig plus Rhubarb Decoction (*guì zhī jiā dà huáng tāng*) is principally for Cinnamon Twig Decoction presentation patients who also have constipation and abdominal pain. This formula can also be used for cinnamon twig constitution patients who have habitual constipation, difficulty with defecation after abdominal surgery, or dysentery accompanied by tenesmus. The presentation for this formula is as follows:

1. Fever or subjective feeling of heat, aversion to wind, spontaneous sweating
2. Constipation, persistent abdominal pain, aversion to pressure on the abdomen, and a thick, dry tongue coating

This formula is not just a laxative. It also can be used to effectively treat cinnamon twig constitution patients with symptoms of stomach pain, cough, wheezing, fever, and headache accompanying constipation with dry stool, abdominal pain, and tongue with a thick, dry coating. Gu treated a patient with recalcitrant urticaria who had already tried Western medicine as well as Chinese medicinals that dispel wind and invigorate the blood, all without effect. At the time when the symptoms would manifest, the patient was freezing and had a dread of cold, along with dry, difficult to pass bowel movements once every two to three days. Using one bag of Cinnamon Twig plus Rhubarb Decoction (*guì zhī jiā dà huáng tāng*) brought about a cure.[11]

Perhaps the reader would like to ask how these three formulas that all treat abdominal pain—Minor Construct the Middle Decoction (*xiǎo jiàn zhōng tāng*), Cinnamon Twig Decoction plus Peony (*guì zhī jiā sháo yào tāng*), and Cinnamon Twig plus Rhubarb Decoction (*guì zhī jiā dà huáng tāng*)—differ from each other. The abdominal pain treated by Minor Construct the Middle Decoction (*xiǎo jiàn zhōng tāng*) is of a chronic and weak nature. The patient's entire body is weak, and the pain is constant. Such patients find that pressure on the abdomen is comfortable, they like sweet foods, and there is no tendency toward interior excess. The abdominal pain treated by Cinnamon Twig Decoction plus Peony (*guì zhī jiā sháo yào tāng*), for the most part, is of an episodic nature that comes and goes. There is somewhat of an interior accumulation. Finally, the abdominal pain for Cinnamon Twig plus Rhubarb Decoction (*guì zhī jiā dà huáng tāng*) is persistent. What is more, in addition to constipation, these patients do not like to have their abdomens pressed upon. The tongue coating is relatively thick and dry. This is clearly a full-on interior condition.

Minor Construct the Middle Decoction (*xiǎo jiàn zhōng tāng*)	Chronic and weak abdominal pain	Likes pressure on the abdomen and sweet foods	No tendency toward exterior excess
Cinnamon Twig Decoction plus Peony (*guì zhī jiā sháo yào tāng*)	Pain is of an episodic nature		Some interior accumulation
Cinnamon Twig plus Rhubarb Decoction (*guì zhī jiā dà huáng tāng*)	Persistent abdominal pain	Does not like pressure on the abdomen; relatively thick and dry tongue coating	Obviously a full-on interior condition

1.5 Cinnamon Twig Decoction plus Dragon Bone and Oyster Shell (桂枝加龍骨牡蠣湯 *guì zhī jiā lóng gǔ mǔ lì tāng*)

SOURCE: *Discussion of Cold Damage*

Cinnamomi Ramulus (*guì zhī*) 5-10g
Paeoniae Radix (*sháo yào*) 6-10g
Glycyrrhizae Radix (*gān cǎo*) 3-6g
Zingiberis Rhizoma recens (*shēng jiāng*) 6g
Jujubae Fructus (*dà zǎo*) 12g

Fossilia Ossis Mastodi (*lóng gǔ*) 10-20g
Ostreae Concha (*mǔ lì*) 10-20g

The Cinnamon Twig Decoction constitution itself includes a subjective upward-gushing sensation and palpitations. If this type of condition is more severe, there will be throbbing sensations in the abdomen and chest, an upward-rushing sensation, a sense of being jumpy and hard to calm down, light sleep or insomnia or many nightmares, and spontaneous sweating or night sweats. For this condition, the formula to use is Cinnamon Twig Decoction plus Dragon Bone and Oyster Shell (*guì zhī jiā lóng gǔ mǔ lì tāng*).

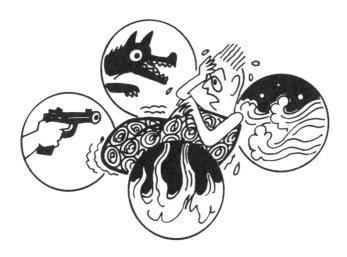

Clinically, it is common to see young children that are pale and thin. Although their eyes have spirit, they are jumpy, have nightmares, and sweat easily. Similarly, thin, pale, delicate adolescent boys and girls also commonly present with palpitations in the chest and pulsations in the abdomen. They readily develop insomnia, and have excessive dreams and night sweats. For these types of kids, the practitioner should pay attention to whether or not they have a Cinnamon Twig Decoction plus Dragon Bone and Oyster Shell presentation.

As he noted in *Essentials from the Golden Cabinet*, Zhang Zhong-Jing originally used this formula to treat people with recurrent seminal emissions whose lower abdomen is tight and irritated, have a cold sensation at the tip of the penis, dizziness, and hair loss. Those with recurrent seminal emissions are mostly gaunt with a pale face, sweat easily, and have frequent nocturnal emissions. This can be considered one type of cinnamon twig constitution.

The 'dragon bone' used in this formula is Fossilia Ossis Mastodi (*lóng gǔ*), which is a substance that has no taste or smell and is exceedingly good at absorbing moisture. It is an important sedative and astringent medicinal that calms the spirit. Clinically, it is effective for throbbing below the navel accompanied by panic with an inability to calm down, irritability and restlessness, seminal emissions, and bleeding.

The medicinal effect of Ostreae Concha (*mǔ lì*) is basically the same as that of Fossilia Ossis Mastodi (*lóng gǔ*), the difference being that Ostreae Concha (*mǔ lì*) is especially targeted toward abdominal and chest pulsations. It can therefore be used to treat stuffiness in the chest, palpitations, dizziness, headaches, night sweats, and nocturnal emissions. Zhang Zhong-Jing always used the combination of Fossilia Ossis Mastodi (*lóng gǔ*) and Ostreae Concha (*mǔ lì*) in Cinnamomi Ramulus (*guì zhī*) and Bupleuri Radix (*chái hú*) formulas to treat pulsation in the chest and abdomen, irritability, and restlessness with an inability to calm down, insomnia, and other such symptoms.

The Cinnamon Twig Decoction plus Dragon Bone and Oyster Shell presentation is as follows:

1. Chest or abdominal pulsation or throbbing, jumpiness, spontaneous sweating or night sweats, insomnia with excessive dreaming
2. A large, floating, and forceless pulse, and a tender and red tongue body with a sparse coating

In my experience, the decision to use this formula is based on key tongue and pulse findings. The pulse must be floating, full, and lacking force. If it is deep and thin, deep and excessive, or large and forceful, it is without exception not the pulse for this formula. This is a very important point. This formula can be used when the tongue is tender and red, moist, and has a thin, white coating. This is indicative of weakness of the normal qi and lack of an internal pathogen. A tongue that is dull, red, tough, and firm indicates heat from constraint in the interior. A pale, white, and puffy tongue suggests internal cold, dampness, and thin mucus. A yellow, greasy, scorched and dry, or thick and greasy coating indicates interior phlegm-heat, heat accumulation, and turbid dampness, respectively. These all impede the actions of this formula: prescribe with caution!

• This formula is commonly used to treat such pediatric illnesses as prolonged pneumonia, rickets, bedwetting, spontaneous sweating or night sweats, night terrors, or low-grade fever. Wang reports using Cinnamon Twig Decoction plus Dragon Bone and Oyster Shell (*guì zhī jiā lóng gǔ mǔ lì tāng*) to treat 13 children with pneumonia who primarily had normal qi deficiency. Of these, eight recovered completely, four showed improvement, and one had no change in condition.[12] Recently this formula, with the addition of untreated Gypsum fibrosum (*shí gāo*) and Paeoniae Radix alba (*bái sháo*), was used to treat a thin, pale child with fever during the summer. The main indications were thirst, irritability and restlessness, and night sweats that occurred just as the child was going to sleep.

- This prescription can also be used to treat insomnia, excessive dreams, palpitations, and stuffiness in the chest from nervous exhaustion. It can be effective for men with seminal emissions, impotence, premature ejaculation, or inability to ejaculate, and for women with irregular menses, frigidity, anxiety, and fear.

I once treated a thin, bookwormish sort of young man with prostatitis, testicular pain, seminal emissions, excessive dreams, and night sweats. This patient had been treated by a specialist who had thrown multiple doses of heat-clearing, blood-invigorating formulas at him, none of which had any effect at all. Observing the patient's thin physique, lively and expressive eyes, tender, red tongue body with a sparse coating, and a pulse that was large and without force, I gave him Cinnamon Twig Decoction plus Dragon Bone and Oyster Shell (*guì zhī jiā lóng gǔ mǔ lì tāng*) with the addition of Schisandrae Fructus (*wǔ wèi zǐ*), Euryales Semen (*qiàn shí*), and Nelumbinis Stamen (*lián xū*). After three packets, the patient slept peacefully and stopped sweating. He was given 30-plus packets in all, and at the end of the treatment was completely cured.

I also frequently use this formula to treat cinnamon twig constitution patients with chronic wheezing, excessive sweating, and a red, tender tongue with sparse coating, or with chronic epigastric or abdominal pain accompanied by excessive dreams, insomnia, night sweats, and dizziness. For this reason, emphysema, bronchial asthma, ulcers of the digestive tract, and gastritis are all opportunities for using this formula, as long as the patient has a cinnamon twig constitution.

1.6 Tangkuei Decoction for Frigid Extremities

(當歸四逆湯 *dāng guī sì nì tāng*)

SOURCE: *Discussion of Cold Damage*

Angelicae sinensis Radix (*dāng guī*) 6-10g

Cinnamomi Ramulus (*guì zhī*) 6-10g
Paeoniae Radix (*sháo yào*) 6-15g
Asari Herba (*xì xīn*) 3-5g
Glycyrrhizae Radix (*gān cǎo*) 3-10g
Tetrapanacis Medulla (*tōng cǎo*) 6g
Jujubae Fructus (*dà zǎo*) 20g

We have already introduced a formula that is excellent for treating stomach and abdominal pain, Minor Construct the Middle Decoction (*xiǎo jiàn zhōng tāng*), and an equally fine one for treating spasmodic pain, Peony and Licorice Decoction (*sháo yào gān cǎo tāng*). Here we will introduce a prescription that excels at treating cold, painful extremities with headache, Tangkuei Decoction for Frigid Extremities (*dāng guī sì nì tāng*).

Tangkuei Decoction for Frigid Extremities (*dāng guī sì nì tāng*) can be regarded as a modification of Cinnamon Twig Decoction (*guì zhī tāng*). The functions of the modifying herbs are as follows:

ANGELICAE SINENSIS RADIX (*dāng guī*)

This herb has a distinctly fragrant aroma, is warm and acrid in nature, and has a sweet taste. Traditionally, it is the herb used to regulate women's menses. It has the ability to sedate, reduce pain, tonify the blood, strengthen the constitution, and moisten the intestines.

Comprehensive Outline of the Materia Medica (本草綱目 *Běn cǎo gāng mù*) states: Angelicae sinensis Radix (*dāng guī*) treats headaches and all kinds of chest and abdominal pain; moistens the intestines and stomach, sinews, bones, and skin; treats abscesses and swelling, expels pus, stops pain, and harmonizes and tonifies the blood. Angelicae sinensis Radix (*dāng guī*) is commonly paired with Paeoniae Radix alba (*bái sháo*) to treat abdominal pain in women as well as irregular menstruation.

ASARI HERBA (*xì xīn*)

This herb is so named because its root is thin (細 *xì*) and its taste is acrid (辛 *xīn*). The nature of Asari Herba (*xì xīn*) is acrid and warm, and it is especially effective at scattering wind-cold and stopping pain. *Divine Husbandman's Classic of the Materia Medica* (神農本草經 *Shén Nóng běn cǎo jīng*) says this herb principally treats cough with ascendant qi, headache with perturbation of the brain, cramping and spasms of all the joints, wind-damp obstruction pain, and muscles that are both nonfunctional and lacking feeling. Clinically, Chinese doctors principally use Asari Herba (*xì xīn*) to:

1. Promote sweating and scatter cold: treats cold damage with a lack of sweating, fever, and a sunken pulse, as in the formula Ephedra, Asarum, and Aconite Accessory Root Decoction (*má huáng xì xīn fù zǐ tāng*)
2. Stop pain: treats headaches from external wind-cold invasion, with body aches and toothache
3. Warm the Lungs and dispel phlegm: treats wind-cold type coughing and wheezing with copious phlegm

Asari Herba (*xì xīn*) is principally used in the formula to scatter wind-cold and warm and open (the yang) to stop pain. Furthermore, when paired with Cinnamomi Ramulus (*guì zhī*), this function is even more clearly pronounced.

Compared with Cinnamon Twig Decoction (*guì zhī tāng*), the ability of Tangkuei Decoction for Frigid Extremities (*dāng guī sì nì tāng*) to warm the channels and stop pain is much stronger. In practice, it is commonly used to treat pain from cold and deficiency. This type of pain principally appears where there is nerve or blood vessel pathology or reduced circulation of blood, especially in those suffering from disorders of the peripheral circulation. Some patients with local inflammation or spasmodic pain can also be seen as fitting this presentation.

Originally, the formula presentation for Tangkuei Decoction for Frigid Extremities (*dāng guī sì nì tāng*) comes from paragraph 351 of *Discussion of Cold Damage*: For those with hands and feet that have inversion [extreme] cold and a pulse that is so thin that it is on the point of exhaustion, Tangkuei Decoction for Frigid Extremities (*dāng guī sì nì tāng*) masters it.

In accordance with what has been written in *Discussion of Cold Damage* and the practical experience of later generations of doctors, this formula's presentation can be summed up as follows:

1. Hands and feet that are extremely cold, numb, and painful, even to the point of turning bluish purple
2. Thin pulse
3. Abdominal pain, headache, or back, foot, or leg pain
4. Pale tongue with a white coating

Cold hands and feet in this formula's presentation refers especially to the tips of the fingers and toes being cold. Even during the summer, they will remain unusually cold. As the four extremities are so severely cold, the formula's name contains the term 'frigid extremities.'

In this presentation, the thin pulse is the result of blood vessel contraction and has nothing to do with a weakening of the heart, so the overall condition of the person is relatively good. To use this formula, pain must be present that will usually worsen on exposure to cold. The symptoms also often worsen for women during menstruation. The pale tongue with a white coating reflects the existence of a cold pattern; in practice, this is an important point of distinction.

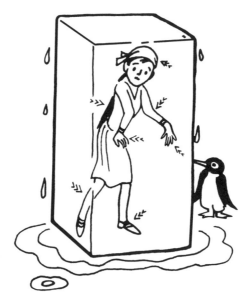

Tangkuei Decoction for Frigid Extremities presentation is often seen in the following pathologic conditions:

• *Problems such as Raynaud's disease, frostbite, and erythematous limb pain.* Raynaud's disease is caused by spasms of the blood vessels at the very end of the extremities. The main clinical sign is that the tips of the fingers and toes intermittently turn pale or cyanotic and become painful. These symptoms are rather close to those of the formula's presentation. To increase its efficacy in treating Raynaud's disease, the formula can be modified with the addition of Evodiae Fructus (*wú zhū yú*), Persicae Semen (*táo rén*), and Carthami Flos (*hóng huā*). Frostbite is usually marked by cold extremities and localized swelling with red and purple discoloration. Tangkuei Decoction for Frigid Extremities (*dāng guī sì nì tāng*) is effective in treating this and can be used both for treating and as a preventative measure. It can be taken orally or used externally as both a steam and a wash. Erythematous limb pain is marked by a burning, excruciating pain due to dilation of the distal blood vessels of the lower extremities: this also can be seen as a Tangkuei Decoction for Frigid Extremities presentation.

- *Headaches.* This formula is effective for treating migraines, cluster headaches, and other headaches from blood deficiency with Liver cold. Migraines are caused by a disruption of the dilation and contraction of blood vessels both inside and outside of the cranium, which leads to periodic headaches. During attacks, the patient will commonly present with a pattern of deficiency-cold.

  In three reports, You stated the results of using this formula with the addition of Chuanxiong Rhizoma (*chuān xiōng*) to treat 70 subjects. Generally, the administration of 15-20 packets of herbs greatly extended the time between headaches. Altogether, 27 subjects had their symptoms controlled, 19 had clear improvement, 16 showed improvement, and for eight subjects, the treatment had no effect.[13, 14]

  Cluster headache pain principally centers around the eye socket, and You reported using this formula to treat 30 subjects. Treatment resulted in control of the symptoms for 11 subjects, clear improvement for seven, some improvement for 11, and for one subject, there was no effect.[15]

  In my experience, Tangkuei Decoction for Frigid Extremities (*dāng guī sì nì tāng*) is effective in treating headaches when accompanied by cold extremities, a pale tongue, and a thin pulse.

- *Thromboangitis obliterans.* This presents with severe pain in the extremities, with some patients being very sensitive to cold and having frigid extremities. If these patients also have aversion to cold and a slow pulse, Aconiti Radix lateralis preparata (*zhì fù zǐ*) can be added. For those with localized infection, add Lonicerae Flos (*jīn yín huā*), Taraxaci Herba (*pú gōng yīng*), and Spatholobi Caulis (*jī xuè téng*). Achyranthis bidentatae Radix (*niú xī*), traditionally used to treat weak legs and knees, can also be added.

- *Sciatica, scapulohumeral periarthritis, rheumatoid arthritis, and joint pain.* Wu reports using this formula to treat 20 subjects with sciatica. They received a course of 6-20 days of treatment, resulting in 18 subjects recovering completely. The remaining two had obvious reduction in their symptoms.[16]

- *Tooth pain.* Zhang reports using this formula plus Evodiae Fructus (*wú zhū yú*) and Zingiberis Rhizoma recens (*shēng jiāng*) to effectively treat tooth pain associated with deficiency-cold in debilitated elderly patients. He believes that without the Evodiae Fructus (*wú zhū yú*) and Zingiberis Rhizoma recens (*shēng jiāng*), there would not have been any obvious effect from the treatment.[17]

- *In women with such problems as menstrual irregularity, dysmenorrhea, or vaginal discharge.* The majority will have frigid extremities during menses, abdominal pain, back pain, and headaches. The discharge usually will be white, thin, and watery and with a fishy odor. In my experience, women who are thin and with a pale complexion often manifest this formula's presentation. If they are overweight and have cold extremities, they have the presentation of a different formula.

MODFICATION

Tangkuei Decoction for Frigid Extremities (*dāng guī sì nì tāng*) plus Evodiae Fructus (*wú zhū yú*) and Zingiberis Rhizoma recens (*shēng jiāng*) is called Tangkuei Decoction for Frigid Extremities plus Evodia and Fresh Ginger (*dāng guī sì nì jiā wú zhū yú shēng jiāng tāng*). In *Discussion of Cold Damage*, it is used to treat long abiding cold in the interior. The nature of Evodiae Fructus (*wú zhū yú*) is hot, and it is excellent for stopping pain and vomiting. It is particularly used for cold-type stomachache, abdominal pain, or headaches. The usual dosage is 2-5g.

Adding Evodiae Fructus (*wú zhū yú*) and Zingiberis Rhizoma recens (*shēng jiāng*) to Tangkuei Decoction for Frigid Extremities (*dāng guī sì nì tāng*) increases its function of reducing pain and stopping vomiting. This is especially appropriate for treating the accompanying symptoms of vomiting, nausea, and headache. It is particularly appropriate for vertex headache.

1.7 **Flow-Warming Decoction** (溫經湯 *wēn jīng tāng*)*

SOURCE: *Essentials from the Golden Cabinet*

Evodiae Fructus (*wú zhū yú*) 3-5g
Angelicae sinensis Radix (*dāng guī*) 10g
Chuanxiong Rhizoma (*chuān xiōng*) 6g
Paeoniae Radix alba (*bái sháo*) 10g
Ginseng Radix (*rén shēn*) 10g
Cinnamomi Ramulus (*guì zhī*) 6-10g

---

* Also translated as Warm the Menses Decoction. It is a famous traditional formula for women's diseases.

Asini Corii Colla (*ē jiāo*)..10g
Moutan Cortex (*mǔ dān pí*)..6-10g
Zingiberis Rhizoma recens (*shēng jiāng*)..................................6g
Glycyrrhizae Radix (*gān cǎo*)...3-6g
Pinelliae Rhizoma preparatum (*zhì bàn xià*)...........................6g
Ophiopogonis Radix (*mài mén dōng*)....................................10g

Flow-Warming Decoction (*wēn jīng tāng*) is a famous traditional formula for women's diseases. From its ingredients, we can see that it is a modification of Cinnamon Twig Decoction (*guì zhī tāng*). Within this formula, Angelicae sinensis Radix (*dāng guī*), Chuanxiong Rhizoma (*chuān xiōng*), and Paeoniae Radix alba (*bái sháo*) function to tonify and invigorate the blood. They are the primary herbs traditionally used to regulate the menses. Asini Corii Colla (*ē jiāo*) can both stop bleeding and tonify the blood and is commonly used to treat menorrhaghia and anemia. The function of Moutan Cortex (*mǔ dān pí*) is to invigorate the blood, transform stasis, and clear heat. Cinnamomi Ramulus (*guì zhī*) and Evodiae Fructus (*wú zhū yú*) warm the menses and stop pain. This formula nourishes the blood, moistens the yin, invigorates the blood and transforms stasis, warms the menses, and stops pain.

There are extensive uses for which this formula is appropriate. It can be considered for irregular menstruation, continuous spotting, cold and painful lower abdomen, and infertility. It has been reported that Flow-Warming Decoction (*wēn jīng tāng*) regulates sex hormones and improves the condition and functioning of the uterus, ovaries, and surrounding tissues.

In my experience, patients for whom this formula is prescribed often have a cinnamon twig constitution. Please note the presentation for this formula:

1. Irregular menstruation, with dark blood and clots
2. Subjective sense of heat in the palms and soles, along with an aversion to wind, spontaneous sweating, feverishness in the afternoon, or headache or nausea
3. Abdominal wall is thin and without strength, lower abdomen is strained, tight, and painful; there may also be bloating
4. Dry lips and a dark, pale tongue body

The signs that lead to a diagnosis of irregular menstruation include irregular periods, or periods with extended bleeding, continuous spotting, or two periods within a month, as well as perimenopausal irregularities. The key to treating these issues is in asking about the color and quality of the blood. Generally, in a Flow-Warming Decoction presentation, the blood is of a dark and pale color, and contains clots. If the color of the blood is fresh red or purple red, and is viscous and sticky, this indicates severe internal heat, for which Flow-Warming Decoction (wēn jīng tāng) is inappropriate. Instead, consider using Augmented Rambling Powder (jiā wèi xiāo yáo sǎn).

In this presentation, there is a subjective sense of feverishness, hot and irritated palms and soles, and dry lips and mouth. While these appear to be signs of heat, there are also obvious signs of cold such as aversion to wind, spontaneous sweating, a dark pale tongue, and lower abdomen that is strained, tight, and painful. Therefore, in practice one should pay close attention to the the process of differentiation.

I once used this formula to treat a woman whose period had not finished after half a month. The menstrual blood was of a dark and pale color, and contained clots. All of her joints were achy and uncomfortable. She couldn't stand cold, but from time to time would have hot flashes that made her sweat. While ordinarily prone to headaches, they had recently become more frequent and severe, to the point of nausea with dry heaves. She was treated by her previous doctor for a heat pattern and prescribed Augmented Rambling Powder (jiā wèi xiāo yáo sǎn). However, this increased her indistinct abdominal pain, which felt better with the application of a hot water bottle. I observed that she had a slim physique and a sallow complexion; her lips were dry, dull, and pale. Her tongue was covered with a greasy coating that was white underneath and yellow on top. The tongue body was dark and pale. After using five packets of Flow-Warming Decoction (wēn jīng tāng), the bleeding stopped and the other symptoms subsided as well.

1.8 Prepared Licorice Decoction (炙甘草湯 zhì gān cǎo tāng)

SOURCE: *Discussion of Cold Damage*

Glycyrrhizae Radix preparata (zhì gān cǎo) 6-15g
Cinnamomi Ramulus (guì zhī) 6-10g
Zingiberis Rhizoma recens (shēng jiāng) 6g
Jujubae Fructus (dà zǎo) 15-25g
Ginseng Radix (rén shēn) 6g
Rehmanniae Radix (shēng dì huáng) 12-20g
Ophiopogonis Radix (mài mén dōng) 10g
Cannabis Semen (huǒ má rén) 10g
Asini Corii Colla (ē jiāo) 10g

Prepared Licorice Decoction (*zhì gān cǎo tāng*) can often be considered for cinnamon twig constitution patients with cardiovascular disease. Paragraph 177 of *Discussion of Cold Damage* states: For cold damage with an irregular pulse and Heart-disturbing palpitations, Prepared Licorice Decoction (*zhì gān cǎo tāng*) masters it.

Supplement to Important Formulas Worth a Thousand Gold Pieces (千金翼方 *Qiān jīn yì fāng*) says to use this formula to treat exhaustion from overwork, sweating with a stuffy feeling in the chest, an irregular pulse, and palpitations. *Arcane Essentials from the Imperial Library* (外台秘要 *Wài tái mì yào*) notes that this formula is used to treat Lung atrophy, excessive saliva, and discomfort in the chest with a slight sense of nausea (心中温温液液 *xīn zhōng wēn wēn yè yè*). All of these symptoms point primarily to Heart disease. The types of Heart disease that Prepared Licorice Decoction (*zhì gān cǎo tāng*) mainly treats usually involve arrhythmia. An irregular pulse, as stated in *Discussion of Cold Damage*, is the pulse that is slow with dropped beats.

Clinical experience indicates that Prepared Licorice Decoction (*zhì gān cǎo tāng*) is effective to varying degrees in treating a variety of cardiac disorders or arrhythmias due to extracardiac factors. From the perspective of Chinese medicine, Prepared Licorice Decoction (*zhì gān cǎo tāng*) is not the only formula that treats arrhythmia. It is not uncommon to see reports of using such formulas as Ephedra, Asarum, and Aconite Accessory Root Decoction (*má huáng xì xīn fù zǐ tāng*), Warm Gallbladder Decoction (*wēn dǎn tāng*), Poria, Cinnamon Twig, Atractylodes, and Licorice Decoction (*líng guì zhú gān tāng*), True Warrior Decoction (*zhēn wǔ tāng*), and Coptis Decoction to Resolve Toxicity (*huáng lián jiě dú tāng*) to treat arrhythmias. A central tenet of practicing Chinese medicine is to treat according to the presentation. It goes without saying, when using Prepared Licorice Decoction (*zhì gān cǎo tāng*) to treat arrhythmias, one must treat according to the differential pattern diagnosis.

From looking at the ingredients of this formula, other than the yang-warming and assisting Cinnamomi Ramulus (*guì zhī*) and Zingiberis Rhizoma recens (*shēng jiāng*), all the others serve to tonify and benefit the qi and blood. It has a stronger ability to tonify, augment, and fortify than Cinnamon Twig and Ginseng Decoction (*guì zhī rén shēn tāng*).

Prepared Licorice Decoction (*zhì gān cǎo tāng*) is an important yin-tonifying formula in *Discussion of Cold Damage*. The yin-moistening and yin-tonifying formulas designed by later generations of physicians mostly originate from this script.

In practice, yin deficiency is a commonly seen presentation. Yin refers to the substances in the body that have form; yang refers to the capabilities of the body that do not have form. Simply stated, yin deficiency means an insufficiency of the substances that have form; yang deficiency is a diminishment of the formless functional capacity. The bones and flesh of the physical body are considered to be formed and substantial. Thus, when there is yin deficiency, these become emaciated, withered, shriveled, and smaller. Yang deficiency is when there is diminishment, weakness, and inhibition of the body's physiological functions. Prepared Licorice Decoction (*zhì gān cǎo tāng*) is most suitable for yin deficient arrhythmia. Specific signs include:

1. A pulse that is deficient, without force, and irregular
2. Emaciation with a drawn and wan complexion, a sparse or nonexistent tongue coating
3. Fatigue, obvious palpitations with a feeling of throbbing in the chest and/or abdomen, deficiency irritability, dizziness, excessive dreaming or insomnia, and constipation

Arrhythmia is the representative sign for Prepared Licorice Decoction (*zhì gān cǎo tāng*); however, the distinguishing feature here is the pulse's weakness and lack of force. If the pulse is slippery and large, this usually represents interior heat and phlegm; use a modification of Warm Gallbladder Decoction (*wēn dǎn tāng*). If the pulse is thready, rough, and with a feeling of not moving smoothly, this represents blood stagnation in the interior; use a modification of Drive Out Stasis from the Mansion of Blood Decoction (*xuè fǔ zhú yū tāng*).

Evaluating the pulse's distinguishing characteristic can be a relatively difficult matter. In my experience, the body type is an important point of differentiation. Prepared Licorice Decoction presentation is commonly seen in those with a cinnamon twig constitution. These people have slim physiques with a drawn and pale complexion. Those who are overweight and with a dark red or oily and greasy complexion have, for the most part, phlegm-heat or phlegm-dampness presentations, and Prepared Licorice Decoction (*zhì gān cǎo tāng*) would be inappropriate for them.

Prepared Licorice Decoction (*zhì gān cǎo tāng*) presentation can be seen in the following types of heart disease:

• *Arrhythmias.* Huang reports using a modification of this formula to treat 25 patients with premature contractions. Treatment resulted in 11 being cured, seven with obvious improvement, three with some improvement, and three having no change in their symptoms.[18] Beijing Jishuitan Hospital reports using this formula to treat 31 subjects with arrhythmia. Among these, 23 had multiple preventricular contractions, four had pre-atrial contractions, and four had junctional premature beats. Treatment resulted in 15 subjects having symptoms completely disappear, three showed obvious improvement, 11 experienced a turn for the better, and two had no change. After taking herbs, the vast majority of subjects within the space of one to two months showed improvement.[19]

- *Coronary artery disease.* Tianjin Hospital of Chinese Medicine reports using Prepared Licorice Decoction (*zhì gān cǎo tāng*) to treat 268 coronary heart disease patients. Of these, 265 had abnormal electrocardiograms, 187 had coronary insufficiency, 39 had remote myocardial infarction, 20 had left bundle branch blockage, nine had myocardial strain, and one suffered atrial fibrillation. Treatment resulted in 93 patients showing obvious improvement, 153 showing some improvement, and 23 having no change. After taking herbs for two weeks, 86 percent of the patients began to get better, and within four weeks, the remaining patients began to show improvement.[20]

- *Sick sinus syndrome.* Gao reports using Prepared Licorice Decoction (*zhì gān cǎo tāng*) plus Aconiti Radix lateralis preparata (*zhì fù zǐ*) to treat 11 patients with sick sinus syndrome. Among these, six had arteriosclerotic cardiopathy, two each had myocarditis and cardiomyopathy, all 11 patients had both conduction blockage and sinus arrest, and four had Adams-Stokes syndrome. Fifteen packets of herbs constituted one course of treatment. After three courses of treatment, four patients had obvious improvement, and the remaining seven showed some improvement. Among these patients, seven had an increase in heart rate to 60 beats per minute, four had an increase to 50 to 60 beats per minute. For nine patients, the conduction blockage was reduced. The sinus arrest disappeared in seven patients and only occasionally occurred in two.[21]

- *Viral myocarditis.* Xu reports using this formula to treat 38 patients with viral myocarditis. Other accompanying symptoms included 28 with palpitations, 19 with shortness of breath, 17 with chest stuffiness, and 26 with dry mouth. The pulse for 15 patients was knotted, for 20 was rapid, and for eight was slow. The others had abnormal electrocardiographs and chest X-rays. Thirty patients were cured completely, four had some improvement, and two showed no change. Two of the patients died from third-degree AV block. The length of treatment was 6-42 days, with an average of 15.6 days.[22]

It is reported that this formula is also effective for rheumatic heart disease complicated by atrial fibrillation and paroxysmal atrial fibrillation.[23]

1.9 Poria, Cinnamon Twig, Atractylodes, and Licorice Decoction
(苓桂术甘湯 *líng guì zhú gān tāng*)

SOURCE: *Discussion of Cold Damage*

Poria (*fú líng*) 10-15g
Cinnamomi Ramulus (*guì zhī*) 6-10g
Atractylodis macrocephalae Rhizoma (*bái zhú*) 10g
Glycyrrhizae Radix (*gān cǎo*) 3g

Poria, Cinnamon Twig, Atractylodes, and Licorice Decoction (*líng guì zhú gān tāng*) is the cinnamon twig family formula for promoting urination. It is appropriate to use for thin mucus problems. Chinese medicine holds that long periods of fatiguing labor, anxiety, and overindulgence in cold foods can cause damage to the yang qi, leading to illness due to stoppage and a lack of transformation of the body's fluids.

The main signs are dizziness, palpitations, sloshing sounds in the stomach, coldness in the middle of the back, a cough with copious thin, clear sputum, fullness and discomfort in the chest and costal regions, urinary difficulty, and a tongue with a slippery coating. When encountering this type of presentation, use Poria, Cinnamon Twig, Atractylodes, and Licorice Decoction (*líng guì zhú gān tāng*).

Within this formula is Poria (*fú líng*), which is traditionally used to treat dizziness and palpitations accompanied by urinary difficulty. It is commonly combined with Atractylodis macrocephalae Rhizoma (*bái zhú*), Cinnamomi Ramulus (*guì zhī*), and Glycyrrhizae Radix (*gān cǎo*); the three latter herbs constitute the formula Cinnamon Twig and Licorice Decoction (*guì zhī gān cǎo tāng*), which treats palpitations, excessive sweating, and stuffiness in the chest. When all four herbs are combined, one obtains Poria, Cinnamon Twig, Atractylodes, and Licorice Decoction (*líng guì zhú gān tāng*), which treats dizziness and palpitations accompanied by urinary difficulty and edema. The presentation for this formula is as follows:

1. Epigastric pulsation, an upward-rushing feeling in the chest, or dizziness
2. Abdomen that is soft and weak, while there is fullness in the chest and costal regions, and gurgling or sloshing sounds in the stomach
3. Urinary difficulty and a tendency toward edema

Other than the already mentioned signs, it is also fairly common to see patients who have an aversion to cold, urinary difficulty, thin and watery stools, lack of appetite along with a reduced sense of taste, constant spitting up of clear saliva, and a white, slippery tongue coating. A distinguishing clinical sign for the presentation of this formula is that the symptoms come and go: there is not a specific time that they are expressed. However, when the symptoms do express themselves, they are severe, and at times come on both fast and furious. Yet after they pass, it is as if nothing has happened. Furthermore, emotional upset and fatigue are common causes that lead to this presentation.

The presentation for this formula is often seen in the following illnesses:

- *Patients with dizziness, for example, aural vertigo and dizziness from hypertension or from nervous exhaustion.* In paragraph 67 of *Discussion of Cold Damage* it is noted: For cold-damage after either [inducing] vomiting or purging with a [feeling of] rebellion and fullness below the Heart, the qi ascends to gush into the chest, so there is dizziness after getting up, and the pulse is sinking and tight. Inducing sweating disrupts the channels, so there is trembling and shaking of the body. Poria, Cinnamon Twig, Atractylodes, and Licorice Decoction (*líng guì zhú gān tāng*) masters it. In Chapter 12 of *Essentials from the Golden Cabinet* it is stated: For phlegm-thin mucus in the epigastrium, fullness in the chest and costal regions, and dizziness, Poria, Cinnamon Twig, Atractylodes, and Licorice Decoction (*líng guì zhú gān tāng*) masters it.

  It is possible to simultaneously see symptoms of dizziness and fullness from rebellion in the chest and ribcage, as well as palpitations and feeling unsteady. Other than this, from the ingredients it can be inferred that urinary difficulty will be part of this presentation. There is a report of the following formula being used to treat 10 patients with aural vertigo: Poria (*fú líng*) 30g, Cinnamomi Ramulus (*guì zhī*) 10g, Atractylodis macrocephalae Rhizoma (*bái zhú*) 30g, and Glycyrrhizae Radix (*gān cǎo*) 6g. After taking an average of 5-10 packets of herbs, the symptoms basically disappeared. Of particular interest was that once the volume of urine increased, the other symptoms disappeared.[24]

- *Patients with palpitations from rheumatic heart disease, coronary artery disease, hypertensive cardiac disease, pulmonary heart disease, or myocarditis.* In practice, what is seen are symptoms of fatigue, profuse sweating, chest stuffiness, floating edema, and urinary difficulty.

- *Patients with sloshing water sounds in the stomach: stomach prolapse, peptic ulcers, chronic gastritis, neurogenic vomiting, and functional gastrointestinal disorders.* At the same time, these patients have symptoms of palpitations, dizziness, and urinary difficulty. Endoscopic examination will reveal evidence of retained fluids.

• *Patients with cough along with chest and costal region fullness as in cases of bronchitis, asthma, and pleurisy.* In practice, patients are seen with coughs that have copious amounts of thin, clear or white sputum and a sensitivity to cold, which is accompanied by dizziness and palpitations.

I have used this formula to treat a young person who was diagnosed with bronchitis and stomach prolapse. The patient presented simultaneously with a cough and a sensation of something rising upward in the chest and abdomen, thin, white sputum, fullness in the costal region, an aversion to wind, and facial edema upon waking in the morning. The previous doctor had tried Minor Bluegreen Dragon Decoction (*xiǎo qīng lóng tāng*) but without any effect. On inspection, the patient had a thin physique, a pale, sallow, lusterless complexion, and a dark tongue body with a white, slippery coating. Using seven packets of Poria, Cinnamon Twig, Atractylodes, and Licorice Decoction (*líng guì zhú gān tāng*) proved effective.

THREE OTHER PRESCRIPTIONS WITH A FUNCTION SIMILAR TO THIS FORMULA

1. The first is the *Discussion of Cold Damage* formula Poria, Cinnamon Twig, Licorice, and Red Date Decoction (*fú líng guì zhī gān cǎo dà zǎo tāng*). This is a modification where Atractylodis macrocephalae Rhizoma (*bái zhú*) is replaced by Jujubae Fructus (*dà zǎo*). Originally, it was used to treat pulsations below the navel that are about to turn into running piglet syndrome. Due to the ability of Jujubae Fructus (*dà zǎo*) to relax tension and calm the spirit, this formula is quite suitable for treating palpitations and rebellious qi presentations such as neuroses, nervous exhaustion, and anemia.

2. Another formula, also from *Discussion of Cold Damage*, is Five-Ingredient Powder with Poria (*wǔ líng sǎn*). It is composed of Polyporus (*zhū líng*) 12g, Poria (*fú líng*) 12g, Alismatis Rhizoma (*zé xiè*) 12g, Atractylodis macrocephalae Rhizoma (*bái zhú*) 10g, and Cinnamomi Ramulus (*guì zhī*) 6g. This formula's ability to improve water metabolism is stronger than that of Poria, Cinnamon Twig, Atractylodes, and Licorice Decoction (*líng guì zhú gān tāng*). It can be considered for problems such as edema, urinary difficulty, vomiting, dizziness, and palpitations.

3. There is also Cinnamon and Poria Sweet Dew Drink (*guì líng gān lù yǐn*)*
   from *Formulas from the Discussion Illuminating the Yellow Emperor's Basic
   Questions* (*Huáng dì sù wèn xuán míng lùn fāng*). Cinnamon and Poria Sweet
   Dew Drink (*guì líng gān lù yǐn*) is generally used for those with febrile disease accompanied by urinary difficulty, vomiting, headache, fever, irritability,
   and thirst.

1.10 Cinnamon Twig and Poria Pill
(桂枝茯苓丸 *guì zhī fú líng wán*)

SOURCE: *Essentials from the Golden Cabinet*

Cinnamomi Ramulus (*guì zhī*) 6-10g
Poria (*fú líng*) 10g
Moutan Cortex (*mǔ dān pí*) 6-10g
Paeoniae Radix (*sháo yào*) 6-15g
Persicae Semen (*táo rén*) 6-10g

Cinnamon Twig and Poria Pill (*guì zhī fú líng wán*) is the cinnamon twig family
formula for invigorating the blood and removing stasis. Static blood is a unique
concept of pathology in Chinese medicine. Under normal conditions, the body's
blood circulates freely, but under the influence of certain pathogenic factors, the
blood encounters obstructions and its proper movement is impeded. This then
becomes static blood, which is both the result of a pathologic mechanism and
the source of secondary pathology. The clinical presentation is as follows:

1. Pain in a fixed location
2. Bleeding of blackish purple blood that congeals easily
3. Restlessness, irritability, and even mania
4. Dark purple tongue body and a dark, lusterless complexion

In *Essentials from the Golden Cabinet*, it is recorded that Cinnamon Twig and
Poria Pill (*guì zhī fú líng wán*) is the gynecology formula that dispels masses.
Chinese medicine believes that, for the most part, masses in the body are
formed from static blood. However, the scope of use of this formula by later
generations of doctors is obviously much broader. It can be used for a wide
variety of gynecological conditions as well as internal and surgical conditions

---

* Cinnamomi Cortex (*ròu guì*), Poria (*fú líng*), Polyporus (*zhū líng*), Atractylodis macrocephalae Rhizoma
(*bái zhú*), Alismatis Rhizoma (*zé xiè*), Gypsum fibrosum (*shí gāo*), Glauberitum (*hán shuǐ shí*), Talcum (*huá
shí*), and Glycyrrhizae Radix (*gān cǎo*).

with blood stasis presentations. Grasping the following signs and symptoms is the key to correctly using this formula:

1. Pain in the lower abdomen that is more intense with pressure or with the presence of nodules or small masses
2. Headaches and dizziness, poor sleep, irritability, and palpitations
3. A red or purplish red complexion and a tongue that is dark and may have purple spots

Pressure pain with masses in the lower abdomen, especially on either side of the navel, is a characteristic sign of blood stasis. Cinnamon twig constitution patients are thin with tight musculature and a dark tongue body; they readily manifest static blood presentations.

In practice, when a patient is seen with a dark yellow complexion and a tongue that is dark and purple, abdominal palpation can be used to confirm the diagnosis. Sometimes, even though there is no obvious pain or palpable masses, there is however a clear feeling of resistance and the patient feels uncomfortable. The area to the left of the navel can also be sensitive to pressure.

Sometimes the presentation for this formula and the Cinnamon Twig Decoction presentation are quite similar. The spasmodic abdominal pain, irritability, and palpitations seen with the Cinnamon Twig Decoction presentation are also seen in the presentation for this formula. The key to differentiating the two lies in inspection and abdominal palpation.

Other than the above-mentioned abdominal signs, a dark and red, or dark and yellow complexion, dark red lips, a dark tongue body, or purple spots on the tongue and bloodshot eyes are all relatively significant signs for diagnosing a Cinnamon Twig and Poria Pill presentation.

Presentations for this formula are for the most part seen with gynecological disorders. Pelvic inflammatory disease, irregular menstruation, dysmenorrhea, postpartum failure of the placenta to descend, tilted uterus, uterine fibroids, infertility, and habitual miscarriage are frequently treated with success using this formula.

In clinical practice, women should be asked about the color and quality of their menstrual blood as well as other related menstrual symptoms. If the color of the blood is dark or black, viscous, and contains clots, and is accompanied by abdominal pain, or if there are premenstrual headaches, breast distention, irritability and bad temper, the practitioner should consider the possibility of a static blood condition.

This formula's presentation can also be seen in lower extremity thrombosis or ulcerations, appendicitis, fluid in the rectouterine pouch, or prostate hypertrophy.

In practice, this formula is commonly modified, as shown in the following chart.

Additional symptoms	Add
For abdominal pain with constipation and a tongue that is dark red	Rhei Radix et Rhizoma (*dà huáng*)
For accompanying discomfort in the costal and hypochondriac regions	Bupleuri Radix (*chái hú*)
For dry skin along with scanty and black menstrual blood	Eupolyphaga/Stelophaga (*tŭ biē chóng*) and Carthami Flos (*hóng huā*)
For lower leg pain	Achyranthis bidentatae Radix (*niú xī*)

In China, Paeoniae Radix (*sháo yào*) is now differentiated into Paeoniae Radix rubra (*chì sháo*) and Paeoniae Radix alba (*bái sháo*). Traditionally, Paeoniae Radix alba (*bái sháo*) is believed to function better in stopping pain and calming spasms. When the abdomen has tight spasmodic pain or there are leg spasms, Paeoniae Radix alba (*bái sháo*) is the herb that is commonly used. Paeoniae Radix rubra (*chì sháo*) has a greater ability to invigorate the blood, and thus for blood stasis presentations, it is used more often or in equal amounts with Paeoniae Radix alba (*bái sháo*).

1.11 Unripe Bitter Orange, Chinese Garlic, and Cinnamon Twig Decoction (枳實薤白桂枝湯 *zhǐ shí xiè bái guì zhī tāng*)

SOURCE: *Essentials from the Golden Cabinet*

Aurantii Fructus immaturus (*zhǐ shí*) 6-10g
Magnoliae officinalis Cortex (*hòu pò*) 6-10g
Allii macrostemi Bulbus (*xiè bái*) 10-15g
Cinnamomi Ramulus (*guì zhī*) 6-10g
Trichosanthis Fructus (*guā lóu*) 10-12g

Unripe Bitter Orange, Chinese Garlic, and Cinnamon Twig Decoction (*zhǐ shí xiè bái guì zhī tāng*) is the cinnamon twig family formula for regulating qi and dispersing clumps. In practice, it is principally used for chest obstruction with chest and back pain, swollen and full hypochondria, and constipation. Chest obstruction (胸痹 *xiōng bì*) is an ancient disease category. Its symptoms are similar to those described by modern medicine for illnesses and symptoms such as obstructive emphysema, angina pectoris, intercostal neuralgia, and stomachache.

Essentials from the Golden Cabinet states: Chest obstruction, obstructed qi that knots up in the chest and creates fullness, qi from below the ribs that rebels upward and strikes against the Heart. Unripe Bitter Orange, Chinese Garlic, and Cinnamon Twig Decoction (*zhǐ shí xiè bái guì zhī tāng*) masters it. Ginseng Decoction (*rén shēn tāng*) also masters it. Here the meaning of 'obstruction' (痹 *bì*) is to be blocked; pain is the primary clinical sign. This is why Chinese doctors like to say, When blocked, there is pain; when unblocked, there is no pain (不通則痛, 通則不痛 *bù tōng zé tòng, tōng zé bù tòng*).

The Trichosanthis Fructus (*guā lóu*) and Allii macrostemi Bulbus (*xiè bái*) in Unripe Bitter Orange, Chinese Garlic, and Cinnamon Twig Decoction (*zhǐ shí xiè bái guì zhī tāng*) are the main medicinals used by Zhang Zhong-Jing to treat chest obstruction. Aurantii Fructus immaturus (*zhǐ shí*) and Magnoliae officinalis Cortex (*hòu pò*) are his must-use substances for distention and fullness of the chest and abdomen. When using Unripe Bitter Orange, Chinese Garlic, and Cinnamon Twig Decoction (*zhǐ shí xiè bái guì zhī tāng*), it is important that there be such signs and symptoms as chest stuffiness, palpitations, and a dark purple tongue. The basic presentation of this formula is as follows:

1. Stuffiness and pain affecting the chest and upper back; epigastric focal distention with fullness
2. Constipation or dry stool that is difficult to pass
3. A thick, greasy, and dry tongue coating with a tongue body that is dark and may have stasis spots

The key to differentiating this formula's presentation is a tongue that tends to be dark, more so than the typical cinnamon twig tongue. If the coating on the tongue is dry and scorched and the tongue body itself is red, this calls for the more appropriate rhubarb family formulas Minor Order the Qi Decoction (*xiǎo chéng qì tāng*) or Major Order the Qi Decoction (*dà chéng qì tāng*). If, however, the surface of the tongue is not dry, but on the contrary is moist and slimy, the tongue body itself is pale and flabby, the patient is overweight with a lusterless complexion, and the stools are either watery or dry at the beginning of the bowel movement, but soft at the end, then even though they have symptoms of chest and upper back pain and focal distention with fullness, this formula cannot be used. In these situations, a formula should be selected from within the dried ginger formula family. For example, Ginseng Decoction (*rén shēn tāng*), also known as Regulate the Middle Pill (*lǐ zhōng wán*), with modifications would be appropriate. *Essentials from the Golden Cabinet* lists both Unripe Bitter Orange, Chinese Garlic, and Cinnamon Twig Decoction (*zhǐ shí xiè bái guì zhī tāng*) and Ginseng Decoction (*rén shēn tāng*) to point out that chest obstruction has both excess and deficiency presentations; one needs to pay close attention to this point of differentiation.

In modern clinical practice, this formula is often used to treat coronary artery disease and angina. In fact, chest obstruction is seen not only in cardiac diseases, but it is common to see respiratory tract diseases with the presentation for this formula as well.

I once treated an elderly woman with chronic asthmatic bronchitis. This problem was induced by her becoming moody and then catching a cold. At the beginning, her chest and diaphragm had a feeling of being distended and full, she had a lack of interest in food or drink, and a slight, productive cough. Following this, she experienced chest and upper back stuffiness and pain as well as focal distention and fullness in the upper abdomen and a cough with wheezing that did not allow her to lay flat. On inspection, she had a thin physique and a sallow complexion. The tongue body was dark and pale and with a thick, dry coating. Palpating the epigastrium proved painful, and her abdomen was flat and rigid. Inquiring into her bowel habits revealed that she had not had a bowel movement in five days. For this patient, I prescribed Unripe Bitter Orange, Chinese Garlic, and Cinnamon Twig Decoction (*zhǐ shí xiè bái guì zhī tāng*) with the addition of Armeniacae Semen (*xìng rén*), Pinelliae Rhizoma preparatum (*zhì bàn xià*), and Perillae Caulis (*zǐ sū gěng*). After three packets, all the symptoms calmed down, and after seven packets, she felt fine.

If the abdominal distention is not as pronounced, the *Essentials from the Golden Cabinet* formula Cinnamon Twig, Ginger, and Unripe Bitter Orange Decoction (*guì zhī shēng jiāng zhǐ shí tāng*) * can be selected instead. This formula was originally used to treat focal distention in the area of the heart, various types of rebellion, and a rising and falling pain behind the lower aspect of the sternum. It is appropriate to prescribe for mild Unripe Bitter Orange, Chinese Garlic, and Cinnamon Twig Decoction presentations that are accompanied by nausea or vomiting.

---

* Cinnamomi Ramulus (*guì zhī*), Zingiberis Rhizoma recens (*shēng jiāng*), and Aurantii Fructus immaturus (*zhǐ shí*).

1.12 Cinnamon Twig, Peony, and Anemarrhena Decoction
(桂枝芍藥知母湯 *guì zhī sháo yào zhī mǔ tāng*)

SOURCE: *Essentials from the Golden Cabinet*

Cinnamomi Ramulus (*guì zhī*) 6-12g

Paeoniae Radix (*sháo yào*) 6-15g

Glycyrrhizae Radix (*gān cǎo*) 3-6g

Ephedrae Herba (*má huáng*) 5-10g

Zingiberis Rhizoma recens (*shēng jiāng*) 5-12g

Atractylodis macrocephalae Rhizoma (*bái zhú*) 6-12g

Anemarrhenae Rhizoma (*zhī mǔ*) 6-10g

Saposhnikoviae Radix (*fáng fēng*) 6-10g

Aconiti Radix lateralis preparata (*zhì fù zǐ*) 6-10g

As we have already discussed, for those with a cinnamon twig presentation that is accompanied by joint pain, Cinnamon Twig plus Aconite Accessory Root Decoction (*guì zhī jiā fù zǐ tāng*) can be used. However, in practice it is common to see patients with joint pain who, while they have the Cinnamon Twig plus Aconite Accessory Root Decoction presentation, also have an aversion to cold, are feverish, have edema, and dizziness. What is more, the joints are severely swollen and painful and there is numbness and a lack of feeling. It feels as though the limbs are about to fall off the body. Their complexion is dark yellow, and they may have facial edema. When presented with this kind of situation, Cinnamon Twig plus Aconite Accessory Root Decoction (*guì zhī jiā fù zǐ tāng*) is not strong enough, and one should consider using Cinnamon Twig, Peony, and Anemarrhena Decoction (*guì zhī sháo yào zhī mǔ tāng*).

Essentials from the Golden Cabinet advises: In all cases of limb and joint pain where the body is emaciated, the feet are swollen to the point that they feel like they are about to fall off, there is dizziness, shortness of breath, and a tendency toward vomiting easily, Cinnamon Twig, Peony, and Anemarrhena Decoction (*guì zhī sháo yào zhī mǔ tāng*) masters it.

Cinnamon Twig, Peony, and Anemarrhena Decoction (*guì zhī sháo yào zhī mǔ tāng*) is composed of the two formulas Cinnamon Twig plus Aconite Accessory Root Decoction (*guì zhī jiā fù zǐ tāng*) and Ephedra Decoction plus Atractylodes (*má huáng jiā zhú tāng*), with the addition of Saposhnikoviae Radix (*fáng fēng*) and Anemarrhenae Rhizoma (*zhī mǔ*). Cinnamon Twig plus Aconite Accessory Root Decoction (*guì zhī jiā fù zǐ tāng*) treats aversion to wind, spontaneous sweating, and joints that are cold and painful. Ephedra and

Atractylodes Decoction (*má huáng bái zhú tāng*) is an ephedra family formula that treats swollen and painful joints. However, its formula presentation and that of Cinnamon Twig plus Aconite Accessory Root Decoction (*guì zhī jiā fù zǐ tāng*) are different. It is appropriate for presentations where there is an aversion to cold, lack of sweating and edema, along with achy and painful joints and muscles. This is why the Cinnamon Twig, Peony, and Anemarrhena Decoction presentation in the original text included swollen feet. Presentations for this formula are as follows:

1. Severe joint pain accompanied by swelling
2. Aversion to wind with feverishness; there may be sweating or only slight sweating
3. Dark yellow complexion or facial edema, along with swollen and edematous feet

Intense joint pain accompanied by swelling is often seen in patients with rheumatoid arthritis. Therefore, the opportunities to use this formula are rather numerous. Furthermore, patients with gout or frozen shoulder can also share the presentations of this formula.

CHAPTER 2

EPHEDRA FORMULA FAMILY

麻黃類方 *má huáng lèi fāng*

EPHEDRAE HERBA (*má huáng*) is composed of the dried twigs and stems of a few plants in the horsetail family. Yellow-green in color, it is slightly fragrant with a bitter and astringent taste. Principally grown throughout most of northern China, Ephedrae Herba (*má huáng*) induces sweating, calms wheezing, promotes urination, and is widely used clinically in Chinese medicine.

This is a large family of related formulas that includes Ephedra Decoction (*má huáng tāng*), Ephedra, Apricot Kernel, Gypsum, and Licorice Decoction (*má xìng shí gān tāng*), Ephedra, Asarum, and Aconite Accessory Root Decoction (*má huáng xì xīn fù zǐ tāng*), and Minor Bluegreen Dragon Decoction (*xiǎo qīng lóng tāng*). Before introducing the members of the ephedra family of formulas, first let us discuss two key concepts as an aid to memory: the ephedra presentation (麻黃證 *má huáng zhèng*) and the ephedra constitution (麻黃體質 *má huáng tǐ zhì*).

Ephedra Presentation (麻黃證 *má huáng zhèng*)

This refers to the key signs for which Ephedrae Herba (*má huáng*) should be used. Just as the cinnamon twig family of formulas all share the distinguishing characteristics of the cinnamon twig presentation, the ephedra family formulas, to a greater or lesser degree, also carry signs associated with the ephedra presentation. Therefore, understanding the ephedra presentation undoubtedly is of great benefit in becoming adept at using the members of the ephedra formula family. The ephedra presentation consists of the following three parts:

1. Fever and chills, headache, joint pain, and body aches
2. Lack of sweating, cough, wheezing, and nasal congestion

3. Edema and urinary difficulty

In practice, it is possible that all three of these groups of signs will be present, or that only one is seen. However, even if just one is present, it is still enough to consider the possibility of an ephedra presentation.

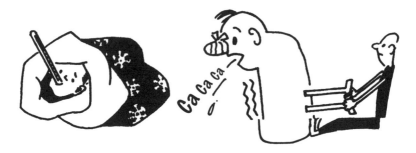

The signs of an ephedra presentation can occur in such diverse illnesses with symptoms such as fever and a lack of sweating and body aches in the common cold; joint pain from rheumatoid arthritis; nasal congestion from allergies, sensitivity to pollen, or asthma; edema from acute nephritis; and atopic skin conditions. As these disorders frequently manifest with the ephedra presentation, it follows that an ephedra family formula is often the appropriate treatment.

Within the ephedra presentation, a lack of sweating is the most important sign. It can be said that this is *the* distinguishing difference between the ephedra and cinnamon twig presentations. As stated previously, a cinnamon twig presentation is a condition of exterior deficiency and indicates that the body's exterior muscle layer is unstable. The sweat glands' production of excessive secretions results in an abnormal condition. The ephedra presentation is exactly the opposite. It is appropriate to see this as a condition of exterior excess where the muscle layer and the exterior are closed shut. It is a situation where the secretions of the sweat glands are inhibited.

The ancients had a saying: "For sweating, use Cinnamomi Ramulus (*guì zhī*); for an absence of sweating, use Ephedrae Herba (*má huáng*)." The lack of appropriate sweating accompanied by either fever with chills, body aches, coughing and wheezing, or edema, should give one cause to consider the presence of an ephedra presentation.

The second item on our list, a lack of sweating with coughing and wheezing or nasal congestion, also can be understood as one type of closed, congested state. Chinese medicine theory holds that the Lung governs the skin and hair and the nose is the orifice of the Lung; this is to say that the skin, Lung, and nose are all part of the same system. So, when the Lung qi is constrained and closed, not only can one see wheezing and fullness in the chest, but also nasal congestion with an inability to breathe through the nose along with chills and a lack of sweating.

A reduction in urinary output is the principal sign of urinary difficulty. The daily amount of urine in a healthy person is 1 to 1.5 liters. In the clinic, patients should be asked how often and how much they urinate. By comparing this with their normal urinary habits, one can judge if there has been any change. Edema in the ephedra presentation is accompanied by urinary difficulty.

There are circumstances we encounter in practice that are quite different from the ephedra presentation: when there is only edema or only urinary difficulty; when the legs are swollen, but there is copious urine; or when there is urinary difficulty, but without edema. One should also carefully consider the presence of a different formula presentation. Ephedrae Herba (*má huáng*) is not to be used in a careless way!

Ephedra Constitution (麻黃體質 *má huáng tǐ zhì*)

The ephedra constitution is the body type that tends to manifest the signs and symptoms of an ephedra presentation. This is determined based on the physician's observation and questions.

- *External appearance.* A slightly fat build with musculature that is either relatively well developed or loose. The color of the skin is yellow, light yellow, or has a shallow dark cast. For people with darker skin, where it is difficult to see the yellow color, or for those with pale skin where the yellow color is washed out, look for a lack of luster in the face and a slight amount of edema. The skin texture is rather coarse and dry. The test for dry skin is to scratch lightly with the fingernail; if it leaves a white mark, it is the dry skin of this presentation. Generally, these people don't sweat easily, and their bodies are relatively robust. They don't have high blood pressure. The lips are dark or purplish red. Their tongues tend to be large, pale red, and with a white coating, and they don't have dry mouths.
- *Commonly expressed symptoms.* These patients do not easily sweat, and when they do, the sweat does not flow smoothly. They readily feel chilled and have a tendency to wheeze. They often have nasal congestion with a clear, runny discharge. The muscles tend to feel

heavy and sore, and the entire body feels tired and worn out. These people are not particularly sensitive to their environment. There is a feeling of heaviness or pressure in the epigastrium or abdominal bloating, and their heads tend to feel heavy. They are inclined to have superficial edema.

Externally-observed features are important evidence for the clinical suitability of using Ephedrae Herba (*má huáng*) and the ephedra formula family. Simply stated, those who are hefty and have a sallow or dark complexion for the most part can be given Ephedrae Herba (*má huáng*) and ephedra family formulas. If the physique is thin, with a tight musculature, red complexion, a body that runs warm and sweats profusely, and there is a red tongue; or for those who have high blood pressure or an elevated heart rate, Ephedrae Herba (*má huáng*) and its family of formulas should be used with caution, if at all. Additionally, careful interviewing to ascertain the patient's tendency to experience the symptoms associated with this formula is an extremely important aspect of concretely confirming the formula presentation.

When we discuss 'increased cold' or 'increased dampness' in relation to the ephedra constitution, we are not saying that the body temperature of the ephedra constitution is low or that the person has an increased amount of internal fluids. It is simply to point to a kind of Chinese medical way of viewing a pathological state. This so-called 'cold' is a description of a bodily state that leads to disease. It is common knowledge that when someone catches a cold, they often have symptoms such as chills, lack of sweating, goosebumps, muscle tension, joint pain, and nasal congestion. Chinese medicine calls this type of condition a 'cold presentation' (寒證 *hán zhèng*). In the same way, people who live in climates where there is a summer rainy season or those who live in damp or humid environments tend to experience superficial edema, a heavy and sluggish body, reduced appetite, joint problems, and reduced urinary output. Put simply, this kind of situation is a 'damp presentation' (濕證 *shī zhèng*), which is just to say that when ephedra constitution patients fall ill, they readily manifest the above-mentioned types of symptoms.

Modern pharmacological research shows that Ephedrae Herba (*má huáng*) has many functions. It can act as a diaphoretic and antipyretic, a significant bronchodilator, an anti-allergic and anti-inflammatory agent, and it has analgesic, diuretic, as well as central and sympathetic nervous system stimulation effects. Looking at the numerous members of the ephedra family of formulas shows that practitioners of Chinese medicine are accustomed to using Ephedrae Herba (*má huáng*) for a wide variety of problems. Although the ancients were unable to separate out the various active compounds within Ephedrae Herba (*má huáng*), they did find ways to elicit and utilize the various functions of Ephedrae Herba (*má huáng*) by applying various ingenious methods of combining it with other medicinals.

2.1 Ephedra Decoction (麻黃湯 *má huáng tāng*)

SOURCE: *Discussion of Cold Damage* (傷寒論 *Shāng hán lùn*)

Ephedrae Herba (*má huáng*) 3-10g
Cinnamomi Ramulus (*guì zhī*) 5-10g
Armeniacae Semen (*xìng rén*) 6-12g
Glycyrrhizae Radix (*gān cǎo*) 3g

Cover up the patient to get a light sweat. It is not necessary to eat congee (rice porridge) with this formula, but it is helpful if the patient rests and avoids drafts and air conditioning.

Ephedra Decoction (*má huáng tāng*) is the representative formula of the ephedra formula family. It is the principal formula from *Discussion of Cold Damage* used for treating *tài yáng* cold damage. Later generations took this as an indispensable formula to scatter wind-cold, promote sweating, and calm wheezing. However, in the Qing dynasty, after the rise of the warm pathogen disease current (溫病派 *wēn bìng pài*), many doctors began to use more medicinals that were cool and acrid; they had real misgivings about using Ephedra Decoction (*má huáng tāng*). In Japan, however, practitioners of Chinese medicine do not have this sort of bias. Not only do they use it to treat the common cold, joint pain, and asthma in adults, but it is also used to treat colds and nasal congestion in children, as well as for difficulties in breast feeding. Therefore, as long as one has a good grasp of the indications, Ephedra Decoction (*má huáng tāng*) can be used without reservation. The Ephedra Decoction presentation is as follows:

1. Chills with fever, headache, and body aches
2. A lack of sweating with the presence of wheezing
3. A floating and tight pulse, and a dark and pale tongue

There is a difference between chills and the Cinnamon Twig Decoction presentation of aversion to wind. Aversion to wind means a sensitivity to drafts. When these are encountered, people feel uncomfortably cold. This sensation, however, goes away if they bundle up or move into a warm environment. Chills is the feeling of being cold and having an aversion to cold even before a fever sets in. Even though one bundles up or puts on more clothes, this does not change the feeling of being cold. Furthermore, these chills must simultaneously be accompanied by fever. Finally, with the Cinnamon Twig Decoction presentation there is sweating and the patient's skin is moist. However, as there is no sweating in the Ephedra Decoction presentation, the patient's skin is dry. One can use this difference as a way to differentiate between the two presentations.

There are some who believe that the fever of an Ephedra Decoction presentation is, for the most part, not particularly high. I agree. In cases where there is a high fever, members of the gypsum, rhubarb, or coptis family formulas are more appropriate.

Zhang investigated the body temperatures of patients with an Ephedra Decoction presentation who had acute fevers (from pneumonia, upper respiratory tract infection, etc.). These patients generally did not have a fever of more than 39°C (102°F), and their white blood cell count did not surpass 12,000/ mm^3.[1] These patients reported that when they had fever and chills and a lack of sweating, there was often accompanying achiness of the entire body or joint pain, and some had particularly sore and painful lower backs.

Lack of sweating with wheezing refers to a passage from *Discussion of Cold Damage*: "For a *tài yáng* disease with headache, fever, body pain, lower back pain, pain in the bones and joints, aversion to wind, lack of sweating and wheezing, Ephedra Decoction (*má huáng tāng*) masters it." Zhang Zhong-Jing uses the character 而 (*ér*) to connect 'lack of sweating' and 'wheezing' to emphasize that within the Ephedra Decoction presentation, these two symptoms must both be present. If sweating does accompany the wheezing, then the formula presentation has undergone a change and the wheezing can be seen as either due to deficiency or excess. One must at this time consider the pulse and the other symptoms to properly distinguish between the two. This cannot be regarded as an Ephedra Decoction presentation.

A floating and tight pulse is one that can be immediately felt when the fingertips lightly touch the pulse. Furthermore, there is strength to the pulse, which indicates the body's resistance is in a state of overdrive. A dark pale tongue indicates a lack of internal heat, and in this situation, Ephedra Decoction (*má huáng tāng*) can be used.

- The Ephedra Decoction presentation is commonly seen in febrile illnesses such as the common cold, influenza, and upper respiratory tract infections. It has been reported that during one summer and fall cold and flu season, some young people with strong constitutions were given Mulberry Leaf and Chrysanthemum Drink (*sāng jú yǐn*) and Honeysuckle and Forsythia Powder (*yín qiào sǎn*) at the beginning of their illnesses. For those with exterior heat patterns, this was effective; for those with exterior cold patterns, the results were poor. After that, Schizonepeta and Saposhnikovia Powder to Overcome Pathogenic Influences (*jīng fáng bài dú sǎn*) was prescribed, but this was not effective for some of the patients. For those who had not recovered, Ephedra Decoction (*má huáng tāng*) was used. Generally, after two to three packets, there was sweating and a reduction of the fever with resulting recovery.[2]

- In another report, this formula was used to treat children with fevers of 39°C (102°F) and above. The study consisted of 167 subjects; among these 44 had tonsillitis, four had parotitis, and nine had a cough. All were given Ephedra Decoction (*má huáng tāng*) in decoction form in order to induce sweating. This resulted in temperatures returning to normal within two days, with 164 subjects being cured.[3] However, it must be pointed out that when using Ephedra Decoction (*má huáng tāng*) in children with a fever, one must pay close attention to both the pattern differentiation and the patient's constitution. Currently, there are quite a few children and young people in our cities that tend to be tall and thin, and they usually are quite active and sweat a lot. Because they eat too many sweet and rich foods, their constitutions have a lot of heat, phlegm, and wind. When they get sick with a cold, most of them have a sudden high fever, a red, swollen, and painful throat, sweating, and wheezing. Some even have convulsions and lose consciousness. These are far from being Ephedra Decoction presentations.

- Cases of asthma where the main manifestations are coughing and wheezing, or bronchitis, can also have an Ephedra Decoction presentation. Because this kind of patient often has a bit of sweating, in practice this often results in the removal of Cinnamomi Ramulus (*guì zhī*) from the formula so as to reduce the diaphoretic effect of Ephedra Decoction (*má huáng tāng*). Ephedra Decoction (*má huáng tāng*) without the Cinnamomi Ramulus (*guì zhī*) is called Three-Unbinding Decoction (*sān ǎo tāng*). In one report, it was found that this formula—consisting of Ephedrae Herba (*má huáng*) 5g, Armeniacae Semen (*xìng rén*) 10g, and Glycyrrhizae Radix (*gān cǎo*) 3g—was steamed with tofu, fresh ginger, and rock sugar, and was then used to treat

196 subjects. Once a day, the tofu was eaten and the fluid was drunk, resulting in 118 subjects being cured and 52 showing significant improvement.[4] In another report, this formula was used with the additions of Mori Ramulus (*sāng zhī*), Lepidii/Descurainiae Semen (*tíng lì zǐ*), Aurantii Fructus (*zhǐ ké*), Perillae Fructus (*zǐ sū zǐ*), Pinelliae Rhizoma preparatum (*zhì bàn xià*), Houttuyniae Herba (*yú xīng cǎo*), and Plantaginis Semen (*chē qián zǐ*) to treat 30 children with coughing and wheezing. In most cases, their clinical symptoms disappeared within one to three days.[5] It should be pointed out that those with coughing and wheezing often have a Cinnamon Twig Decoction plus Magnolia Bark and Apricot Kernels presentation.

In my experience, the primary key to differentiation is the constitution. With the ephedra constitution, the face is dark, the body is robust, and there is an absence of sweating. With the cinnamon twig constitution, the face is fair, the body is thin and weak, and there is a tendency to sweat.

MODIFICATIONS

Ephedra Decoction (*má huáng tāng*) with the addition of 12g of either Atractylodis macrocephalae Rhizoma (*bái zhú*) or Atractylodis Rhizoma (*cāng zhú*) is called Ephedra Decoction plus Atractylodes (*má huáng jiā zhú tāng*), which has the ability to induce sweating and promote urination. It treats an Ephedra Decoction presentation with accompanying edema, arthritis with achy muscles, nephritis, or the common cold. Generally, for those with significant edema and unformed stools, use Atractylodis macrocephalae Rhizoma (*bái zhú*). For those with abdominal fullness and a white, greasy tongue coating, use Atractylodis Rhizoma (*cāng zhú*).

I once used this formula with the addition of Zingiberis Rhizoma (*gān jiāng*) to treat a young man who worked in a refrigeration unit. It was summertime, and he had been sweating. He then contracted a cold due to his work environment. He had a lack of sweating and chills, body aches, abdominal fullness, and a thick white, greasy tongue coating. After taking the herbs, he sweated and was cured.

The strength of this formula's ability to promote sweating is relatively strong. If it is used inappropriately, it can induce side effects of nervousness, excessive sweating, and muscle spasms. This is especially true for some middle-aged or elderly women who are slightly overweight and with fair skin. Because they present with sore joints, edema, and muscle aches, this formula is sometimes erroneously prescribed. In practice, close attention must be paid to this (see Chapter 5 on the astragalus formula family).

Discussion of Cold Damage forbids the use Ephedra Decoction (*má huáng tāng*) in patients who have ongoing tendencies of having sores, urinary dribbling, nosebleeds, or bleeding of any kind. It should never be used for patients with exterior deficiency and spontaneous sweating, those with a slow proximal pulse or palpitations and a heavy-feeling body due to having been improperly purged. Generally speaking, this formula should not be used for patients with wasting diseases, bleeding disorders, high blood pressure, ischemic heart disease, as well as those with a weak constitution who easily fall ill, those who are debilitated and of advanced age, or postpartum women with sweating.

2.2 Ephedra, Asarum, and Aconite Accessory Root Decoction
(麻黃細辛附子湯 *má huáng xì xīn fù zǐ tāng*)

SOURCE: *Discussion of Cold Damage*

Ephedrae Herba (*má huáng*)......................................3-10g
Asari Herba (*xì xīn*) 3-6g
Aconiti Radix lateralis preparata (*zhì fù zǐ*) 5-10g

In practice, we see some patients with a cold and fever, joint pain, coughing or wheezing, heart disease, or allergic rhinitis who will manifest with the Ephedra Decoction presentation signs of chills with fever, body aches, a lack of sweating, and a pale tongue with a white coating. Additionally, these patients are listless and dispirited, significantly fatigued, have a dark and lusterless complexion, cold hands and feet, clear and thin nasal discharge, and copious amounts of urine. The pulse is not floating and tight, but instead is sinking and weak, sinking and minute, or sinking and thin, like that of the aconite and asarum presentation (see Chapter 9 on the aconite formula family). For these types of patients, simply giving Ephedra Decoction (*má huáng tāng*) would be inappropriate. The strong diaphoretic action of Ephedra Decoction (*má huáng tāng*) would likely give such patients unwanted side effects. For these patients, Chinese doctors often use the formula Ephedra, Asarum, and Aconite Accessory Root Decoction (*má huáng xì xīn fù zǐ tāng*).

This formula is found in paragraph 301 of *Discussion of Cold Damage*. As stated in the original text: "*Shào yīn* illness, when one has just begun to get it and yet is feverish with a submerged pulse, Ephedra, Asarum, and Aconite Accessory Root Decoction (*má huáng xì xīn fù zǐ tāng*) masters it."

A sinking pulse is the distinguishing sign that Zhang Zhong-Jing used for prescribing this formula. As already noted, the floating and tight pulse seen in the Ephedra Decoction presentation reflects the body's resistance being in overdrive. By contrast, a sinking pulse, especially one that is sinking and slow, sinking and weak, or sinking and thin, is the reflection of the body's low resistance. In Chinese medicine, this sort of resistance is commonly referred to as 'yang qi', and thus pulses such as sinking and weak are considered manifestations of 'yang qi deficiency'.

Therefore, an Ephedra Decoction presentation accompanied by a sinking and slow pulse (aconite presentation) is the distinctive feature of an Ephedra, Asarum, and Aconite Accessory Root Decoction presentation. In the technical language of Chinese medicine, this presentation is one of 'exterior excess with interior deficiency'. Specific signs include the following:

1. Lack of sweating, obvious feeling of chills; may or may not have a fever
2. Listless and dispirited, significant fatigue, a dark and lusterless complexion, cold hands and feet
3. Sinking and weak pulse, or one that is sinking and thin or sinking and slow
4. Pale tongue body with a wet, white coating

A lack of sweating, significant feeling of chills, and the presence or absence of a fever, even though it may be low-grade, resemble an Ephedra Decoction presentation. However, the condition of the spirit and the complexion are not at all what one would see in an Ephedra Decoction presentation. Being dispirited is a symptom of reduced function, a manifestation of a decline in the body's ability to respond to the outside world.

Discussion of Cold Damage often uses the phrase "a pulse that is faint and thin with a tendency toward somnolence" to describe this type of condition. These are the typical signs and symptoms of *shào yīn* conditions. Somnolence refers to the condition in which one appears to be half asleep, fatigued, and listless. A minute and thin pulse is indicated by the pulse being sinking and weak, sinking and thin, or sinking and late, as all of these are weak pulses. A pale tongue body with a wet, white coating is representative of a decline in the digestive function.

• This formula's presentation can be seen in cases of the common cold, influenza, bronchitis, and pharyngitis marked by chills and fever. The learned Japanese practitioner Fujihara Ken believes this formula is especially good for treating sore throat from the common cold, and in 60 percent of the patients that took this formula at the very onset of illness, it controlled the progression of the illness to bronchitis.[6] Cao reported that this formula is effective in treating the common cold in those who are debilitated and of advanced age, or those who are weak after an illness. It is especially effective for those patients in whom the distinctive feature is that they have a hard to describe dread of cold over their entire upper back.[7]

• Cold-type coughing and wheezing, laryngitis, and allergic rhinitis can also be treated with this formula. Japanese doctors reported that 5 to 15 minutes after taking this formula, patients with allergic rhinitis felt like their symptoms began to disappear, and that the effect lasted for three to four hours.[8] Allergic rhinitis for the most part manifests as nasal congestion and sneezing, with a large amount of clear watery discharge; these symptoms are similar to those in the presentation of this formula.

• This formula's presentation is often seen in patients who have chills and body aches with problems such as back pain, bone spurs, osteoarthritis, sciatica, trigeminal neuralgia, headache, or toothache. Chills and body aches are part of the Ephedra Decoction (*má huáng tāng*) presentation. However, Ephedra, Asarum, and Aconite Accessory Root Decoction (*má huáng xì xīn fù zǐ tāng*) can be used if the pulse is sinking and weak in those who are listless and dispirited with cold extremities. It has been reported that a modification—Ephedrae Herba (*má huáng*) 6g, Asari Herba (*xì xīn*) 6g, and Aconiti Radix lateralis preparata (*zhì fù zǐ*) 15g—was used to treat a case of renal colic with cold extremities. Within an hour after administering the herbs, the pain disappeared. However, this method is not effective for pain from stones in general.[9]

• Ephedra, Asarum, and Aconite Accessory Root Decoction (*má huáng xì xīn fù zǐ tāng*) was used, with the addition of Gentianae Radix (*lóng dǎn cǎo*), Chuanxiong Rhizoma (*chuān xiōng*), and Bombyx batryticatus (*bái jiāng cán*), to treat 20 subjects with trigeminal neuralgia. All were cured, and it was reported in follow-up interviews over the course of many years that there were no recurrences.[10] To treat sciatica and improve the analgesic effect, I often add Peony and Licorice Decoction (*sháo yào gān cǎo tāng*) with a large dose of 30g of Paeoniae Radix alba (*bái sháo*).

• More than a few patients with cardiovascular disease have a deep and slow, or deep and weak pulse, and many have a pale tongue body with a moist, white coating. Liu reports that this formula, with the addition of Zingiberis Rhizoma (*gān jiāng*), can be used to preventatively treat frigid extremities and yang deficiency-type Keshan disease, especially when there is a minute pulse that is on the point of being impalpable.[11] This formula was also used to treat five cases of sick sinus syndrome, with three having coronary heart disease and two suffering from the sequelae of viral myocarditis. Their pulses were significantly slow; slow and lax; or deep, slow, and thin. A few also had a knotted pulse. After the treatment, the heart rhythm returned to normal and symptoms basically disappeared. On average, the speed of the heart increased 10 beats or more per minute. Patients with sick sinus syndrome are, for the most part, quite debilitated. In addition to using this formula, they can also be given Ginseng Radix (rén shēn) and Cervi Cornu pantotrichum (lù róng), to be taken separately as a powder. Alternatively, it may also be combined with Astragalus Decoction to Construct the Middle (huáng qí jiàn zhōng tāng), All-Inclusive Great Tonifying Decoction (shí quán dà bǔ tāng), or Tonify the Middle to Augment the Qi Decoction (bǔ zhōng yì qì tāng).

- The presentation for this formula can be seen in conditions where the primary symptom is frigidly cold extremities. It has been reported that this formula has been used with a large dosage of Aconiti Radix lateralis preparata (zhì fù zǐ) up to 60g [cooked first for two hours], Ephedrae Herba (má huáng) 10g, and Asari Herba (xì xīn) 6g to treat 21 cases of deficiency-cold type sloughing ulcer (脱疽 tuō jū), which is roughly the equivalent of arteritis obliterans. Of these, 15 were cured.[12]

- This formula can also be prescribed for those with a weak constitution and whose primary symptoms are feeling listless and dispirited, along with nervous exhaustion. The Japanese practitioner Nakamura discovered that using this formula with the addition of Glycyrrhizae Radix (gān cǎo) was effective in treating patients whose main complaint was throat pain and fatigue from summer colds. He discovered that after taking these herbs, both the cold and the fatigue disappeared. From this came the inspiration to use the formula for those who have a weak constitution with fatigue, those with autonomic dystonia, and those recovering from surgery. This formula can be effective for treating all of these problems.[13]

The pharmacological effects of the constituents of Ephedra, Asarum, and Aconite Accessory Root Decoction (má huáng xì xīn fù zǐ tāng) are extensive. Ephedrae Herba (má huáng) has significant diaphoretic, antipyretic, anti-asthmatic, antitussive, anti-inflammatory, anti-allergic, analgesic, and central nervous system stimulatory effects. It also has epinephrine-like effects on the nervous system, thus raising the blood pressure, heart rate, and blood sugar levels. Aconiti

Radix lateralis preparata (*zhì fù zǐ*) dilates the peripheral vasculature and also has significant cardiotonic, anti-inflammatory, analgesic, adrenocortical stimu-lating, and antihypothermal effects. Asari Herba (*xì xīn*) has notable analgesic, anti-inflammatory, antipyretic, bronchiodilating, antihistamine, and anti-allergic effects. It enhances Ephedrae Herba's (*má huáng*) antipyretic, anti-asthmatic, anti-inflammatory, and anti-allergic properties. It also increases the ability of Aconiti Radix lateralis preparata's (*zhì fù zǐ*) to stimulate the metabolism, strengthen the heart, dilate the peripheral blood vessels, raise blood glucose levels, and reduce pain and inflammation. Used together, these three medicinals are rather good at warming the yang and scattering the cold.

2.3 Minor Bluegreen Dragon Decoction
(小青龍湯 *xiǎo qīng lóng tāng*)

SOURCE: *Discussion of Cold Damage*

Ephedrae Herba (*má huáng*)..3-6g
Cinnamomi Ramulus (*guì zhī*)..3-6g
Asari Herba (*xì xīn*)..3-6g
Paeoniae Radix (*sháo yào*)...6-10g
Zingiberis Rhizoma (*gān jiāng*)..3-6g
Glycyrrhizae Radix (*gān cǎo*)...3-6g
Schisandrae Fructus (*wǔ wèi zǐ*)..3-5g
Pinelliae Rhizoma preparatum (*zhì bàn xià*)..............................6-10g

In the ephedra family of formulas, Minor Bluegreen Dragon Decoction (*xiǎo qīng lóng tāng*) is recommended as being the best for stopping coughing and calming wheezing. This ancient prescription, which has been used countless times over thousands of years to good effect, is named for the deity of an ancient East Asian myth. Today it is still used as a primary formula in Chinese medicine to treat respiratory tract illnesses.

Minor Bluegreen Dragon Decoction (*xiǎo qīng lóng tāng*) is a derivative of Ephedra Decoction (*má huáng tāng*) from which the Armeniacae Semen (*xìng rén*) has been removed and Asari Herba (*xì xīn*), Zingiberis Rhizoma (*gān jiāng*), Schisandrae Fructus (*wǔ wèi zǐ*), and Paeoniae Radix (*sháo yào*) have been added. Zhang Zhong-Jing frequently used the combination of Asari Herba (*xì xīn*), Zingiberis Rhizoma (*gān jiāng*), and Schisandrae Fructus (*wǔ wèi zǐ*) to treat coughs.

Concerning the Minor Bluegreen Dragon Decoction presentation, paragraph 40 of *Discussion of Cold Damage* states: "Cold damage with an unresolved exterior and water qi (水氣 *shuǐ qì*) in the epigastrium will have dry heaves, fever, and coughing. There may also be thirst, diarrhea, dysphagia, urinary difficulty, lower abdominal distention, or wheezing. Minor Bluegreen Dragon Decoction (*xiǎo qīng lóng tāng*) masters it." *Essentials from the Golden Cabinet* (金匱要略 *Jīn guì yào lüè*) has this indication: "coughing rebellion where one needs support to breathe and an inability to recline."

Cold damage with an unresolved exterior implies that the symptoms of chills with fever, a lack of sweating, and body aches are still present. Water qi is also called 'phlegm and thin mucus' (痰飲 *tán yǐn*) or 'water and thin mucus' (水飲 *shuǐ yǐn*), indicating stagnation of the body fluids, which in turn leads to further pathogenic changes. These can manifest as edema, thin, clear sputum, gurgling sounds in the abdomen, dizziness, urinary difficulty, a cold feeling in the middle of the back, or abdominal fullness. Water qi in the epigastrium implies that the patient either has a cough with copious amounts of watery sputum, back that feels cold, or gurgling sounds in the abdomen. Because the clinical manifestation of water qi is complicated, *Discussion of Cold Damage* records several possible symptoms. From looking at the description in *Essentials from the Golden Cabinet*, the degree of coughing and wheezing is relatively severe. Consequently, the Minor Bluegreen Dragon Decoction presentation should reflect a combination of both the Ephedra Decoction presentation and signs of a problem due to phlegm and thin mucus. The specifics of the formula presentation are as follows:

1. Coughing and wheezing with a relatively copious amount of sputum that can be either watery or sticky, or nasal congestion with sneezing and a clear, watery discharge
2. Chills, with the back being particularly sensitive to cold. There may or may not be fever; usually there is a lack of sweating, but there may be sweating during episodes of coughing or wheezing
3. A white and slippery tongue coating

When diagnosing for this formula's presentation, discerning the character of the sputum and nasal discharge is extremely important. These secretions must be copious, thin, and clear as well as either viscous or watery. At the same time, the tongue has a white, slippery coating that is sticky and covers the entire tongue. As an aid to memory, this is jokingly called 'bluegreen dragon water.' This is because in folklore, the bluegreen dragon causes a great tumult in the

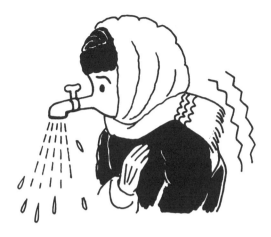

oceans and rivers, stirs up wind, and makes waves. However, sputum that is yellow, sticky, and hard to expectorate, or coughing and wheezing along with a tongue that has a greasy, dried-out coating, are not a Minor Bluegreen Dragon Decoction presentation.

Chills is the symptom that must be present; however, there will not necessarily be a fever or a lack of sweating. Some patients will have a fever, while others will not. Some will even have lower than normal body temperatures, especially the elderly and debilitated, whose body temperatures on the average are lower. It is common to see a lack of sweating with these patients, especially in the winter. However, during episodes of coughing with an inability to lay flat, some patients will sweat a little. This will not be a strong sweat, however, and in no way will they be drenched. Furthermore, although there is ceaseless coughing and wheezing, the mind is usually clear, not like the dispirited listlessness seen in the Ephedra, Asarum, and Aconite Accessory Root Decoction presentation. Additionally, the aforementioned ephedra constitution is frequently seen in patients who present with a Minor Bluegreen Dragon Decoction presentation. Knowing the commonly manifested symptoms for these patients is a big help with the differential diagnosis.

A Minor Bluegreen Dragon Decoction presentation is commonly seen in patients with respiratory illness where the main symptoms are coughing and wheezing. In the 1970s I was working in the hospital wards, and every year during the winter when a cold front would come through, a significant number of elderly patients with chronic asthmatic bronchitis would come into the hospital, one after the other, as their long-term unresolved illnesses began to act up. Quite a few of these patients had Minor Bluegreen Dragon Decoction presentations.

I followed the methods of the old Chinese doctor Xia Wu-Ying in treating many patients. What I saw were patients who were feverish and with chills; others without fever but who complained of coldness in the middle of the back; and still others with headaches and dry heaves. The commonly shared symptoms were copious amounts of thin, clear sputum, and most also had a white, slippery tongue coating. Minor Bluegreen Dragon Decoction (*xiǎo qīng lóng tāng*) had a distinct ability to improve the symptoms in these patients.

- In Japan, Morishima Akira used this formula in granulated form to treat Lung cold-type bronchial asthma in 31 children. This treatment resulted in a significant effect in stopping the asthma attacks for four children (12.9 percent), had some effect for 12 children (38.7 percent), slight improvement for another four children (12.9 percent), and no effect for eight children (25.8 percent); for three children (9.7 percent), it was unclear if there was any effect, but there was no increase in the frequency or severity of the attacks after taking the herbs. Furthermore, in those subjects for whom the herbs were effective, there was a drop in their blood level of IgE (immunoglobulin E).[14]

- Wang reports that readjusting the dosages of the herbs within this formula, increasing the amounts of Ephedrae Herba (*má huáng*), Asari Herba (*xì xīn*), Pinelliae Rhizoma preparatum (*zhì bàn xià*), and Paeoniae Radix alba (*bái sháo*), resulted in improvement in clinical efficacy. From 1980 to 1981, he treated six asthmatic patients. Within 30 to 60 minutes after administering the herbs, their asthma calmed down. Auscultation of both lungs found either a great reduction in rales or complete lack thereof. After taking two to three packets of herbs, the patients' condition stabilized.[15] The prescription he used was Honey-Fried Ephedrae Herba (*zhì má huáng*) 15g, Cinnamomi Ramulus (*guì zhī*) 9g, Schisandrae Fructus (*wǔ wèi zǐ*) 9g, Zingiberis Rhizoma (*gān jiāng*) 6g, Pinelliae Rhizoma preparatum (*zhì bàn xià*) 30g, Asari Herba (*xì xīn*) 6-9g, and Glycyrrhizae Radix (*gān cǎo*) 9-15g.

After publishing this first report, he again used the same treatment method to treat 24 subjects. The average length of illness was 11.4 years. Fifteen subjects had cold-type asthma, nine had hot-type, one case also had right ventricular hypertrophy, and two also had emphysema. Among 20 of the subjects, after taking one packet of herbs, their asthma either gradually subsided or did not flare up that evening. The remaining four subjects required six to 10 packets of herbs before an effect was seen. After the course of treatment, only one subject had a relapse. All the other 23 basically had their symptoms controlled.[16] From this it can be deduced that this formula is reliably effective for the treatment of asthma.

- The main presenting symptoms of allergic rhinitis are sneezing and watery nasal discharge, which also are the primary signs of a Minor Bluegreen Dragon Decoction presentation. It is common to see the Minor Bluegreen Dragon Decoction presentation with cases of allergic rhinitis. Clinical reports from Japan concerning this topic are relatively abundant. Okazaki treated 60 subjects, 33 of whom had intractable allergic rhinitis and 27 had recent attacks. Treatment resulted in significant clinical effect for 18 subjects, some effect for 14 subjects, no effect for 25 subjects, and a worsening of the condition for three. Interestingly, 85.7 percent of those with severe symptoms had some benefit from the treatment. For those whose symptoms were of moderate or mild severity, the efficacy rates were 49.9 and 28.6 percent, respectively. Of those patients who had previously received desensitization treatment, 52 percent had a positive response to this treatment. Those for whom the herbs were effective continued to feel the effect for four to eight weeks after discontinuing the herbs, with the longest maintaining an effect for two years.[17]

- Imai Nao used a granulated form of Minor Bluegreen Dragon Decoction (*xiǎo qīng lóng tāng*) to treat 20 patients with sinus infections. Among these, 16 had allergic rhinitis, two had an acute upper respiratory tract infection, one had sinusitis, and one had acute rhinitis. Treatment resulted in one patient having significant improvement, 12 patients showing some improvement, five patients with a little improvement, and no improvement for two patients. Cessation of nasal discharge was the improvement that occurred most quickly.[18]

- Kuriyama used Minor Bluegreen Dragon Decoction (*xiǎo qīng lóng tāng*) in granulated form to treat 29 subjects for allergic rhinitis from household dust who had previously undergone one to three years of unsuccessful desensitization treatments. The formula was administered for three weeks, and resulted in 21 subjects reporting a subjective sense of improvement. Fourteen of the subjects showed improvement when examined with a rhinoscope. Furthermore, blood levels of IgE and histamine decreased, while cAMP (cyclic AMP, an important second messenger) levels went up.[19]

  Additionally there are reports of Minor Bluegreen Dragon Decoction (*xiǎo qīng lóng tāng*) being effective for such diverse illnesses as the common cold, hayfever, spring conjunctivitis, pleurisy, and acute nephritis. Most of these cases, however, underwent differential diagnosis, and the formula was only used if the patient had signs of a Minor Bluegreen Dragon Decoction presentation.

- Although this formula is mostly made up of acrid and warm herbs, as long as one confirms its use through differential diagnosis, generally speaking, there are no significant side effects. Miyata reports treating 53 children.[20] He discovered that in 25 children who were given the formula without regard to its presentation, five had side effects of nausea and headache. When the herbs were discontinued, these symptoms promptly disappeared. However, when the medicine was administered to 33 children in accord with the formula's presentation, it was used for an average of over 2.5 years without side effects. This formula should be used only with caution in patients whose presentations do not match that of this formula. Examples of this include a red tongue with a dry coating, a tendency toward bleeding, dryness in the throat and mouth, hacking cough without phlegm, or an elevated temperature along with excessive sweating. Using it with such patients can easily lead to side effects such as headaches, palpitations, profuse sweating, insomnia, and bleeding. One must pay particular attention to this.

2.4 Ephedra, Apricot Kernel, Gypsum, and Licorice Decoction
(麻杏石甘湯 *má xìng shí gān tāng*)

SOURCE: *Discussion of Cold Damage*

Ephedrae Herba (*má huáng*)... 5-10g
Armeniacae Semen (*xìng rén*) 6-12g
Gypsum fibrosum (*shí gāo*).. 10-20g
Glycyrrhizae Radix (*gān cǎo*).. 3-6g

Readers with clinical experience perhaps already know that not every patient with coughing and wheezing has an aversion to cold with a lack of sweating, clear, thin sputum, and a pale tongue with a moist coating. On the contrary, more than a few patients are feverish and sweating, have sticky, yellow sputum, a dry mouth, are thirsty, and have a red tongue with a yellow coating. For this type of patient, it is inappropriate to use Minor Bluegreen Dragon Decoction (*xiǎo qīng lóng tāng*) or Ephedra Decoction (*má huáng tāng*) because this is a heat wheezing (熱喘 *rè chuǎn*) type of cough and wheezing. Chinese doctors call this 'Lung heat' (肺熱 *fèi rè*) or 'phlegm-heat' (痰熱 *tán rè*). Ephedra, Apricot Kernel, Gypsum, and Licorice Decoction (*má xìng shí gān tāng*), with its primary pairing of Ephedrae Herba (*má huáng*) and Gypsum fibrosum (*shí gāo*), is most appropriate for this type of heat wheezing.

The ingredients of Ephedra, Apricot Kernel, Gypsum, and Licorice Decoction (*má xìng shí gān tāng*) and Ephedra Decoction (*má huáng tāng*) are similar, the only difference being the substitution of Gypsum fibrosum (*shí gāo*) for Cinnamomi Ramulus (*guì zhī*), which brings about a significant change in the formula's presentation.

The passages concerning this formula from *Discussion of Cold Damage* include the following: "One cannot again use Cinnamon Twig Decoction (*guì zhī tāng*) after inducing sweating. If there is sweating and wheezing without intense fever, Ephedra, Apricot Kernel, Gypsum, and Licorice Decoction (*má xìng shí gān tāng*) can be used." (paragraph 63) In addition, paragraph 162 states: "After purging, Cinnamon Twig Decoction (*guì zhī tāng*) cannot be used again. If there is sweating with wheezing, without intense fever, Ephedra, Apricot Kernel, Gypsum, and Licorice Decoction (*má xìng shí gān tāng*) can be used."

The key points for differential diagnosis are sweating with wheezing and lack of intense fever. The Cinnamomi Ramulus (*guì zhī*) in Ephedra Decoction (*má huáng tāng*) strengthens its ability to induce sweating; therefore, the Ephedra Decoction presentation includes wheezing without sweating. Ephedra, Apricot Kernel, Gypsum, and Licorice Decoction (*má xìng shí gān tāng*), however, pairs Ephedrae Herba (*má huáng*) with Gypsum fibrosum (*shí gāo*), so its ability to clear heat is quite strong; its presentation therefore includes wheezing with sweating.

Gypsum fibrosum (*shí gāo*) is an important medicinal used to clear heat in Chinese medicine. It is used to treat heat diseases with such symptoms as high fevers, thirst with desire to drink, irritability, heat wheezing, headache, tooth pain, and the development of maculae on the skin. The gypsum fibrosum presentation includes fever with skin that is hot to the touch, thirst, and sweating. These types of symptoms are similar to the body's natural physiologic reaction to a scorchingly hot summer day or to taking a sauna. The Ephedra, Apricot Kernel, Gypsum, and Licorice Decoction presentation, metaphorically speaking, is basically like being in these situations, but with the addition of coughing and wheezing. As sweating dissipates the heat, the exterior of the body is not scorchingly hot, and thus there is no intense fever. Commonly, some upper respiratory tract infections and allergies that lead to fever, coughing, and wheezing manifest the Ephedra, Apricot Kernel, Gypsum, and Licorice Decoction presentation of sweating and wheezing without intense fever. The specifics of the presentation include the following:

1. Fever with sweating that at times is heavy and at other times is mild, a body temperature that could be either higher or lower than normal, and thirst

2. Coughing and wheezing, even to the point of panting, with flaring nostrils and chest stuffiness
3. A slippery and rapid pulse, and a thin, greasy, and rather dry tongue coating

Specific markers that help differentiate between the presentation of this formula and that of Ephedra Decoction (*má huáng tāng*) are as follows: for both formulas, the presentation includes wheezing, but in the Ephedra Decoction presentation, there is no sweating and the patient's complexion at times flushes red and other times has an ashen pallor. The patient has goose bump-like eruptions under the skin, which is dry to the touch, and a complete absence of sweating. At the same time, there is ceaseless coughing and wheezing. By contrast, the Ephedra, Apricot Kernel, Gypsum, and Licorice Decoction presentation includes wheezing with sweating. Although there is not a lot of sweating, the skin is moist to the touch, but not hot. The patient's complexion is red, but not lacking moisture. Additionally, the Ephedra Decoction presentation has a lack of thirst and a coating on the tongue that is moist, while the Ephedra, Apricot Kernel, Gypsum, and Licorice Decoction presentation has thirst with a desire to drink and a dry tongue coating.

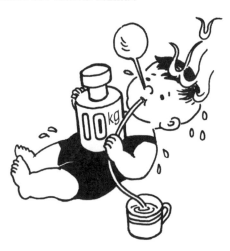

The Ephedra, Apricot Kernel, Gypsum, and Licorice Decoction presentation should also be differentiated from that of Minor Bluegreen Dragon Decoction (*xiǎo qīng lóng tāng*). In addition to the differences already noted between the Ephedra, Apricot Kernel, Gypsum, and Licorice Decoction presentation and the Ephedra Decoction presentation, there are also important differences in the character of the phlegm and fluids. The sputum in the Minor Bluegreen

Dragon Decoction presentation is watery and relatively copious, while in the Ephedra, Apricot Kernel, Gypsum, and Licorice Decoction presentation it is thick and sticky, and yellowish white in color.

Within the cinnamon twig family of formulas there is a modification of Cinnamon Twig Decoction (*guì zhī tāng*) called Cinnamon Twig Decoction plus Magnolia Bark and Apricot Kernels (*guì zhī jiā hòu pò xìng zǐ tāng*) that also treats coughing and wheezing. Because the Cinnamon Twig presentation includes sweating and an aversion to wind, it can therefore be used clinically to treat sweating with wheezing. The point that distinguishes the two presentations is that the Cinnamon Twig Decoction plus Magnolia Bark and Apricot Kernels Decoction presentation includes sweating, an aversion to wind, and a lack of thirst, while the Ephedra, Apricot Kernel, Gypsum, and Licorice Decoction presentation includes thirst as well as sweating and wheezing. The presence or absence of thirst is the most important indicator of whether or not there is internal heat.

- The Ephedra, Apricot Kernel, Gypsum, and Licorice Decoction presentation is often seen in patients with asthmatic bronchitis, bronchial asthma, and some types of allergies, as well as acute bronchitis, pneumonia, and other such respiratory tract infections where the main symptoms are coughing and wheezing. The Tianjin College of Chinese Medicine reported treating 229 cases of pediatric asthma. A modification of this formula was given to 184 subjects with heat-type asthma, of which 168 were cured. Minor Bluegreen Dragon Decoction (*xiǎo qīng lóng tāng*) was given to 45 subjects with cold-type asthma, of which 31 subjects were cured.[21] Pang used this formula to treat 50 children with acute bronchitis, resulting in 26 children being cured, five showing some improvement, and 19 experiencing no effect. While the rate of efficacy when using this formula by itself was slightly over 62 percent, if it is combined with a modification of Minor Decoction [for Pathogens] Stuck in the Chest (*xiǎo xiàn xiōng tāng*), the rate increased to 88 percent.[22]

In another report, 172 subjects were treated for bronchitis, with 34 subjects being cured, 62 experiencing significant improvement, and 63 subjects experiencing some improvement. The curative effect was more pronounced for those subjects whose wheezing was of a hot and dry variety.[23] It was observed that in a group of boys and girls under the age of seven with coughing and wheezing, 50 percent had an Ephedra, Apricot Kernel, Gypsum, and Licorice Decoction presentation. Ephedra, Apricot Kernel, Gypsum, and Licorice Decoction (*má xìng shí gān tāng*) was especially effective for treating the fever, followed by its effectiveness at calming the wheezing, its ability to stop the

67

coughing, and, lastly, its ability to resolve the inflammation. The researchers report that, although coughs with fever are this formula's main presentation, it is also effective for patients without a fever.[24]

• Clinical manifestations of pneumonia are often similar to the Ephedra, Apricot Kernel, Gypsum, and Licorice Decoction presentation. As a result, this formula is often used to treat many types of pneumonia such as pediatric pneumonia, bronchopneumonia, measles pneumonia, infectious asthma, lobar pneumonia, and eosinophilic pneumonia. There is a report of treating 136 children with measles. Of those within the group who had the dangerous condition of measles pneumonia, all benefited from being treated with this formula.[25]

• This formula can be used to treat pertussis. A combination of this formula and Descurainia and Jujube Decoction to Drain the Lungs (tíng lì dà zǎo xiè fèi tāng)* was used to treat 228 subjects. Of these, 195 subjects were cured, and 25 showed improvement. Regardless of whether the patients were in the earlier acute inflammatory stage or in the later spasmodic coughing stage, both responded well to the treatment, with those in the acute infectious stage responding particularly well.[26]

• This formula can be used to effectively treat all kinds of rhinitis. However, it is necessary to match the herbs to the presentation. These symptoms should include nasal congestion with yellow discharge and headache. There is a report of this formula, modified with the addition of Pheretima (dì lóng), being used to treat 11 subjects with paranasal sinusitis. Of these, three were cured, four showed obvious improvement, and four showed some improvement. The least amount of herbs given was four bags and the most was 60 bags.[27]

• There are also reports of using this formula to treat urticaria.

2.5 Maidservant from Yue's Decoction plus Atractylodes
(越婢加朮湯 Yuè bì jiā zhú tāng)

SOURCE: *Essentials from the Golden Cabinet*

Ephedrae Herba (má huáng)...5-10g
Gypsum fibrosum (shí gāo)..10-15g
Zingiberis Rhizoma recens (shēng jiāng)..............................3-10g
Glycyrrhizae Radix (gān cǎo)..3-5g

---

* Lepidii/Descurainiae Semen (tíng lì zǐ) and Jujubae Fructus (dà zǎo).

Jujubae Fructus (*dà zǎo*) 12g

Atractylodis macrocephalae Rhizoma (*bái zhú*) 12g

Maidservant from Yue's Decoction plus Atractylodes (*Yuè bì jiā zhú tāng*) is composed of the *Essentials from the Golden Cabinet* formula Maidservant from Yue's Decoction (*Yuè bì tāng*) with the addition of Atractylodis macrocephalae Rhizoma (*bái zhú*). Maidservant from Yue's Decoction plus Atractylodes presentation includes "aversion to wind, whole body edema, a floating pulse, lack of thirst, continuous sweating, and no intense fever." Maidservant from Yue's Decoction plus Atractylodes (*Yuè bì jiā zhú tāng*) treats internal water (裡水 *lǐ shuǐ*) disease, which manifests as yellowness and swelling of the entire body, face, and eyes, a sinking pulse, and urinary difficulty. From looking at its ingredients, it can be seen that this formula is a modification of Ephedra, Apricot Kernel, Gypsum, and Licorice Decoction (*má xìng shí gān tāng*), with the removal of Armeniacae Semen (*xìng rén*) and the addition of Atractylodis macrocephalae Rhizoma (*bái zhú*), Zingiberis Rhizoma recens (*shēng jiāng*), and Jujubae Fructus (*dà zǎo*). Of these changes, the substitution of Atractylodis macrocephalae Rhizoma (*bái zhú*) for Armeniacae Semen (*xìng rén*) causes the most significant change in the presentation for which the formula should be used. Armeniacae Semen (*xìng rén*) is the medicinal that Zhang Zhong-Jing chose to treat patients with coughing, wheezing, and fullness with stuffiness in the chest. For this reason, it is used in the formulas Ephedra Decoction (*má huáng tāng*), Ephedra, Apricot Kernel, Gypsum, and Licorice Decoction (*má xìng shí gān tāng*), and Cinnamon Twig Decoction plus Magnolia Bark and Apricot Kernels (*guì zhī jiā hòu pò xìng zǐ tāng*).

The formula Maidservant from Yue's Decoction plus Atractylodes (*Yuè bì jiā zhú tāng*) does not contain Armeniacae Semen (*xìng rén*), and so its presentation does not include coughing, wheezing, chest stuffiness, or other respiratory tract symptoms. In addition, as gleaned from Zhang Zhong-Jing's experience, there must be urinary difficulty for Atractylodis macrocephalae Rhizoma (*bái zhú*) to be used.

After undergoing this modification, that is, the substitution of Atractylodis macrocephalae Rhizoma (*bái zhú*) for Armeniacae Semen (*xìng rén*), Ephedra, Apricot Kernel, Gypsum, and Licorice Decoction (*má xìng shí gān tāng*) is transformed from a prescription that treats wheezing with sweating, thirst, irritability, and restlessness by clearing heat and calming wheezing, into a formula that clears heat and promotes urination in order to treat swelling with sweating and urinary difficulty. Its presentation includes the following signs and symptoms:

1. Fever, an aversion to wind, sweating that can be either mild or severe, and thirst
2. Edema, achy and heavy muscles or joints that are swollen and painful, and urinary difficulty

The Maidservant from Yue's Decoction plus Atractylodes presentation is a pathology that includes elements of both wind and dampness. The symptoms are primarily concentrated in the muscle layer, resulting in signs such as fever, aversion to wind, painful joints, and achy muscles. It is possible to see aspects of the ephedra presentation within this formula's presentation. Signs of a gypsum presentation, namely, sweating, thirst, and fever, are also relatively clear. Urinary difficulty and edema are signs of stagnation of the internal fluids; this would fall into both the ephedra and atractylodis presentations.

Note that *Divine Husbandman's Classic of the Materia Medica* (神農本草經 *Shén Nóng běn cǎo jīng*) does not differentiate between Atractylodis macrocephalae Rhizoma (*bái zhú*) and Atractylodis Rhizoma (*cāng zhú*). It was not until the Northern Song Dynasty that Tao Hong-Jing (陶弘景) distinguished between two types of 术 (*zhú*), one being white and the other red. The red variety we know as Atractylodis Rhizoma (*cāng zhú*). *Materia Medica Arranged According to Pattern* (證類本草 *Zhèng lèi běn cǎo*) was the first materia medica to describe this difference. This must be taken into account when reading pre-Song texts.

Divine Husbandman's Classic of the Materia Medica states that Atractylodis Rhizoma (*cāng zhú*) "treats wind, cold, damp obstruction with nonfunctioning muscles, ... stops sweating, and gets rid of heat." *Miscellaneous Records of Famous Physicians* (名醫別錄 *Míng yī bié lù*) says that it "eliminates phlegm and [pathogenic] water, and eliminates clumps and swellings from wind and [pathogenic] water in the skin." *Bag of Pearls* (珍珠囊 *Zhēn zhú náng*) says that it can "eliminate foot and lower leg dampness and swelling, and when combined with Ephedrae Herba (*má huáng*), can treat such symptoms as swollen and painful joints, muscle weakness, and edema."

Zhang Zhong-Jing used Ephedra Decoction plus Atractylodes (*má huáng jiā zhú tāng*) specifically to treat those with an ephedra presentation and painful and swollen joints, along with achy, heavy-feeling muscles, and edema. The combination of Ephedrae Herba (*má huáng*) and Gypsum fibrosum (*shí gāo*) restrains the diaphoretic function of Ephedrae Herba (*má huáng*), thereby more fully bringing into play its analgesic and diuretic functions, while not activating its ability to calm wheezing, as occurs when Ephedrae Herba (*má huáng*) is matched with Armeniacae Semen (*xìng rén*). In comparison to Ephedra Decoction plus Atractylodes (*má huáng jiā zhú tāng*), while Maidservant from Yue's Decoction plus Atractylodes (*Yuè bì jiā zhú tāng*) does not have Cinnamomi Ramulus (*guì zhī*), it does contain Gypsum fibrosum (*shí gāo*). With one herb removed and another added, the warming and cooling nature of the prescription changes. These two formulas can both treat the symptoms of swollen and painful joints with edema. However, because Ephedra Decoction plus Atractylodes (*má huáng jiā zhú tāng*) uses both Ephedrae Herba (*má huáng*) and Cinnamomi Ramulus (*guì zhī*), it is designed for presentations that lean toward cold, with signs of aversion to cold and a lack of both sweating and thirst. The Maidservant from Yue's Decoction plus Atractylodes presentation calls for combining Ephedrae Herba (*má huáng*) and Gypsum fibrosum (*shí gāo*); it is designed for presentations that lean toward heat, with signs of fever with an aversion to wind along with sweating and thirst.

- The Maidservant from Yue's Decoction plus Atractylodes presentation is frequently seen in cases where the joints are swollen and painful and there is a fever, which is seen in diseases such as rheumatic fever and rheumatoid arthritis. This type of presentation is referred to in Chinese medicine as 'wind-damp-heat painful obstruction' (風濕熱痹 *fēng shī rè bì*). There is a report of using this formula to treat 32 subjects with painful obstruction from wind, dampness, and heat. The treatment resulted in eight subjects recovering completely, 17 showing significant improvement, five taking a turn for the better, and two subjects experiencing no effect.[28]

- The presentation for this formula is commonly seen in cases of acute nephritis that manifest with signs of fever, aversion to wind, and full body edema. It is common for those with acute edema who fit this formula's presentation to sweat heavily after taking the herbs, with a corresponding decrease in the extent of the edema.

An experimental treatment case is presented, which, although it cannot definitely be said to be a case of nephritis, nonetheless shows the ability of Maidservant from Yue's Decoction plus Atractylodes (*Yuè bì jiā zhú tāng*) to reduce edema by diaphoresis. A 25-year-old male tailor had gone to a neighboring village the previous month to visit family. While on the road home, a sudden rainstorm left him completely soaked. When he got home, he took a shower, changed his clothes, and did not think much about it. Three days later he developed a fever with chills, headache, body aches, and a feeling of heaviness with movement. His doctor prescribed diaphoretic herbs, which caused him to sweat lightly, but the exterior was not completely resolved, and he discontinued taking the herbs. After a few days, his entire body was edematous, and any place that was pressed would leave a depression that remained for some time. He had an aversion to wind, body aches, and a lack of sweating. The previous doctor prescribed Apricot Kernel, Perilla Leaf Powder, and Five-Peel Drink (xìng sū wǔ pí yǐn). Because this did not reduce the swelling, the formula was changed to Five-Ingredient Powder with Poria (wǔ líng sǎn), but the patient's condition remained as before.

An examination of the pulse showed it to be floating and tight, and the patient had an aversion to wind with a lack of sweating, his body felt heavy, and the mouth and tongue were dry. A large preparation of Maidservant from Yue's Decoction plus Atractylodes (Yuè bì jiā zhú tāng)* was prescribed. One entire bag was taken warm in a single dose; the patient was asked to lie down and was covered up. He became drenched in sweat, and the edema was reduced by more than half. Another large preparation of this formula was given, which quickly and completely eliminated all the edema.[29]

It should be pointed out that, in this case, the cold presentation signs of aversion to wind with a lack of sweating and body aches were particularly clear. Therefore, the amount of Ephedrae Herba (má huáng) used in the prescription was quite large, considerably more than the standard amount used in normal circumstances. This means that the practitioner here had unique experience in this regard. When treating the usual kinds of edema or joint pain, it is generally appropriate to stick to the standard dosage.

• Some cases of eczema and swelling of the vocal cords also share this formula's presentation.

2.6 Balmy Yang Decoction (陽和湯 yáng hé tāng)

SOURCE: Complete Compendium of Patterns and Treatments in External Medicine (外科證治全生集 Wài kē zhèng zhì quán shēng jí)

Ephedrae Herba (má huáng)..5g
Cinnamomi Cortex (ròu guì) 5g
Fried Zingiberis Rhizoma (bāo gān jiāng) 5g
Glycyrrhizae Radix (gān cǎo)..6g
Rehmanniae Radix preparata (shú dì huáng) 30g
Sinapis Semen (bái jiè zǐ)...6g
Cervi Cornus Colla (lù jiǎo jiāo) 10g

---

* Ephedrae Herba (má huáng), Atractylodes Rhizoma (cāng zhú), Zingiberis Rhizomatis Cortex (shēng jiāng pí), Gypsum fibrosum (shí gāo), Jujubae Fructus (dà zǎo), and Glycyrrhizae Radix (gān cǎo).

Balmy Yang Decoction (*yáng hé tāng*) is the famous Chinese external medicine formula for treating yin flat abscesses (陰疽 *yīn jū*), which are a type of relatively serious skin or subdermal pus-filled infection with a yin-cold type presentation. It manifests clinically as a localized headless swelling without any changes in skin color and lacking a sensation of heat. These patients have lusterless complexions, favor warmth, are not thirsty, and have copious amounts of clear urine. The tongue has a white coating and is accompanied by a pulse that is sinking and lax, or slow, or thin. These types of symptoms indicate that the body's internal yang qi is insufficient, and on the surface of the muscle layer is a condition of overflowing yin-cold (陰寒瀰漫 *yīn hán mí màn*). Balmy Yang Decoction (*yáng hé tāng*) can certainly be relied upon to treat this type of presentation.

As the famous Qing-dynasty external medicine doctor Ma Pei-Zhi observed, "This formula treats yin disease, is unsurpassed [in effectiveness], and when used appropriately, the disease is cured with a flick of the hand." Because this formula is used for yin-type symptoms, it is like the sun that comes out and drives away a dense fog, thus it is called Balmy Yang Decoction (*yáng hé tāng*). The Balmy Yang Decoction presentation is as follows:

1. Locally, the skin lacks a feeling of warmth, has an ashen pallor or is purple and dark in color, and there are flat, headless abscesses lacking well-defined borders. When pressed, they could feel hard like stone, or the center could feel soft like cotton. The patients themselves feel either little or no pain, numbness, or achiness.

2. Generally, listless and dispirited, is averse to cold and favors warmth, the spine may feel weak and painful, there may be shortness of breath and wheezing, and there may also be impotence and frigidity. The person appears emaciated and anemic, with skin that has an ashen pallor. There is a lack of thirst along with copious and clear urination. The pulse is sinking, slow, and thin, and the tongue is both pale and tender.

The presentation for this formula is seen in such illnesses as deep-seated abscesses, bone or joint tuberculosis, chronic osteomyelitis, chronic lymphadenitis, thromboangitis obliterans, rheumatoid arthritis, sciatica, herniated lumbar disks, and frostbite. These generally will not manifest with ulcers on the skin.

It has been reported that the use of a modified version of this formula—

Rehmanniae Radix preparata (*shú dì huáng*) 30g, Aconiti Radix lateralis preparata (*zhì fù zǐ*) 30g, Cervi Cornus Colla (*lù jiǎo jiāo*) 10g, Ephedrae Herba (*má huáng*) 10g, Asari Herba (*xì xīn*) 10g Glycyrrhizae Radix (*gān cǎo*) 10g, Cinnamomi Ramulus (*guì zhī*) 20g, Zingiberis Rhizoma preparata (*páo jiāng*) 15g, Scorpio (*quán xiē*) 3g—was used to treat five patients with Raynaud's disease.[30]

Shang reports using a modification of this formula with good effect to treat yin-cold type thromboangiitis obliterans in 25 patients.[31] There is also a report of adding Angelicae sinensis Radix (*dāng guī*) and Astragali Radix (*huáng qí*) to this formula to treat 63 subjects with peripheral neuritis. Treatment resulted in 43 subjects being completely cured, 14 subjects experiencing significant effects, and six having no effect. Those with mild cases were cured with taking just six packets. Those with severe cases took the herbs for up to 1.5 months.[32]

The Balmy Yang Decoction presentation is frequently seen in cases of cold-type asthma, dysmenorrhea, uterine bleeding, and cardiac disease where the body is in a debilitated condition. There is a report of using a modification of this formula to treat 40 patients with sick sinus syndrome. During the time the herbs were administered, the use of atropine and isoproterenol were discontinued. Treatment resulted in a significant effect (heart rate of 70 beats per minute and above) in four patients, and some effect (heart rate of 60 beats per minute and above) in 34 patients.[33]

A trace of the ephedra presentation is seen within this formula's presentation, that is, body aches, aversion to cold, and a lack of sweating. This formula's presentation is, however, an ephedra presentation with a weakened physical condition that has been brought on by chronic illness. As a result, the person is wan and thin, listless, and has sagging skin with an ashen pallor. Furthermore, due to the long-term depleting nature of the illness, the body becomes progressively thin and anemic. In the Ephedra, Asarum, and Aconite Accessory Root Decoction presentation, there is damage only to the yang qi without significant depletion of the physical body, and for this reason, there are no signs of anemia or emaciation. However, with the Balmy Yang Decoction presentation, there is damage to both the yin and yang, most notably the rather severe depletion of the yin and blood.

CHAPTER 3

BUPLEURUM FORMULA FAMILY

柴胡類方 *chái hú lèi fāng*

BUPLEURI RADIX *(chái hú)* is the root of an herbaceous perennial that can be found throughout much of China. Although it lacks the variety and color of delicate flowers and beautiful foliage, people have come to love and trust this herb due to its outstanding curative powers. In Japan, Minor Bupleurum Decoction *(xiǎo chái hú tāng)* was taken in the early 1990s on an average of a million times a year and still remains a very popular medicinal. Similarly, Bupleuri Radix *(chái hú)* formulas such as Bupleurum and Cinnamon Twig Decoction *(chái hú guì zhī tāng)*, Major Bupleurum Decoction *(dà chái hú tāng)*, Bupleurum, Cinnamon Twig, and Ginger Decoction *(chái hú guì zhī gān jiāng tāng)*, and Frigid Extremities Powder *(sì nì sǎn)* are other commonly used formulas in the Japanese Kampō tradition. In China, as well, Bupleuri Radix *(chái hú)* based prescriptions are an important class of formulas used in the clinic.

There has been a great deal of discussion about the function and efficacy of Bupleuri Radix *(chái hú)* by our predecessors. *Rectification of the Meaning of Materia Medica* (本草正義 *Běn cǎo zhèng yì*) says that Bupleuri Radix *(chái hú)* is an exterior-resolving medicinal; *Encountering the Sources of the Classic of Materia Medica* (本經逢原 *Běn jīng féng yuán*) says that it is a foot *shào yáng* Gallbladder channel herb; *Origins of Medicine* (醫學啟源 *Yī xué qǐ yuán*) says that it is an herb that enters the *shào yáng* and *jué yīn* channels; and *One Hundred Records of the Classic of Materia Medica* (本草經百種錄 *Běn cǎo jīng bái zhōng lù*) says that it is an herb for the Stomach and Intestines. From the point of view of those beginning the study of Chinese medicine, understanding this kind of complicated technical terminology is indeed difficult. Clinicians, though, are most concerned with those signs that directly lead to the clinical application of Bupleuri Radix *(chái hú)*. Pay close attention to the following three key aspects of the clinical presentation for using Bupleuri Radix (*chái hú*).

Bupleurum Presentation (柴胡證 *chái hú zhèng*)

This, like the ephedra and cinnamon twig presentations, consists of the basic signs for which Bupleuri Radix (*chái hú*) is appropriately used. In addition, each of the various presentations of the bupleurum family formulas, to a greater or lesser degree, has the markings of the bupleurum presentation. The bupleurum presentation consists of the following three aspects:

1. Chest and hypochondriac fullness and discomfort
2. Alternating fever and chills, or episodic expression of symptoms
3. Symptoms appearing in the bupleurum zone

CHEST AND HYPOCHONDRIAC FULLNESS AND DISCOMFORT (胸脅苦滿 *xiōng xié kǔ mǎn*)

This is the 'must-see' sign for a bupleurum presentation. It is a feeling in the chest and hypochondria of distention and pain, distention and fullness, firm fullness, or tenderness when palpated; for women, swollen and painful breasts or nodules in the breasts; or what in modern medicine is referred to as biliary colic and intercostal neuralgia. All are included as signs in the bupleurum presentation. Chinese medicine traditionally holds that chest and hypochondriac fullness and discomfort is a symptom that the patients themselves experience. However, Japanese practitioners believe that this is a feeling of resistance that the practitioner feels against their fingertips when palpating along the costal margin toward the chest cavity, with the patient responding to this palpation with a feeling of discomfort including distention and pain. Honsono Shiro thinks that, for patients with chest and hypochondriac fullness and discomfort, palpation by gathering and pinching the skin can be employed. This is done by using the thumb and index finger to gather and pinch the skin and subcutaneous tissues in the subcostal area, which can feel swollen and thickened. At the same time, the patient is sensitive to this type of touch and experiences pain. This area of reactivity can be wide or narrow, and has a direct relation to the severity of the chest and hypochondriac fullness and discomfort.[1]

Alternating Fever and Chills (寒熱往來 *hán rè wǎng lái*)

In addition to changes in the measurable body temperature, this also includes a subjective sense of alternating cold and heat on the part of the patient where at times they may have a real aversion to wind and feel cold, while at other times they might have a reddish complexion and feel hot and irritable. Or, the upper part of the body could be feverish, while there is an aversion to cold in the lower body. Or, it might be that one side of the body is hot, while the other side is cold. Likewise, the chest could feel hot and irritable, while the four extremities are icy cold. When covered up, they may immediately feel feverish and agitated, as if they are sweating, although they are not. Furthermore, if they throw off the covers, they feel chilled to the bone and get goose bumps. Along with all this, they are very sensitive to changes in the temperature.

'Alternating' (往來 *wǎng lái*) and 'episodic' (休作有時 *xiū zuō yǒu shí*) indicate that there is a definite regularity, a particular cycle, or alternation in the expression of the illness. The famous late-Qing-dynasty physician Fei Bo-Xiong used a modification of Rambling Powder (*xiāo yáo sǎn*) to cure a strange case of insomnia that would last the entire night and manifest every other day. The modern practitioner Yue Mei-Zhong used Minor Bupleurum Decoction (*xiǎo chái hú tāng*) to cure a child whose entire body would become numb everyday right at noon. There are also reports from Japan of using Bupleurum and Cinnamon Twig Decoction (*chái hú guì zhī tāng*) to treat epilepsy. All of these cases regarded the alternating or episodic nature of the problem as the basis for the differential diagnosis.

I believe that in looking at chest and hypochondriac fullness and discomfort and alternating fever and chills, the former is more important. In clinical manifestations of a bupleurum presentation, it is possible for there not to be alternating fever and chills or episodic symptoms, however, chest and hypochondriac fullness and discomfort *must* be present.

Bupleurum Zone (柴胡帶 *chái hú dài*)

This term indicates the areas on the surface of the body that reflect the bupleurum presentation. Chinese doctors frequently use phrases such as "areas traversed by the *shào yáng* channel" and "the boundary of the Liver channel" to describe it. To make it easier to understand and remember, here we will use the term 'bupleurum zone' as a way to refer to this area. The bupleurum zone primarily includes the regions of the chest and hypochondria, the shoulders and nape of the neck, forehead, hips and lower abdomen, and the groin, as well as the lateral aspects of the body. When these regions manifest distending pain, feel achy, have unusual sensations, or lumps, one can usually consider the possibility of a bupleurum presentation, or any of the various bupleurum decoction-type presentations. This would include the following:

> Distention and pain, achiness, a dragging sensation, odd sensations, swellings, lumps or nodules in the area of the chest and hypochondria, neck and shoulders, forehead, hips and lower abdomen or groin

Bupleurum Constitution (柴胡體質 *chái hú tǐ zhì*)

By bupleurum constitution, we mean a body type that frequently manifests a bupleurum presentation or a bupleurum family formula presentation. Due to the complex nature of bupleurum family formula presentations, patients can have numerous main complaints. By being able to differentiate constitutional types, the complex can be simplified and one can more quickly grasp the nature of an illness.

- *Distinctive external features.* A medium to slightly thin physique with a complexion that is dark yellow, greenish yellow, or greenish pale, and lacking luster. The skin tends to be relatively dry, and the muscle tone is firm. The tongue characteristically looks tough and firm, dark and with purple spots; the tongue body is neither pale nor flabby; and the coating is either normal or a little dry. The pulse is generally wiry or thin.

- *Easily manifested symptoms.* The main complaints consist mostly of subjective symptoms such as a sensitivity to temperature changes or at times feeling cold while at other times feeling hot, mood swings, and an appetite that is easily affected by the emotions. There could be a stuffy and full sensation in the chest and hypochondria, which can be painful to the touch. The neck and shoulders often feel achy or have spasms, with cold extremities and a lower abdomen that readily becomes distended and is painful. Women may experience irregular periods and are commonly seen with premenstrual symptoms such as stuffiness in the chest, breast distention, and irritability, along with abdominal pain with menstruation and dark menstrual blood or clots in the menstrual blood.

- *Constitutional proclivities.* Tendency toward qi stagnation as well as blood stasis.

A dark complexion is an important external distinction. This darkness is an external manifestation of qi and blood stagnation. Apart from the complexion, the tongue can also be dark or purple. Due to the stagnation of blood, it is common to see dry skin. Chest and hypochondriac fullness and discomfort and extremities that are often cold are also important signs. In practice, other than interviewing the patient, abdominal palpation can also be used to determine the presence of the chest and hypochondriac signs. Menstruation is an important clue in determining a woman's constitution; one should use the interview to gather plenty of information about this.

These are the most basic elements of the bupleurum presentation. Furthermore, distinguishing the bupleurum zone and bupleurum constitution is done by considering the location of physical manifestations as well as one's clinical gaze, including visual examination, interviewing, and palpation. This perspective aids one in determining the presence of a bupleurum or Minor Bupleurum Decoction presentation.

Modern pharmacological experimentation and research has found evidence that Bupleuri Radix (*chái hú*) resolves fever by sedating the central nervous system fever centers and has other inhibitory effects on the central nervous system including sedation, prevention of spontaneous movement, prolongation of sleep, analgesia, and antispasmodic actions. Research also indicates that Bupleuri Radix (*chái hú*) can promote the synthesis of liver proteins, has significant hepatoprotective and anti-inflammatory functions, and strengthens the production of adrenocortical anti-inflammatory hormones. Beyond that, it also has anti-allergic, anti-ulcer, and antitussive properties. The various pharmacological functions of Bupleuri Radix (*chái hú*) are expressed in different degrees when combined with other medicinals within the bupleurum family of formulas.

3.1 **Minor Bupleurum Decoction** (小柴胡湯 *xiǎo chái hú tāng*)

SOURCE: *Discussion of Cold Damage* (傷寒論 *Shāng hán lùn*)

Bupleuri Radix (*chái hú*)..10-20g
Scutellariae Radix (*huáng qín*)..6-10g
Pinelliae Rhizoma preparatum (*zhì bàn xià*)........................6-15g
Ginseng Radix (*rén shēn*)..5-10g

Glycyrrhizae Radix (*gān cǎo*)..10g
Zingiberis Rhizoma recens (*shēng jiāng*)...........................10g
Jujubae Fructus (*dà zǎo*)..12g

Minor Bupleurum Decoction (*xiǎo chái hú tāng*) is one of the most used formulas in clinical practice. *Discussion of Cold Damage* devoted many lines of text to recounting the presentation, modifications, related formulas, and associated presentations of Minor Bupleurum Decoction (*xiǎo chái hú tāng*). Later generations of practitioners also have, from both the perspectives of standard clinical practice and pharmacological research, made a great many inquiries into this formula. Especially in Japan, the application of and research into Minor Bupleurum Decoction (*xiǎo chái hú tāng*) is quite common. In 1989, the Japanese Kampō pharmaceutical industry manufactured 143,450,000,000 yen (roughly one billion dollars) worth of products, and of this sum, the value of Minor Bupleurum Decoction (*xiǎo chái hú tāng*) accounted for 36,000,000,000 yen ($250 million). Unlike in China, the Japanese commonly use Minor Bupleurum Decoction (*xiǎo chái hú tāng*) to treat hepatitis, and there is quite a bit of pharmacological research and clinical study of this issue. There was a big news story in the Japanese media in 1989 that reported a medical study had found that Minor Bupleurum Decoction (*xiǎo chái hú tāng*) could harm liver function. This caused quite a panic among the population, resulting in the Ministry of Health and Welfare ordering further investigation into the side effects of manufactured Kampō formulas. After this, Kampō practitioners emphasized the use of the fundamentals of differential diagnosis in prescribing. As is common knowledge, basing the treatment on a differentiation of illness patterns is the very soul of Chinese medical thought. The propriety of using Minor Bupleurum Decoction (*xiǎo chái hú tāng*) is not based on the name of the disease, whether it be hepatitis or cholecystitis, but rather is dependent on whether or not there is a Minor Bupleurum Decoction presentation.

In *Discussion of Cold Damage*, Minor Bupleurum Decoction (*xiǎo chái hú tāng*) is used to treat a large number of illnesses:

• Paragraph 96 states that it is for "alternating chills and fever, a sense of discomfort and fullness in the chest and ribs, being dejected with no desire to eat, irritability of the Heart and a tendency to vomit." This paragraph also includes several other possible symptoms, such as irritability in the chest without vomiting, thirst, abdominal pain, focal distention and firmness below the ribs, epigastric palpitations, urinary dysfunction, lack of thirst, slight fever, or coughing.

- Paragraph 149: "vomiting and feverishness …."
- Paragraph 97: "alternating chills and fever with times of respite and [they are] dejected with no desire to eat" along with abdominal pain and vomiting.
- Paragraph 266: "When what was originally a *tài yáng* disease is not resolved and shifts into the *shào yáng*, there is firmness and fullness beneath the ribs, dry heaves with an inability to eat, and alternating chills and fever. When neither vomiting nor purging has yet been done and the pulse is sinking and tight, give Minor Bupleurum Decoction *(xiǎo chái hú tāng)*."
- Paragraph 99: "body heat, aversion to wind, stiff nape and neck, fullness below the ribs, warm hands and feet, and thirst …."
- Paragraph 229: "tidal feverishness, loose stools, urine that is all right, and fullness in the chest and ribs that does not go away …."
- Paragraph 230: "hardness and fullness below the ribs, no bowel movements, along with vomiting and a white coating on the tongue."

From the above, the key signs and symptoms for the Minor Bupleurum Decoction presentation as described in *Discussion of Cold Damage* can be summarized as follows:

1. Chest and hypochondriac fullness and discomfort, or stiffness and fullness beneath the ribs, or focal distention and fullness in the subcostal region
2. Alternating fever and chills
3. Vomiting and lack of desire or inability to eat

To more completely understand the Minor Bupleurum Decoction presentation, let us take a moment to analyze the presentations of Scutellariae Radix *(huáng qín)*, Pinelliae Rhizoma preparatum *(zhì bàn xià)*, and Ginseng Radix *(rén shēn)*.

- Scutellariae Radix *(huáng qín)* is traditionally used as an herb to clear heat. It can treat illnesses with high fever, irritability and thirst, fevers with cough, diarrhea, jaundice, headache, abdominal pain, turbid urination, red swollen eyes, restless fetus syndrome, and abscesses and furuncles. Additionally, it treats bleeding disorders such as vomiting of blood, nosebleeds, and uterine bleeding. Modern pharmacological research has found that Scutellariae Radix *(huáng qín)* functions as an anti-inflammatory, anti-allergenic, antibacterial, antipyretic, diuretic, and antihypertensive medicinal; it also promotes biliary function and acts as a sedative.

Scutellariae Radix (*huáng qín*) is frequently paired with Bupleuri Radix (*chái hú*) and is used to treat such symptoms as alternating fever and chills, chest and hypochondriac fullness with focal distention and pain, and vomiting with a bitter taste in the mouth. In addition to Minor Bupleurum Decoction (*xiǎo chái hú tāng*), the *Discussion of Cold Damage* formulas Major Bupleurum Decoction (*dà chái hú tāng*), Bupleurum and Cinnamon Twig Decoction (*chái hú guì zhī tāng*), and Bupleurum plus Dragon Bone and Oyster Shell Decoction (*chái hú jiā lóng gǔ mǔ lì tāng*) all make use of this two-herb combination. Scutellariae Radix (*huáng qín*) is also commonly paired with Coptidis Rhizoma (*huáng lián*) to treat symptoms such as epigastric focal distention with firmness, irritability, and fever with diarrhea. The *Discussion of Cold Damage* formulas Pinellia Decoction to Drain the Epigastrium (*bàn xià xiè xīn tāng*), Kudzu, Scutellaria, and Coptis Decoction (*gé gēn huáng qín huáng lián tāng*), and Ginger, Coptis, Scutellaria, and Ginseng Decoction (*gān jiāng huáng lián huáng qín rén shēn tāng*) also utilize this combination. Therefore, generally when using Scutellariae Radix (*huáng qín*), the must-see symptoms are upper abdominal focal distention and fullness, or abdominal pain.

- Pinelliae Rhizoma preparatum (*zhì bàn xià*) is a medicinal traditionally used to stop vomiting and transform phlegm. It primarily treats symptoms such as nausea, vomiting, coughing with copious amounts of sputum, chest and diaphragm fullness, epigastric focal distention, loss of consciousness due to phlegm, dizziness, headache, and insomnia. Zhang Zhong-Jing commonly used Pinelliae Rhizoma preparatum (*zhì bàn xià*) together with Zingiberis Rhizoma recens (*shēng jiāng*) to synergistically increase both herbs' ability to stop vomiting. For stomach and intestinal symptoms of nausea with vomiting, epigastric focal distention with bloating and pain, and irritability, the combination of Pinelliae Rhizoma preparatum (*zhì bàn xià*) with Scutellariae Radix (*huáng qín*) is also commonly used.

- In *Discussion of Cold Damage* there are three aims in using Ginseng Radix (*rén shēn*). The first is as a rescue treatment after there has been sweating, vomiting, or diarrhea, or for those with a minute pulse due to collapse from loss of blood or dehydration, along with a dry tongue. The second is to treat debility and shortness of breath in the aftermath of an illness. The third use is to treat epigastric focal distention with firmness. Minor Bupleurum Decoction (*xiǎo chái hú tāng*) belongs to the second and third categories, especially the latter. This type of epigastric focal distention with firmness refers to a sense of distention but without actual bloating. Palpation reveals the abdominal muscles to be thin and with a relatively high degree of tension. This is commonly seen in patients who are debilitated or have chronic gastrointestinal illness.

The upper abdomen focal distention, fullness, and pain of the scutellaria presentation, the nausea and vomiting of the pinellia presentation, and the epigastric focal distention and firmness of the ginseng presentation can all be viewed as symptoms of gastrointestinal illness. For the Minor Bupleurum Decoction presentation, other than the signs of the bupleurum presentation, there are the relatively obvious stomach and intestinal symptoms of vomiting and abdominal pain simultaneously accompanied by alternating fever and chills. Its specific signs include:

1. Chest and hypochondriac fullness and discomfort, or upper abdominal focal distention and pain, or significant tenderness in the area of the gallbladder
2. Fever or persistent low-grade fever, with alternating fever and chills
3. Irritability in the chest with a desire to vomit, or vomiting with a bitter taste in the mouth, and feelings of dejection, with lack of interest in food or drink
4. A wiry, thin and wiry, slippery and wiry, or sinking and wiry pulse; a tongue coating that is yellow, yellow and white mixed together, pale yellow, or yellow and greasy

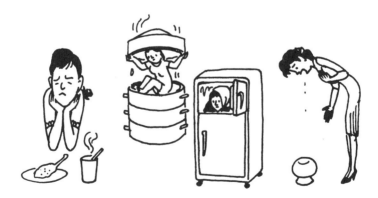

The symptoms of alternating fever and chills and chest and hypochondriac fullness and discomfort here have already been discussed in the bupleurum presentation. However, here there is a significant elevation of body temperature, the presence of remittent fever, or persistent low-grade fever, while at the same time, the patient experiences alternating fever and chills.

Simultaneous manifestations of chest and hypochondriac fullness and discomfort along with abdominal pain and distention, irritability in the chest with a desire to vomit, and stomach and intestinal symptoms can be said to be the primary signs of a Minor Bupleurum Decoction presentation. This is also the basis for the use of Scutellariae Radix (*huáng qín*), Pinelliae Rhizoma preparatum (*zhì bàn xià*), and Zingiberis Rhizoma recens (*shēng jiāng*) in this formula. The words irritability (煩 *fán*), desire/inclination (喜 *xǐ*), and dejected (默默 *mò mò*) in the phrases 'irritability in the chest, with an inclination to vomit' (心煩喜嘔 *xīn fán xǐ oǔ*) and 'dejected with a lack of interest in food or drink' (默默不欲飲食 *mò mò bù yù yǐn shí*) reflect the relatively strong subjective feelings expressed by the patient when describing their main complaint, and at the same time reflect the patient's bad mood.

The bitter taste in the mouth is a subjective feeling of the patient that there is a bitter sensation in the mouth, especially upon waking from sleep and when eating. The appetite and emotions are frequently influenced by this bitter taste. Chinese medicine regards a bitter taste in the mouth as a sign of internal heat. Likewise a yellow tongue coating is also representative of heat in the interior. A wiry pulse refers to a pulse that, when pressed, feels like a piece of bamboo or a piano string and is clearly felt during both systole and diastole. This type of pulse frequently appears with the Minor Bupleurum Decoction presentation.

The amount of Bupleuri Radix (*chái hú*) used in this formula is relatively large. In one report that claimed to treat acute pyelonephritis due to *shào yáng* heat from constraint, the amount of Bupleuri Radix (*chái hú*) used was 15-30g.[2] There are those who use Minor Bupleurum Decoction (*xiǎo chái hú tāng*) to treat intermittent fevers from unknown origins, and in these cases, the amount of Bupleuri Radix (*chái hú*) can reach 30g.[3] Large amounts of Bupleuri Radix (*chái hú*) can perhaps increase the antipyretic function of Minor Bupleurum Decoction (*xiǎo chái hú tāng*). That being said, a large dosage of Bupleuri Radix (*chái hú*) could lead to toxicity, especially if using southern Bupleuri Radix (*chái hú*), the root of *Bupleurum scorzonerifolium*. Some have pointed out that using large doses can cause a rise in blood pressure, nausea, vomiting, and edema with a reduction, or even a complete lack, of urination.

I believe that the amount of Bupleuri Radix (*chái hú*) used in Minor Bupleurum Decoction (*xiǎo chái hú tāng*) cannot be based on the original [large] amounts set forth in *Discussion of Cold Damage* and that a dosage of 10-20g is acceptable. Northern Bupleuri Radix (*chái hú*), the root of *B. Chinense*, is regarded as the best.

Based on clinical reports, it can be seen that Minor Bupleurum Decoction (*xiǎo chái hú tāng*) certainly is effective for treating feverish-type infectious illness. Gu reports using the prescription Bupleuri Radix (*chái hú*) 10-14g, Scutellariae Radix (*huáng qín*) 10-30g, Codonopsis Radix (*dǎng shēn*) 10-30g, Glycyrrhizae Radix (*gān cǎo*) 10-20g, Pinelliae Rhizoma preparatum (*zhì bàn xià*) 10-20g, Zingiberis Rhizoma recens (*shēng jiāng*) 10-20g, and Jujubae Fructus (*dà zǎo*) 10-30g to treat 86 patients with high fever. Among these were 36 patients who had respiratory tract infections, 20 with bile duct infections, nine with urinary tract infections, four with postpartum infections, two with septicemia, three with hepatitis, two with epidemic encephalitis B, two with the common cold, five who had the mumps, and three with bacterial dysentery. The length of time the patients had been ill varied from one to 30 days, with an average of 15 days. It took from one to five days, with an average of three days, for the fever to recede. The development of the illness from the point of view of their fevers was such that in the beginning, there were fever and chills that would come and go. However, this progressed to fever without chills but with specific occurrences of tidal fever. After that, alternating fever and chills set in with episodic, or concurrent, symptoms of headache with dizziness and coughing with chest stuffiness; a bitter taste in the mouth with reduced food intake; or sweating with an aversion to wind and urinary difficulty; or chest irritability and stuffiness; or nausea and vomiting.[4]

Wana Tadashi used Minor Bupleurum Decoction (*xiǎo chái hú tāng*) plus Gypsum fibrosum (*shí gāo*) to treat four subjects with fever, three of whom were exposed to wind and cold; they characteristically had a normal body temperature of 37°C (98.6°F) in the morning that would rise in the evening to 38.5°C to 39.8°C (101.3°F to 103.6°F). Additionally, there was headache, a thick white tongue coating, and accompanying chest and hypochondriac fullness and discomfort. After two to five days of treatment, the patients recovered.[5]

Shen reports using a modification of Minor Bupleurum Decoction (*xiǎo chái hú tāng*) to treat eight patients, all of whom were young, robust women with postpartum fever. Their fevers for the most part were 38°C (100.4°F) and above, with the highest reaching 39.6°C (103.3°F). These fevers were all due to postpartum infection, with white blood cell counts ranging from 12,000/mm³ and above, with one patient having a count of 32,000/mm³. These fevers had persisted for three to six days without interruption. Before using the Chinese herbs, all the patients had been prescribed a variety of antibiotics. Within this group, five had no significant effect from the Western medicine, while the body temperature of three patients trended downward, but they still complained of dizziness or headache, or chest stuffiness accompanied by a bitter taste in the mouth, complete lack of appetite, and nausea with fluid in the mouth. After these eight were switched to the Chinese herbs, the fastest resolution of the fever came about after taking just two packets and the slowest required five packets. The herbs comprising this formula were Minor Bupleurum Decoction (*xiǎo chái hú tāng*) with the addition of Angelicae sinensis Radix (*dāng guī*), Paeoniae Radix alba (*bái sháo*), Chuanxiong Rhizoma (*chuān xiōng*), Leonuri Herba (*yì mǔ cǎo*), and Salviae miltiorrhizae Radix (*dān shēn*). For those whose fever was accompanied by a slight aversion to cold, joint discomfort, and spontaneous sweating, Cinnamomi Ramulus (*guì zhī*) was added. Those with abdominal pain who disliked having pressure applied to their abdomen were given a modification with the Paeoniae Radix alba (*bái sháo*) and Zingiberis Rhizoma recens (*shēng jiāng*) removed and the formula Generating and Transforming Decoction (*shēng huà tāng*)* added.[6]

The Minor Bupleurum Decoction presentation can be seen in such illnesses as bronchitis, pleurisy, pulmonary tuberculosis, nephritis, hepatitis, and dermatological diseases. There are quite a few reports from Japan on these conditions. For example, Yashiki Michiaki frequently used this formula to improve the constitution of pediatric patients with a tendency to contract upper respiratory tract infections, diarrhea, or hives, and manifest chest and hypochondriac fullness and discomfort.[7] Hasegawa Hiashi effectively used this formula, combined with Five-Ingredient Powder with Poria (*wǔ líng sǎn*), to treat chronic nephritis.[8] Ogawa Yukio combined this formula with Cinnamon Twig and Poria Pill (*guì zhī fú líng wán*), with satisfactory results, to treat three patients with systemic lupus erythematosus.[9] Wada Tadashi used it for chronic eczema,[10] and Yashiki Michiaki used it as well to treat erythematic scaly eczema,[11] both with good results.

Zhang used Minor Bupleurum Decoction (*xiǎo chái hú tāng*) to treat a case of chronic nephritis. The patient had full body edema, ascites, and very poor kidney function. Urinary output in a single day was only 600 to 700ml. He had a fever of 40°C (104°F) as a result of catching a cold after taking a bath. He had already taken a course of both synthomycin and penicillin, but the fever did not recede, his urinary output became even more reduced, while the edema and ascites were even more pronounced. Furthermore, there was flushing in the face, a yellow-coated tongue, and immediate vomiting of any ingested fluids. The patient was thirsty and had a bitter taste in the mouth, with a slight amount of sweating, alternating fever and chills, and loose stools. Minor Bupleurum Decoction (*xiǎo chái hú tāng*) with the addition of Trichosanthis

---

* Angelicae sinensis Radix (*dāng guī*), Chuanxiong Rhizoma (*chuān xiōng*), Armeniacae Semen (*xìng rén*), Zingiberis Rhizoma preparata (*páo jiāng*), and Prepared Licorice Decoction (*zhì gān cǎo tāng*).

Fructus (*guā lóu*) and Citri reticulatae Pericarpium (*chén pí*) was prescribed. After taking two packets, the body temperature returned to normal, urinary output increased to 3,200ml, and both the edema and ascites were significantly reduced. Zhang says in the three months prior to using formulas where the focus was on improving the patient's kidney function and increasing urinary output, the largest amount of urine excreted was 1,200ml, which was surpassed after using this formula. This is an example of Minor Bupleurum Decoction's (*xiǎo chái hú tāng*) ability to promote urination.[12] It must be pointed out that for Minor Bupleurum Decoction (*xiǎo chái hú tāng*) to be effective in promoting urination, it must be used only when there is a Minor Bupleurum Decoction presentation in patients with edema. Should edema accompany a Cinnamon Twig Decoction presentation, it would be very difficult to see improvement in the urinary output by using Minor Bupleurum Decoction (*xiǎo chái hú tāng*). This underlines the point that to successfully treat using Chinese medicine, one must employ differential diagnosis. The principle here is that formulas and herbs must be chosen in accordance with the presentation.

There is the example of the famous contemporary practitioner Yashiki Michiaki who once used Minor Bupleurum Decoction (*xiǎo chái hú tāng*) to treat a patient with reticuloendotheliosis. The patient was four years old when this illness first struck, the original diagnosis was leukemia, and only later was it correctly diagnosed as reticuloendotheliosis. The patient frequently had high fevers, with a body temperature of 38°C to 40°C (100.4°F to 104°F), and at times the joints would be red and swollen. The patient's complexion had an ashen pallor, and was obviously anemic. The lymph nodes in the neck, axilla, and groin were all swollen, and the entire abdomen was distended, especially in the upper epigastrium, which was resistant when pressed and painful when palpated. The stools were normal, and the pulse was floating and rapid. Both the spleen and liver were enlarged by 5 centimeters, the hemoglobin content increased by 45 percent, with a red blood cell count of 27,200,000/mm^3, and the white blood cell count was 6,700/mm^3. Undergoing both antibiotic and hormone therapy proved ineffective. After one month of treatment using Minor Bupleurum Decoction (*xiǎo chái hú tāng*), the patient's condition had steadily improved. After two months, the body temperature returned to normal, the lymph nodes shrunk, and the patient's energy and complexion improved. Afterwards, this formula was combined with String of Pearls Drink (*lián zhū yǐn*),*

---

* This consists of Angelicae sinensis Radix (*dāng guī*), Chuanxiong Rhizoma (*chuān xiōng*), Paeoniae Radix alba (*bái sháo*), Rehmanniae Radix preparata (*shú dì huáng*), Atractylodis macrocephalae Rhizoma (*bái zhú*), Poria (*fú líng*), Cinnamomi Ramulus (*guì zhī*), and Glycyrrhizae Radix (*gān cǎo*).

and after eight months, the patient was cured. Examination of this patient 13 years after discontinuing the herbs revealed no relapse.[13]

The names of the illnesses in the above two cases were completely different: one was a case of nephritis and the other a blood disease. Even so, both had the Minor Bupleurum presentation. The first case had alternating fever and chills, vomiting, and a bitter taste in the mouth with a yellow-coated tongue. Although chest and hypochondriac discomfort and fullness was not explicitly mentioned, it must have existed due to the fullness and distention from the ascites. In the second case, there was significant chest and hypochondriac discomfort and fullness accompanied by fever, and enlargement of the lymph nodes in the 'bupleurum zones' of the neck, axilla, and groin. Because there were no clear digestive symptoms, String of Pearls Drink (*lián zhū yǐn*) was added later. For these types of illnesses, although quite different, the same formula could be prescribed because they had the same kind of presentation. Or as we say in Chinese medicine, "The same treatment can be effective for different illnesses" (異病同治 *yì bìng tóng zhì*).

MODIFICATIONS

- Minor Bupleurum Decoction (*xiǎo chái hú tāng*) combined with Minor Decoction [for Pathogens] Stuck in the Chest (*xiǎo xiàn xiōng tāng*) is called Bupleurum Decoction [for Pathogens] Stuck in the Chest (*chái hú xiàn xiōng tāng*). It is used to treat those who have coughing with sticky phlegm accompanied by chest and hypochondriac discomfort and fullness with pressure pain when the epigastrium is palpated. It is often used to treat patients who have respiratory tract infections accompanied by inflammation of the digestive tract.

- When combined with Pinellia and Magnolia Bark Decoction (*bàn xià hòu pò tāng*), it is called Bupleurum and Magnolia Bark Decoction (*chái pò tāng*). It is used to treat those with chest stuffiness and rib pain, a feeling of something being caught in the throat, an unsettled spirit, poor appetite, nausea and vomiting, and a greasy, white tongue coating. It is often used to treat those with bronchitis, asthma, and neurosis.

- When combined with Five-Ingredient Powder with Poria (*wǔ líng sǎn*), it becomes the formula Bupleurum and Poria Decoction (*chái líng tāng*). This is used to treat those with a Minor Bupleurum Decoction presentation accompanied by a reduction in urinary output, edema, and thirst. Often, it is used to treat patients with nephritis, acute gastroenteritis, summerheat, and edema.

• When combined with Calm the Stomach Powder (*píng wèi sǎn*), it becomes the formula Bupleurum and Calm the Stomach Decoction (*chái píng tāng*) from *Collected Treatises of [Zhang] Jing-Yue* (景岳全書 *Jing-Yuè quán shū*). This formula treats those with a Minor Bupleurum Decoction presentation, abdominal fullness, and a white, greasy tongue coating.

3.2 **Bupleurum and Cinnamon Twig Decoction**
(柴胡桂枝湯 *chái hú guì zhī tāng*)

SOURCE: *Discussion of Cold Damage*

Bupleuri Radix (*chái hú*) 5-12g
Cinnamomi Ramulus (*guì zhī*) 5-10g
Paeoniae Radix (*sháo yào*) 6-12g
Scutellariae Radix (*huáng qín*) 6-10g
Ginseng Radix (*rén shēn*) 3-6g
Glycyrrhizae Radix (*gān cǎo*) 3g
Pinelliae Rhizoma preparatum (*zhì bàn xià*) 6-10g
Jujubae Fructus (*dà zǎo*) 10g
Zingiberis Rhizoma recens (*shēng jiāng*) 6g

Bupleurum and Cinnamon Twig Decoction (*chái hú guì zhī tāng*) is made by combining Minor Bupleurum Decoction (*xiǎo chái hú tāng*) with Cinnamon Twig Decoction (*guì zhī tāng*); its original presentation was for those who had fever with a slight aversion to cold, nonspecific joint pain (支節煩疼 *zhī jié fán téng*), slight vomiting, clumping below the heart (心下支結 *xīn xià zhī jié*), and an exterior condition that had not completely resolved. Fever with a slight aversion to cold and nonspecific joint pain can be seen as the fever with aversion to cold, joint pain, and agitation typical of a Cinnamon Twig Decoction presentation. The slight nausea and clumping below the Heart can be seen as the chest and hypochondriac fullness and discomfort, and the irritability in the chest with a desire to vomit, typical of the Minor Bupleurum Decoction presentation. Nonspecific joint pain refers to joints that seem achy and painful but have no fixed location; at the same time, the patient is irritable and in a bad mood. Epigastric focal distention refers to a sensation of something pushing upward in the area between the ribs in the chest, a subjective feeling on the part of the patient of focal distention and fullness that seems to have form, and a feeling of resistance against the practitioner's fingertips when palpating, or discomfort on the part of the patient. The Bupleurum and Cinnamon Twig

Decoction presentation is in fact a complex of both the Minor Bupleurum Decoction and Cinnamon Twig Decoction presentations, at a comparatively mild level however. This formula's presentation is as follows:

1. Fever with aversion to wind, alternating fever and chills, sweating, sore and painful joints
2. Chest and hypochondriac pain and discomfort, or abdominal pain, poor appetite, irritability in the chest with a desire to vomit
3. The tongue body is dark red or dark and pale, with a thin white or yellow, greasy coating

To me, this formula's presentation can be seen as either a person with a cinnamon twig constitution experiencing chest and hypochondriac pain and discomfort, alternating fever and chills, and vomiting with a bitter taste in the mouth, or as a person with a bupleurum constitution having spontaneous sweating, nasal congestion, abdominal pain, joints that are achy and painful, and muscle spasms. Alternatively, it can appear as a mix of the bupleurum and cinnamon twig presentations. Especially for some patients with chronic conditions, differentiating the constitution is quite important. Aside from this, the tongue body tends to be dark. If the tongue body is shiny red and without a coating, or pale and flabby with a white, greasy coating, then one should consider another formula presentation.

• In Japan, Bupleurum and Cinnamon Twig Decoction (*chái hú guì zhī tāng*) has gained quite a bit of attention for its use in treating epilepsy. The Japanese practitioner Soumi Ichiro has on numerous occasions reported on the striking clinical results of this formula when appropriately prescribed.[14, 15, 16, 17] Laboratory studies have also proven this formula's anti-epileptic and sedative functions are not the same as those of commonly used anti-epileptic and sedative drugs.[18, 19, 20] According to Soumi Ichiro's report, among 433 patients, there were 125 who were completely cured, and 79 patients had a significant reduction in their symptoms. The remaining patients discontinued treatment for various reasons, so it is impossible to comment on them. Among the above-discussed cases, 181 patients had previously undergone an electro-encephalogram (EEG) examination. Two months prior, 123 patients had an epileptic episode. After taking this formula, the seizures stopped, EEG signs of 'epilepsy wave' disappeared for 46 percent, while for 38 percent of the patients, although the EEG showed waveforms for epilepsy, clinically, there were no epileptic episodes.[21] Soumi Ichiro noticed that most patients experienced chest and hypochondriac pain and discomfort along with tight and spasmodic rectus abdominus muscles. He believes that in the treatment process, as long as this abdominal presentation still exists, even if the EEG is clean and the seizures have stopped, the patient should continue using the herbs.

• The chest and hypochondriac pain and discomfort, lack of appetite, irritability in the chest with a desire to vomit, and abdominal pain symptoms of the Bupleurum and Cinnamon Twig Decoction presentation are symptoms that are often seen in patients with digestive system disorders. Therefore, this formula can be used to treat such illnesses as peptic ulcers, cholecystitis, choledocholithiasis, chronic colitis, and pancreatitis.

I have used this formula to treat many cases of chronic colitis accompanied by aversion to wind, spontaneous sweating, and a sensitivity to temperature changes. Subjective symptoms disappear on average after a week of treatment.

Patients with liver disease also frequently manifest with chest and hypochondriac pain and discomfort, and thus in Japan, bupleurum formulas are the medicinals most commonly used to treat chronic hepatitis and cirrhosis of the liver, and Bupleurum and Cinnamon Twig Decoction (*chái hú guì zhī tāng*) is one of the most commonly used prescriptions. However, this formula's presentation should be rigorously confirmed because in the course of the changes that occur in chronic liver disease, many patients do not manifest with a bupleurum presentation, but rather with a cinnamon twig presentation; in those cases, Minor Construct the Middle Decoction (*xiǎo jiàn zhōng tāng*), Cinnamon Twig Decoction plus Peony (*guì zhī jiā sháo yào tāng*), and Peony and Licorice Decoction (*sháo yào gān cǎo tāng*) should perhaps be given instead.

The Bupleurum and Cinnamon Twig Decoction presentation is seen quite often in such illnesses as functional disruption of the autonomic nervous system, nervous exhaustion, neurosis, and premenstrual syndrome. This formula is effective for improving the conditions of spontaneous sweating, chest stuffiness, abdominal pain, poor appetite, and depression.

I once treated a middle-aged woman who had been diagnosed with cervical spondylosis. Her main complaint was neck and shoulder pain with accompanying spontaneous sweating, aversion to wind, and significant sternal pain tenderness. Otherwise, her physical condition was fine. At that time, it was not possible to conclusively say whether or not this was a case of cervical spondylosis. However, as all the parts of the Bupleurum and Cinnamon Twig Decoction presentation were present, I just gave her five packets of this formula. After taking the herbs, the symptoms disappeared. Later, she again became ill, this time with abdominal fullness, pain, and diarrhea accompanied by a lot of gas. Because of the spontaneous sweating, aversion to wind, and chest and hypochondriac pain and discomfort, three packets of Bupleurum and Cinnamon Twig Decoction (*chái hú guì zhī tāng*) were prescribed, which promptly led to her recovery.

- Some patients with allergic illnesses, such as allergic rhinitis, intractable urticaria, and allergic purpura, also have the presentation for this formula. These patients, for the most part, manifest with aversion to wind, spontaneous sweating, sensitivity to temperature changes and pain, along with irritability and chest and hypochondriac pain and discomfort. Modern pharmacological research has found evidence that both Cinnamon Twig Decoction (*guì zhī tāng*) and Minor Bupleurum Decoction (*xiǎo chái hú tāng*) have significant anti-allergy functions.[22, 23]

- Symptoms such as fevers of unknown origin, alternating fever and chills, and aversion to wind with sweating can all be considered part of this formula's presentation.

3.3 Bupleurum, Cinnamon Twig, and Ginger Decoction
(柴胡桂枝乾薑湯 *chái hú guì zhī gān jiāng tāng*)

SOURCE: *Discussion of Cold Damage*

Bupleuri Radix (*chái hú*) 6-12g
Cinnamomi Ramulus (*guì zhī*) 6-12g
Zingiberis Rhizoma (*gān jiāng*) 3-6g
Scutellariae Radix (*huáng qín*) 5-10g
Trichosanthis Fructus (*guā lóu*) 10-12g
Ostreae Concha (*mǔ lì*) 10-15g
Glycyrrhizae Radix (*gān cǎo*) 3-6g

Bupleurum, Cinnamon Twig, and Ginger Decoction (*chái hú guì zhī gān jiāng tāng*) is the buplerurum family formula for calming and restoring energy for those with fatigue from overwork. The Japanese practitioner Honsono Shiro, author of *Ten Discussions on the Study of Kampō* (漢方醫學十講 *kanpo igaku jukko*), believes that the Bupleurum, Cinnamon Twig, and Ginger Decoction presentation is appropriate for addressing emotional symptoms from fatigue, which are seen more often in women. For instance, these patients can be quite full of enthusiasm and energy when entertaining guests or being out and about, but afterward they suddenly lose all their energy and feel completely worn out. These types of patients can frequently manifest the Bupleurum, Cinnamon Twig, and Ginger Decoction presentation. Honsono says this kind of body type falls within the Bupleurum constitution, which is to say, the fluctuation in energy levels is quite large. The Bupleurum, Cinnamon Twig, and Ginger Decoction presentation readily develops in situations of extreme emotional stress and irregular dietary habits with the additional stressors of excessive physical labor or excessive sweating.

Discussion of Cold Damage describes the presentation for this formula as "cold damage for five or six days that has already been sweated and purged, chest and hypochondriac pain with slight binding, urinary difficulty and thirst without vomiting, sweating only from the head, alternating fever and chills, and irritability in the chest." The chest and hypochondriac pain with slight clumping and alternating fever and chills is part of the bupleurum presentation. The slight binding (微結 *wēi jié*) is similar to, but less intense than, the clumping (支結 *zhī jié*) of the Bupleurum and Cinnamon Twig Decoction presentation. Fever and chills with sweating, irritability, and simultaneous aversion to wind are cinnamon twig presentations. Urinary difficulty and thirst are originally symptoms of the poria and atractylodis presentations, while thirst without vomiting, a lack of dizziness, and palpitations accompanying chest and hypochondriac pain and discomfort are not the presentations treated by poria and atractylodis. Based on the original text, this formula's presentation is not that clear. That being said, in line with the clinical experience of later generations of doctors, the presentation of this formula can be described as follows:

1. Chest and hypochondriac pain, or coughing, or sternal pain, especially when palpated
2. Alternating fever and chills, or aversion to wind, night sweats or spontaneous sweating, especially from the neck up
3. Poor appetite, thirst without drinking much, urinary difficulty, loose stools
4. Irritability, pulsation in the chest and abdomen, insomnia or vivid dreaming, tinnitus
5. Dry tongue with a thick white coating

The differences between the Bupleurum, Cinnamon Twig, and Ginger Decoction presentation and that of the Minor Bupleurum Decoction presentation are as follows:

- The Bupleurum, Cinnamon Twig, and Ginger Decoction presentation includes spontaneous sweating.

- The Bupleurum, Cinnamon Twig, and Ginger Decoction presentation does not include vomiting, but there is urinary difficulty, with a dry mouth and lack of desire to drink.

- The Minor Bupleurum Decoction presentation includes being dejected and without a desire for food or drink, while this formula's presentation includes irritability with a lack of desire to drink, palpitations, and insomnia or light sleeping. Because there is sweating, Cinnamomi Ramulus (*guì zhī*) is added, and because there is no vomiting, Pinelliae Rhizoma preparatum (*zhì bàn xià*) is omitted. Ostreae Concha (*mǔ lì*) is used to treat the irritability, and Zingiberis Rhizoma (*gān jiāng*) functions to treat the thick white tongue coating and poor appetite.

The presentations for this formula and that of Bupleurum and Cinnamon Twig Decoction both include spontaneous sweating. However, there are more significant nervous system symptoms with this formula's presentation. The Bupleurum and Cinnamon Twig Decoction presentation has more abdominal pain, and palpation reveals that the muscles of the abdomen are relatively tight. By contrast, in this formula's presentation, the abdomen is soft, nor is there any pain. The lack of appetite here is also an important distinction. Looking at the tongue, in a Bupleurum, Cinnamon Twig, and Ginger Decoction presentation, the coating is white and rather thick with the tongue itself being dry, while the coating in the Minor Bupleurum Decoction presentation is thin and white, or thick and yellow, with a moist tongue body. Furthermore, while both presentations include fever, the Bupleurum and Cinnamon Twig Decoction presentation is usually accompanied by joint pain, whereas that is not the case for Bupleurum, Cinnamon Twig, and Ginger Decoction (*chái hú guì zhī gān jiāng tāng*).

Signs of nervous exhaustion, neurosis, allergic colitis, chronic cholecystitis, dysmenorrhea, and menopausal syndrome often accompany this formula's presentation. As long as the diagnosis is correct, the treatment results in quick relief.

3.4 **Bupleurum plus Dragon Bone and Oyster Shell Decoction**
(柴胡加龍骨牡蠣湯 *chái hú jiā lóng gǔ mǔ lì tāng*)*

SOURCE: *Discussion of Cold Damage*

Bupleuri Radix (*chái hú*)... 6-12g
Fossilia Ossis Mastodi (*lóng gǔ*)..................................10-20g
Scutellariae Radix (*huáng qín*)......................................5-10g
Zingiberis Rhizoma recens (*shēng jiāng*)........................... 5g
Ginseng Radix (*rén shēn*)..5g
Cinnamomi Ramulus (*guì zhī*)..5-10g
Poria (*fú líng*)...5-12g
Pinelliae Rhizoma preparatum (*zhì bàn xià*)..................... 6-10g
Rhei Radix et Rhizoma (*dà huáng*)............................... 5-10g
Ostreae Concha (*mǔ lì*)...10-20g
Jujubae Fructus (*dà zǎo*)..15g

Chronic illness, advanced age, long-term psychological stress, and external injury all can lead to patients with a bupleurum constitution losing their psycho-emotional and neurological equilibrium, which can manifest with serious neuropsychiatric symptoms. Problems are expressed in aspects of the behavior, emotions, speech and thought processes, perceptions, consciousness, memory, focus, and sleep. In addition, there may be neurological pathologies such as epilepsy, tremors, headaches, tinnitus, and increased muscle tension.

Paragraph 107 of *Discussion of Cold Damage* describes it this way: "Cold damage for eight or nine days, which is purged. If there is then fullness in the chest, irritability and fright, urinary dysfunction, incoherent speech, the body feels completely and thoroughly heavy with an inability to turn to [either] side, Bupleurum plus Dragon Bone and Oyster Shell Decoction (*chái hú jiā lóng gǔ mǔ lì tāng*) masters it." The "chest fullness" here can be seen as the bupleurum presentation's principal sign of chest and hypochondriac fullness and discomfort. "Panic and anxiety" refers to the psycho-emotional and nervous system symptoms of anxiety, insomnia, and palpitations. "Incoherent speech" can be seen as an impediment to both the speech and thought processes, and "heaviness throughout the entire body" can be understood as a pathology of the nerves and muscles. "Urinary difficulty" can be understood as symptoms of edema, incontinence, and constipation in patients with psychosomatic illness. Bupleurum plus Dragon Bone and Oyster Shell Decoction (*chái hú jiā lóng gǔ*

---

* Note that the original formulation contains Minium (*qiān dān*), which is not included at present.

mǔ lì tāng) has been used by doctors in China for thousands of years with good effect to treat countless patients with psychological and neurological illnesses.

The Bupleurum plus Dragon Bone and Oyster Shell Decoction presentation is as follows:

1. Bupleurum presentation
2. Psycho-emotional and nervous system symptoms, especially for those with strong pulsations around the naval, who are easily startled, or have incoherent speech
3. Red tongue with a thick, greasy, yellow coating

Strong pulsations in the area around the navel are an important sign for which Zhang Zhong-Jing prescribed Fossilia Ossis Mastodi (*lóng gǔ*) and Ostreae Concha (*mǔ lì*). It therefore stands to reason that those with the presentation for this formula commonly have these symptoms. When the symptoms are severe, these are frequently the patient's main complaint. When the symptoms are less severe, the patient will have no obvious sensation. However, when the practitioner palpates the abdomen, it will be flat and the pulsation of the aorta will be obvious. 'Easily startled' can manifest as excessive dreaming, being easily awakened, or being easily subject to palpitations, while 'incoherent speech' is the sign of a confused or deranged mind.

The differences between the presentation for this formula and that of Cinnamon Twig Decoction plus Dragon Bone and Oyster Shell (*guì zhī jiā lóng gǔ mǔ lì tāng*) include the following:

• *Thickness of the tongue coating.* The coating in the Cinnamon Twig Decoction plus Dragon Bone and Oyster Shell presentation is thin, white, and moist, while that associated with the Bupleurum plus Dragon Bone and Oyster Shell Decoction presentation is thick and yellow, or may even be dry and scorched. Many patients have accompanying abdominal fullness and constipation.

• *Severity of the psycho-emotional symptoms.* The psycho-emotional symptoms of the Cinnamon Twig Decoction plus Dragon Bone and Oyster Shell presentation are merely insomnia or excessive dreaming, while for this formula, there are more severe mental problems such as insanity.

• *Constitutional difference.* These are the aforementioned differences between the bupleurum and cinnamon twig constitutions.

This formula's presentation is often seen in cases of epilepsy. The famous Qing-dynasty doctor Xu Ling-Tai noted: "This formula can reduce Liver and

Gallbladder fright-phlegm and will definitely be effective in the treatment of epilepsy." The renowned contemporary doctor Yue Mei-Zhong reports using a modification of this formula to treat a case of recalcitrant pediatric epilepsy.[24] And the famous contemporary Japanese physician Sakaguchi also reports this formula is effective for treating epilepsy.[25]

This formula can be effective in treating schizophrenia. Ge reports treating 67 subjects where one patient completely recovered, 35 showed significant improvement, 15 experienced some improvement, and 16 experienced no effect.[26] Zhou reports using the formula, with the additions of Persicae Semen (*táo rén*), Carthami Flos (*hóng huā*), Moutan Cortex (*mǔ dān pí*), Paeoniae Radix rubra (*chì sháo*), Salviae miltiorrhizae Radix (*dān shēn*), Citri reticulatae viride Pericarpium (*qīng pí*), and Cyperi Rhizoma (*xiāng fù*), to treat 40 subjects. Of these, 10 were cured, another 10 showed improvement, and 20 showed no change.[27]

Bupleurum plus Dragon Bone and Oyster Shell Decoction (*chái hú jiā lóng gǔ mǔ lì tāng*) may be effective in the treatment of hyperthyroidism. Yu reports using this formula, with the addition of Gypsum fibrosum (*shí gāo*), Puerariae Radix (*gé gēn*), Uncariae Ramulus cum Uncis (*gōu téng*), Bombyx batryticatus (*bái jiāng cán*), and Cinnabaris (*zhū shā*), to treat 100 patients. Treatment resulted in significant effect for 50 patients, some improvement for 40, and no effect for nine.[28]

There is ongoing research into the efficacy of this formula in treating senile dementia. According to reports by Zhou, this formula, combined with Iron Filings Drink (*tiě luò yǐn*), was used to treat 13 patients with early-stage senile dementia (of these, 10 had cerebral atrophy). Three patients were completely cured, eight experienced significant improvement, one improved slightly, and there was no improvement at all for one.[29]

This formula is effective for treating high blood pressure accompanied by neurological symptoms. Reports on the treatment of this type of presentation with Bupleurum plus Dragon Bone and Oyster Shell Decoction (*chái hú jiā lóng gǔ mǔ lì tāng*) are mostly from Japan.[30, 31] Additionally, this formula can be effective in treating illness involving hair loss, tremors, Meniere's syndrome, insomnia, dizziness, and headaches.

3.5 Frigid Extremities Powder (四逆散 *sì nì sǎn*)

SOURCE: *Discussion of Cold Damage*

Bupleuri Radix (*chái hú*) 6-10g

Paeoniae Radix (*sháo yào*) 6-30g

Aurantii Fructus immaturus (*zhǐ shí*) 6-10g

Glycyrrhizae Radix (*gān cǎo*) 3-10g

Minor Construct the Middle Decoction (*xiǎo jiàn zhōng tāng*) is the Cinnamomi Ramulus (*guì zhī*) formula family's most effective prescription for stopping abdominal pain. In the Bupleuri Radix (*chái hú*) formula family, Frigid Extremities Powder (*sì nì sǎn*) is best for treating chest, rib, and abdominal pain. In this formula, Bupleuri Radix (*chái hú*) clearly has sedative and analgesic effects. The combination of Paeoniae Radix alba (*bái sháo*) and Glycyrrhizae Radix (*gān cǎo*), which constitutes the well-known formula Peony and Licorice Decoction (*sháo yào gān cǎo tāng*), is known for relieving spasms and stopping pain. It is also one of the principal components of Minor Construct the Middle Decoction (*xiǎo jiàn zhōng tāng*). Aurantii Fructus immaturus (*zhǐ shí*) primarily treats chest and abdominal fullness and distention, constipation, and prolapse of the stomach and uterus. In *Essentials from the Golden Cabinet* (金匱要略 *Jīn guì yào lüè*), Aurantii Fructus immaturus (*zhǐ shí*) and Paeoniae Radix alba (*bái sháo*) are specifically used together to treat "postpartum abdominal pain, irritability, and fullness in the chest such that the patient is unable to lie down." The clinical effectiveness of these two herbs has already been proven by many years of use. The four herbs of Frigid Extremities Powder (*sì nì sǎn*)—Bupleuri Radix (*chái hú*), Paeoniae Radix alba (*bái sháo*), Aurantii Fructus immaturus (*zhǐ shí*), and Glycyrrhizae Radix (*gān cǎo*)—primarily target chest, rib, and abdominal pain. The formula is suitable for a wide range of internal medicine, gynecological, and surgical complaints where pain is the primary symptom. According to various reports, this formula can treat cholecystitis, cholelithiasis, biliary ascariasis, hepatitis, gastritis, peptic ulcers, gastric hypertrophy, gastric neurosis, prolapse of the stomach, recalcitrant stomach pain, allergic colitis, diarrhea, dysentery, hiccup, appendicitis and appendicular abscess, intestinal obstruction, intestinal adhesions, pancreatitis, cough, coronary heart disease, premenstrual syndrome, menopausal syndrome, irregular periods, dysmenorrhea, fallopian tube obstruction, acute mastitis, intercostal neuralgia, costal condritis, neurogenic headache, trigeminal neuralgia, epilepsy, plum pit qi, urinary tract stones, autonomic dystonia, impotence, seminal emissions, allergic rhinitis, dermatitis, cold extremities following a fever, and shock from infectious hemorrhagic illness. No other formula comes close to the extensive scope of uses for which this formula may be employed. This requires that practitioners be rigorous in their grasp of the Frigid Extremities Powder presentation.

Paragraph 318 of *Discussion of Cold Damage* states: "*shào yīn* disease, disease with frigid extremities—the person may have cough or palpitations or urinary dysfunction or pain in the abdomen or draining diarrhea with downbearing; Frigid Extremities Powder (*sì nì sǎn*) masters it." The term 'four reversals' (四逆 *sì nì*) indicates that the extremities of the four limbs are cold. The manifestation of frigid extremities can be due to yang deficiency, as in the presentations for Cinnamon Twig plus Aconite Accessory Root Decoction (*guì zhī jiā fù zǐ tāng*) and Frigid Extremities Decoction (*sì nì tāng*). Frigid extremities can also arise from heat constraint, as in the presentations for White Tiger Decoction (*bái hǔ tāng*), Major Order the Qi Decoction (*dà chéng qì tāng*), and this formula. In these cases, the coldness of the extremities is not at all due to an insufficiency of yang qi, but rather to the yang qi becoming knotted and constrained in the interior, thus being unable to disperse outward. The coldness of the extremities associated with a Frigid Extremities Powder presentation will often be accompanied by many other signs or symptoms of heat. Moreover, the key indication is abdominal pain that is of a distending nature and tends to be located either in the chest and hypochondria or on either side of the lower abdomen. It can be said that the abdominal, chest, and hypochondriac pain of the Frigid Extremities Powder presentation is exactly that of the bupleurum presentation. The Frigid Extremities Powder presentation is as follows:

1. Bupleurum presentation or a bupleurum constitution with a sensitivity to pain, hands that are often cold, and a tendency to have anxiety and muscle spasms
2. Chest and hypochondriac fullness and discomfort with pain, and distending abdominal pain
3. A wiry pulse and a stiff, dark tongue, or a tongue with purple spots

A wiry pulse is one where the pulse is long and felt clearly in all positions, as if one were pressing down on a piano wire. This type of pulse often appears in presentations where there is pain. Furthermore, it is often seen in patients with a bupleurum constitution.

Abdominal pain is the primary symptom of both the Frigid Extremities Powder and Minor Construct the Middle Decoction presentations, yet these two presentations have significant differences:

• *Constitutional types.* Differentiate between the bupleurum and cinnamon twig body types.

- *Pulse and tongue.* The Minor Construct the Middle Decoction (*xiǎo jiàn zhōng tāng*) pulse is floating, large, and without force. The tongue body is tender, red, and moist, and in most cases, it has a thin white coating, whereas the Frigid Extremities Powder (*sì nì sǎn*) pulse is wiry and forceful and accompanied by a stiff, dry tongue that could have either a thin and white or yellow coating, or in many cases, a dry and greasy coating.

- *Quality of the abdominal pain.* The abdominal pain of Frigid Extremities Powder (*sì nì sǎn*) is usually continuous and centered in the area of the chest and hypochondria, and when pressed, it increases. The abdominal pain of Minor Construct the Middle Decoction (*xiǎo jiàn zhōng tāng*), by contrast, is usually intermittent, and pressure feels good to these patients.

Some individual case reports of the use of Frigid Extremities Powder (*sì nì sǎn*) may be quite helpful in understanding the rules for using this formula. Xie treated a case where the patient had suffered four years of intractable abdominal pain. Visual inspection found the face to be dark and lusterless, the pulse was moderate, and there was thirst, but without much desire to drink. The pain was located about an inch above the navel and involved an area about the size of a teacup. When the pain occurred, the extremities would become cold. Frigid Extremities Powder (*sì nì sǎn*) with a large dose of Paeoniae Radix alba (*bái sháo*) was prescribed, and after 12 packets, the patient was cured.[32]

I once treated a 37-year-old school teacher who had abdominal pain for three years. When the pain came on, she would get hot, but her extremities were cold, and there usually were accompanying leg spasms and constipation. She had been to the hospital for a Western medical examination where she was diagnosed as having tuberculous peritonitis. The patient had a thin build and pale complexion, the tongue had a thin, white coating, and the pulse was thin and wiry. Frigid Extremities Powder (*sì nì sǎn*) with 30g of Paeoniae Radix alba (*bái sháo*) was prescribed, and after taking five packets, the pain stopped. Although it later returned, the severity of the abdominal pain was reduced, and could be stopped by using the original formula. This is an example of a case where pain was the main complaint, but where cold limbs were the distinguishing feature.

There also are cases where abdominal pain is not the main complaint within the symptom set, but Frigid Extremities Powder (*sì nì sǎn*) can also have a significant effect. For example, Fan treated a 36-year-old female elementary school teacher who had suffered from impeded urination for 10 years. When severe, her urine was yellow and difficult to pass, and she felt as if she could not completely void her bladder. There was burning pain in the urethra and incomplete, dribbling urination. She had undergone all kinds of examinations and treatments, but none had any significant effect. At her consultation, her main complaint was that she would urinate 10 times in the course of 24 hours, but that it was always scanty, at times just a dribble, and accompanied by pain. She had lower back and lower abdominal pain, erosions on the lower part of her vagina, copious amounts of leukorrhea, and cold extremities. The tongue had a red tip with a slippery, white coating. She was given four packets of Frigid Extremities Powder *(sì nì sǎn)*, modified as follows: Bupleuri Radix *(chái hú)*, Paeoniae Radix alba *(bái sháo)*, Aurantii Fructus immaturus *(zhǐ shí)* 24g each, Glycyrrhizae Radix *(gān cǎo)* 9g, Platycodi Radix *(jié gěng)* 30g, and Poria *(fú líng)* 30g. Additionally, she was given a powder that Fan devised to spread topically on the lower vagina. After taking the herbs, her ability to urinate improved and all her symptoms resolved.[33]

Chest, hypochondriac, and abdominal pain, cold extremities, and a bupleurum constitution are the fundamental conditions I use to diagnose a Frigid Extremities Powder presentation. Furthermore, although these patients frequently experience abdominal pain, they are vigorous and appear neither wan nor sallow. What is more, they do not have a rhubarb, cinnamon twig, or aconite presentation. These are all important indications for consideration.

Due to the extensive scope of problems for which this formula can be used, clinical applications of Frigid Extremities Powder *(sì nì sǎn)* usually require some modification. Examples of such modifications are detailed in the accompanying table.

Sign / Symptom	Addition
Chest and hypochondriac pain	Melia Toosendan Powder *(jīn líng zǐ sǎn)*
Distention	Chuanxiong Rhizoma *(chuān xiōng)*, Cyperi Rhizoma *(xiāng fù)*, Citri reticulatae Pericarpium *(chén pí)*
Headache	Chuanxiong Rhizoma *(chuān xiōng)*
Dysmenorrhea	Angelicae sinensis Radix *(dāng guī)*
Gastroenteritis with abdominal pain	Coptidis Rhizoma *(huáng lián)*, Scutellariae Radix *(huáng qín)*, Aucklandiae Radix *(mù xiāng)*
Constipation with abdominal pain	Rhei Radix et Rhizoma *(dà huáng)*
Acid reflux with abdominal pain	Left Metal Pill *(zuǒ jīn wán)*

Thick, greasy, yellow tongue coating with abdominal pain	Coptidis Rhizoma (*huáng lián*), Scutellariae Radix (*huáng qín*), Gardeniae Fructus (*zhī zǐ*)
Abdominal pain with a pale tongue and sinking pulse	Aconiti Radix lateralis preparata (*zhì fù zǐ*)
Dark purple tongue	Paeoniae Radix rubra (*chì sháo*), Carthami Flos (*hóng huā*), Persicae Semen (*táo rén*), Salviae miltiorrhizae Radix (*dān shēn*)
Shiny tongue with no coating	Ophiopogonis Radix (*mài mén dōng*), Dendrobii Herba (*shí hú*)
Abdominal pain with masses	Paeoniae Radix rubra (*chì sháo*), Persicae Semen (*táo rén*), Salviae miltiorrhizae Radix (*dān shēn*), Notoginseng Radix (*sān qī*)
Abdominal pain with nausea and vomiting	Pinelliae Rhizoma preparatum (*zhì bàn xià*), Zingiberis Rhizoma recens (*shēng jiāng*)
Impotence	Scolopendra (*wú gōng*)
Palpitations with abdominal pain	Cinnamomi Ramulus (*guì zhī*)
Chest stuffiness with abdominal pain	Allii fistulosi Bulbus (*cōng bái*)

If a Frigid Extremities Powder presentation is accompanied by recalcitrant psychological or neurological symptoms such as stubborn headaches, insomnia, abdominal pain, or hiccup, or the patient has a dark purple tongue body and a dark and lusterless complexion, one should use Drive Out Stasis from the Mansion of Blood Decoction (*xuè fǔ zhú yū tāng*).

3.6 Drive Out Stasis from the Mansion of Blood Decoction
(血府逐瘀湯 *xuè fǔ zhú yū tāng*)

SOURCE: *Correction of Errors among Physicians* (醫林改錯 *Yī lín gǎi cuò*)

Bupleuri Radix (*chái hú*)..............5-10g
Paeoniae Radix (*sháo yào*)..............6-20g
Aurantii Fructus immaturus (*zhǐ shí*)..............6-10g
Glycyrrhizae Radix (*gān cǎo*)..............3g
Persicae Semen (*táo rén*)..............6-12g
Carthami Flos (*hóng huā*)..............5-10g
Angelicae sinensis Radix (*dāng guī*)..............6-12g
Chuanxiong Rhizoma (*chuān xiōng*)..............5-10g

Rehmanniae Radix (*shēng dì huáng*) 12g
Platycodi Radix (*jié gěng*) 5g
Achyranthis bidentatae Radix (*niú xī*) 12g

This formula is a combination of Frigid Extremities Powder (*sì nì sǎn*) and Four-Substance Decoction with Safflower and Peach Pit (*táo hóng sì wù tāng*), which is the representative formula for treating blood stasis. Chinese medicine regards blood stasis as both the product as well as a cause of illness. Infections, fever, bleeding, getting chilled, long-term psycho-emotional upset (especially depression), trauma, and chronic illness can all lead to disharmonies of the qi and blood, resulting in the formation of blood stasis. The distinguishing clinical manifestations of blood stasis are:

1. Pain that is usually in a fixed location
2. When bleeding occurs, the blood readily congeals and is purple or black in color
3. Irritability and restlessness, with an unsettled spirit, and mania in extreme cases
4. The tongue is purple and dark, along with a dark complexion

Blood stasis frequently occurs in those with a bupleurum constitution. The Drive Out Stasis from the Mansion of Blood Decoction presentation is often seen in cases where there is recalcitrant insomnia, headaches, abdominal pain, or fever. Therefore, in the process of treating chronic illness in bupleurum constitution patients, one must be aware of signs of blood stasis. Once any of the aforementioned blood stasis signs appears, Drive Out Stasis from the Mansion of Blood Decoction (*xuè fǔ zhú yū tāng*) can be used. This formula can also be applied if there is a Frigid Extremities Powder presentation accompanied by signs of blood stasis. The following are several types of illnesses where a Drive Out Stasis from the Mansion of Blood Decoction presentation is commonly seen:

- *Headaches.* Wang Qing-Ren, the early nineteenth-century creator of Drive Out Stasis from the Mansion of Blood Decoction (*xuè fǔ zhú yū tāng*), said: "In examining patients with headaches where there are no exterior signs or internal symptoms, no signs of qi deficiency or phlegm, where headaches suddenly come and go, and many prescriptions have been tried to no avail, using one packet of this formula will resolve the problem." This formula can be used for neurogenic headaches, headaches from high blood pressure, headaches from cerebrovascular disease or trigeminal neuralgia, traumatic headaches,

headaches as a sequelae of a concussion, migraines, epilepsy, or headaches that have become chronic and recalcitrant.

Wang reports using this formula to treat 100 children who had suffered chronic headaches for a month or longer (not including those with head injuries or organic illnesses of the eyes, ears, nose, or throat). Among these young patients, there were 83 cases of neurogenic headaches, 14 suffered from vascular headaches, two had nervous exhaustion, and one had epilepsy. After taking the herbs for between four to 28 days, 76 of the children were completely cured, 20 took a turn for the better, and four experienced no effect.[34] Tian reports using a modification of this formula to treat 24 patients with critical head injuries. Of these patients, 17 recovered fully within an average of 20 days.[35]

- *Chest and hypochondriac pain.* This includes coronary heart disease with angina, cardiopulmonary disease, pleurisy, costochondritis, trauma to the thorax, intercostal neuralgia, or silicosis. Chest and hypochondriac fullness and discomfort is a primary sign of the bupleurum presentation. If there is unceasing pain with a dark tongue, then this formula must be used. There is a report of using this formula together with Trichosanthes Fruit, Chinese Chive, and Pinellia Decoction (*gūa lǒu xiè bái bàn xià tāng*) to treat 53 patients suffering from coronary heart disease with stable angina. Using the herbs for three days led to visible results.[36] Zhang reports using this formula to treat 14 patients with nonsuppurative costochondritis, resulting in a complete recovery for all.[37]

- *Spasms.* This formula can be used for illnesses such as hiccups and neurogenic vomiting. I have used this formula to treat quite a few patients with persistent hiccups. The course of the disease lasted anywhere from five to 30 days, and all had been treated unsuccessfully with conventional methods. Most of these patients had a dark tongue and a wiry pulse, and were cured after taking three to five packets of herbs.

- *Digestive diseases.* This formula can be used for such problems as intestinal obstruction due to adhesions, chronic hepatitis, cirrhosis of the liver, or enlargement of the spleen. There is a report of using a modification of Drive Out Stasis from the Mansion of Blood Decoction (*xuè fǔ zhú yū tāng*) in pill form, which was used to treat 18 patients who had suffered for two to 15 years from cirrhosis with ascites. The modified formula consisted of Bupleuri Radix (*chái hú*), Aurantii Fructus immaturus (*zhǐ shí*), Chuanxiong Rhizoma (*chuān xiōng*), red Ginseng Radix (*hóng rén shēn*) 40g each, Persicae Semen (*táo rén*), Carthami Flos (*hóng huā*), Paeoniae Radix rubra (*chì sháo*),

Rehmanniae Radix *(shēng dì huáng)* 60g each, Achyranthis bidentatae Radix *(niú xī)* 80g, Glycyrrhizae Radix *(gān cǎo)* 30g, Angelicae sinensis Radix *(dāng guī)*, Salviae miltiorrhizae Radix *(dān shēn)* 150g each, ground into a powder and made into 8g honey pills. Three pills were taken three times per day. Laboratory tests showed a reversal of the albumin and globulin levels and blood serum total protein levels of 6g or less for 14 of the patients, while 15 patients had abnormal liver function studies. Treatment resulted in the complete recovery of seven patients: their symptoms disappeared, their livers softened, and spleens shrunk to varying degrees, and their liver functions returned to normal; three months after stopping the herbs, there was no recurrence of symptoms.[38]

• *OB/Gyn diseases.* This formula can be used for irregular periods, dysmenorrhea, pelvic inflammation, fallopian tube obstruction, infertility, ectopic pregnancy, amenorrhea, menopausal syndrome, bleeding and back pain after a miscarriage, and breast hyperplasia. When diagnosing, aside from paying attention to the patient's overall condition, symptoms related to the menstrual cycle must not be overlooked. The diagnosis of this formula's presentation can be aided by the presence of such symptoms as early or late periods, painful swelling or lumps in the breast before the period, a sore lower back that feels heavy and weighed down, or menstrual blood that is dark or with clots.

• *Vascular problems.* This formula can be used for such problems as high blood pressure, coronary artery disease, arrhythmia, heart valve disease, arteritis, or phlebitis. In practice, these patients often have dark complexions, dark red lips, dark purple tongues, wiry, rough pulses, and dry skin.

• *Neuropsychiatric disorders.* This formula is used for such problems as intractable insomnia, neurosis, sleepwalking, epilepsy, or autonomic dystonia. The main complaints of these patients are usually serious and complicated, and the course of illness relatively long. The condition of their spirit and energy, however, does not appear to be compromised.

The renowned contemporary doctor from Ningbo, Fan Wen-Hu, has a case in which he used this formula to cure intractable insomnia. The patient was a local businessman in the prime of his life. Due to overwork and worry, he became exhausted, and after a long time, he finally developd insomnia. While he sought out all kinds of treatment, none was effective. When he came for his consultation, he had not slept in three nights. He was foggyheaded, wore more clothes than one would think appropriate, and had no interest in food. When patients wear more clothes than seems appropriate, it can be a sign that they experience alternating fever and chills.

Fan noticed that although the patient's complexion was pale, he seemed in good spirits and was talking and laughing as if nothing was amiss, and that his eyes were slightly bloodshot. Furthermore, his pulses on both sides in the middle position were wiry and long, and the sides of his tongue had bluish lines. He diagnosed the patient as having static blood clumped in the interior, and gave him Drive Out Stasis from the Mansion of Blood Decoction (*xuè fǔ zhú yū tāng*), omitting Platycodi Radix (*jié gěng*) and adding Notoginseng Radix (*sān qī*). After one packet, the patient promptly slept through the night.[39]

I have used this formula to cure a patient with bruxism. The patient did not have any particular problems or symptoms from this, but there were signs of dry skin, hard and tight muscles, and a dark red tongue. After seven packets of herbs, the teeth grinding was brought under control. From this, we can see that Drive Out Stasis from the Mansion of Blood Decoction (*xuè fǔ zhú yū tāng*) functions as a relatively good sedative.

- *Other.* This formula has also been used for obstinate dermatological problems such as chronic urticaria, eczema, and dermatitis with purple spots, stasis spots, pigmented spots, areas where the pigment is fading, or where there is pain or hypertrophy. Finally, it is also an important formula for ophthalmo-logical diseases such as fundal hemorrhage, retinal periphlebitis, and retinal vein occlusion.

The scope of appropriate uses for Drive Out Stasis from the Mansion of Blood Decoction (*xuè fǔ zhú yū tāng*) is quite extensive. In practice, one should watch for the presence of the Drive Out Stasis from the Mansion of Blood Decoction presentation in the following situations:

- The disease process has persisted for a long time, and conventional methods of treatment have not yielded any significant results. There is a saying in Chinese medicine: "Long-term illness enters the blood" (久病入血 *jiǔ bìng rù xuè*). When there has been treatment for a long period of time and the patient does not appear to be weak or debilitated, one can often consider the presence of blood stasis.

- There are odd symptoms and complicated main complaints that tend toward neurosis or other psycho-emotional illnesses.

- The spirit and vigor are intact, and there is no debilitation or listlessness, especially in those who have chronic pain or those who have suffered with their illness for a long time.

- Patients who have hard and tight muscles.

• There are signs of blood stasis.

If differential pattern diagnosis has been properly applied, this method brings about results rather quickly and without any side effects. However, if the formula is overused with patients who do not have any signs of blood stasis, some people might manifest with such problems as a feeling of weakness throughout the body or with lax muscles with no strength.

3.7 **Rambling Powder** (逍遙散 *xiāo yáo sǎn*)

Source: *Formulary of the Pharmacy Service for Benefiting the People in the Taiping Era* (太平惠民和劑局方 *Tài píng huì mín hé jì jú fāng*)

Bupleuri Radix (*chái hú*)	5-10g
Paeoniae Radix (*sháo yào*)	6-15g
Atractylodis macrocephalae Rhizoma (*bái zhú*)	6-12g
Poria (*fú líng*)	10g
Angelicae sinensis Radix (*dāng guī*)	6-12g
Zingiberis Rhizoma recens (*shēng jiāng*)	5g
Menthae haplocalycis Herba (*bò hé*)	5g

If Aurantii Fructus immaturus (*zhǐ shí*) is removed from Frigid Extremities Powder (*sì nì sǎn*) and Angelicae sinensis Radix (*dāng guī*), Atractylodis macrocephalae Rhizoma (*bái zhú*), Poria (*fú líng*), and Menthae haplocalycis Herba (*bò hé*) are added, it becomes the well-known gynecology formula Rambling Powder (*xiāo yáo sǎn*). Angelicae sinensis Radix (*dāng guī*) is the medicinal traditionally used to regulate the menses, while Paeoniae Radix alba (*bái sháo*), Atractylodis macrocephalae Rhizoma (*bái zhú*), and Poria (*fú líng*) are used together as the principal ingredients in the *Essentials from the Golden Cabinet* formula Tangkuei and Peony Powder (*dāng guī sháo yào sǎn*). Tangkuei and Peony Powder (*dāng guī sháo yào sǎn*) was originally used to treat abdominal pain during pregnancy. Because it has the ability to tonify and augment the qi and blood, the scope of this formula has expanded beyond pregnancy and postpartum illnesses, and can be used for various types of anemia, abdominal pain, low back pain, achy low back, edema, urinary difficulty, and irregular menstruation. Rambling Powder (*xiāo yáo sǎn*) is good for treating the chest or abdominal pain that Frigid Extremities Powder (*sì nì sǎn*) or a similar formula would treat; thus, it can be used for women with an anemic appearance and a wan or sallow complexion who also experience irregular menstruation. The Rambling Powder presentation is as follows:

1. Chest and hypochondriac fullness and discomfort or pain, abdominal pain and distention, dysmenorrhea, premenstrual breast distention or headache
2. A feeling of alternating fever and chills, or irregular periods
3. Poor appetite, and edema
4. Pale red tongue with a thin, white coating

There are reports that Rambling Powder (*xiāo yáo sǎn*) is effective for treating irregular periods, dysmenorrhea, excessive menstrual bleeding and spotting, and amenorrhea. It can be used for premenstrual problems such as breast distention, flaring of facial acne, and tension. It is also used for headaches, fevers, and fainting during the period. It treats vaginal discharge, endometriosis, breast hyperplasia, bleeding nipples, as well as irritability during pregnancy, postpartum insomnia, postpartum galactorrhea, insufficient lactation, uterine leiomyoma, menopausal syndrome, infertility, low libido, abdominal pain after tubal ligation, and nervous exhaustion.

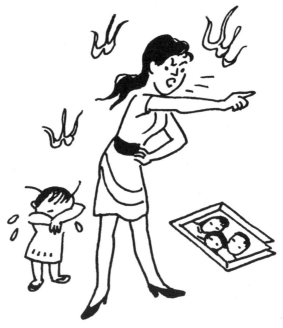

In practice, the formula is often used in women who do not have much interest in or feel inhibited about sex, or for whom intercourse is painful. They do not have much enthusiasm for being involved in social activities with other people and tend to keep their feelings inside, sulk in anger, and are nervous. The meaning of 'rambling' (逍遙 *xiāo yáo*) in Rambling Powder (*xiāo yáo sǎn*) is to be free and unrestrained. For this reason, changing a patient's sullen and unhappy feelings into optimistic ones with a feeling of ease is the primary function of Rambling Powder (*xiāo yáo sǎn*). There is a report of using a modification of this formula to treat 20 patients with psycho-emotional illness. The treatment resulted in a significant effect for 16 patients, some effect for seven, and none for three.[40] There are other reports that this formula is effective for the treatment of insomnia from nervous exhaustion, gastrointestinal neurosis, and unusual feelings in the throat.

Rambling Powder (*xiāo yáo sǎn*) with the addition of Gardeniae Fructus (*zhī zǐ*) and Moutan Cortex (*mǔ dān pí*) is called Augmented Rambling Powder (*jiā wèi xiāo yáo sǎn*). It is used for the Rambling Powder presentation accompanied by a red complexion, red eyes with blurry vision, headache, fever, irritability, bleeding, and painful, yellow urination.

3.8 **Major Bupleurum Decoction** (大柴胡湯 *dà chái hú tāng*)

SOURCE: *Discussion of Cold Damage*

Bupleuri Radix (*chái hú*)	10-15g
Scutellariae Radix (*huáng qín*)	6-10g
Paeoniae Radix (*sháo yào*)	6-20g
Pinelliae Rhizoma preparatum (*zhì bàn xià*)	6-10
Zingiberis Rhizoma recens (*shēng jiāng*)	3-6g
Aurantii Fructus immaturus (*zhǐ shí*)	6-10g
Jujubae Fructus (*dà zǎo*)	10-20g
Rhei Radix et Rhizoma (*dà huáng*)	5-10g

Because it contains Rhei Radix et Rhizoma (*dà huáng*), Major Bupleurum Decoction (*dà chái hú tāng*) is the bupleurum family formula used for purging. This formula is not only a laxative, but also functions as an antipyretic, has hepatic-protective and biliary-strengthening effects, reduces blood pressure and blood lipid levels, acts as an anticoagulant, antispasmodic, and muscle relaxant, and has anti-inflammatory and anti-allergic properties. Its scope of use is similarly extensive. What can be said about the statements regarding the Major Bupleurum Decoction (*dà chái hú tāng*) presentation?

This formula appears three times in *Discussion of Cold Damage*. In paragraph 103 it is stated that "for those who have a bupleurum presentation, first use

Minor Bupleurum Decoction (*xiǎo chái hú tāng*); if [however] there is incessant vomiting, a gripping pain and tenderness in the upper epigastrium, and a sense of constraint and slight irritability, [the illness has] not yet resolved. Giving Major Bupleurum Decoction (*dà chái hú tāng*) to purge it will bring about the cure." Paragraph 165 says: "For cold damage with feverishness and sweating without resolution [of the condition] with focal distention and hardness in the chest, vomiting, and diarrhea, Major Bupleurum Decoction (*dà chái hú tāng*) masters it." Finally, in paragraph 136, it states: "For those with cold damage for more than 10 days when heat has clumped in the interior and there are repeated bouts of alternating chills and fever, give Major Bupleurum Decoction (*dà chái hú tāng*)." Based on what has been recorded in *Discussion of Cold Damage*, the primary Major Bupleurum Decoction presentation symptoms of fever, vomiting, chest and hypochondriac fullness and discomfort are more severe than those of the Minor Bupleurum Decoction presentation. In addition, there are symptoms of heat clumped in the interior and constraint with a slight feeling of agitation.

Heat clumped in the interior refers to an interior excess heat presentation, which then leads to constipation, abdominal distention, abdominal pain, and heat clumping with circumfluence (熱結旁流 *rè jié páng liú*) where green, watery, and foul-smelling diarrhea form as a result of hard stool retained in the colon. These are accompanied by other heat signs: fever, dry mouth, dry tongue, irritability, and a red tongue with a yellow coating. Depression with a slight feeling of agitation is also a manifestation of heat clumped in the interior.

In accordance with these classic signs from *Discussion of Cold Damage* and modern day uses of this formula, the Major Bupleurum Decoction presentation can be defined as follows:

1. Fever, or alternating fever and chills
2. Chest and hypochondriac fullness and discomfort with upper abdominal pain from contracted muscles, and other localized muscle tightness
3. Constipation with yellow urine, or watery, smelly diarrhea or vomiting, jaundice, or headache
4. A dry tongue with a white or yellow coating and a slippery, rapid pulse

This formula is commonly used to treat cholelithiasis, cholecystitis, and pancreatitis. These diseases all have clinical manifestations of fever or alternating fever and chills, chest and hypochondriac fullness and discomfort, epigastric focal distention with firmness, tightness in the epigastrium, and vomiting. As patients with these diseases often have a Major Bupleurum Decoction presentation, this formula should be considered when treating them. Huang reports using this formula modified with Melia Toosendan Powder (*jīn líng zǐ sǎn*)* to treat acute cholecystitis in 40 patients, of whom 35 were cured. Of the 35 patients that had fevers, all had their temperatures return to normal within 72 hours. In subsequent follow-ups, three patients had relapses.[41] Wang reports using a modification of this formula to treat biliary colic in 324 patients. Chinese herbs alone resolved the pain for 306 of the patients, a combination of Chinese herbs and Western drugs stopped the pain for 13, and five subjects required surgery. Of these 319 patients whose condition resolved either with the use of Chinese herbs alone or in combination with Western medication, the pain stopped after passing gallstones in 112 cases, and continued use of the herbs resulted in the passage of stones in 35 cases.[42]

Zheng reports a study comparing treatments for acute pancreatitis using a combination of Western and Chinese medicine with a group that only received Western medicine. The Chinese medicine group of 300 patients was given a modified combination of Major Bupleurum Decoction (*dà chái hú tāng*) and Virgate Wormwood Decoction (*yīn chén hāo tāng*). The group receiving only Western medicine consisted of 113 subjects. A comparison of surgery and mortality rates as well as the time it took for major symptoms such as abdominal pain, muscle tension, and fever to disappear showed the clinical effectiveness for the group receiving Chinese medicine to be superior in all cases.[43]

In recent years, there have been quite a number of clinical reports concerning the ability of Major Bupleurum Decoction (*dà chái hú tāng*) to treat pathologies of the gallbladder and pancreas. A review of the prescriptions showed that most of them were modified. Bupleuri Radix (*chái hú*), Rhei Radix et Rhizoma (*dà huáng*), Scutellariae Radix (*huáng qín*), Paeoniae Radix (*sháo yào*), and Aurantii Fructus immaturus (*zhǐ shí*) within Major Bupleurum Decoction (*dà chái hú tāng*) are the principal herbs employed, while medicinals such as Artemisiae scopariae Herba (*yīn chén*), Aucklandiae Radix (*mù xiāng*), Coptidis Rhizoma (*huáng lián*), Curcumae Radix (*yù jīn*), Lysimachiae Herba (*jīn qián cǎo*), Natrii Sulfas (*máng xiāo*), Toosendan Fructus (*chuān liàn zǐ*), and Corydalis Rhizoma (*yán hú suǒ*) are frequently used as modifications.

Reports on the use of Major Bupleurum Decoction (*dà chái hú tāng*) to treat high blood pressure, diabetes, and gout mostly come from Japan. Of course, one

---

* Toosendan Fructus (*chuān liàn zǐ*) and Corydalis Rhizoma (*yán hú suǒ*).

must use differential diagnosis when employing this formula. Japanese Kampō doctors emphasize that this formula should be used for those with strong constitutions and physiques, and those with severe chest and hypochondriac fullness and discomfort along with constipation. These are the same signs noted in *Discussion of Cold Damage*.

RHUBARB FORMULA FAMILY

大黃類放 dà huáng lèi fāng

RHEI RADIX ET RHIZOMA (*dà huáng*) is one of the main herbs used in clinical practice. Its use was first recorded in *Divine Husbandman's Classic of the Materia Medica* (神農本草經 *Shén Nóng běn cǎo jīng*). There are 60 varieties of Rhei Radix et Rhizoma (*dà huáng*), most of which are produced in China, particularly in Sichuan, Qinghai, Tibet, Gansu, Yunnan, and Guizhou provinces. Good quality Rhei Radix et Rhizoma (*dà huáng*) is yellowish brown with striations and dots; it is heavy, compact, oily, and fragrant with a bitter and nonastringent taste.

Since ancient times, Rhei Radix et Rhizoma (*dà huáng*) has been used as a purgative and heat-clearing medicinal. In *Discussion of Cold Damage* (傷寒論 *Shāng hán lùn*), there are 16 prescriptions that use Rhei Radix et Rhizoma (*dà huáng*); its range of use is extensive. Clinically, Rhei Radix et Rhizoma (*dà huáng*) is often used for, and effectively treats, patients with acute febrile diseases manifesting with high fever, constipation, coma, delirium, and tetanic collapse (痙厥 *jīng jué*, a traditional term for convulsions and loss of consciousness). Additionally, it treats dysentery with blood and pus in the stool, repeated bouts of tenesmus, headache with red eyes, throat, and tooth pain, mouth and tongue ulcers, or irritability and irascibility. Furthermore, it treats vomiting of blood and nosebleeds, fever with jaundice, scanty reddish urine, amenorrhea, postpartum, prolonged lochia, sores and toxic swellings, and wounds from traumatic injuries. All of these kinds of symptoms, which are described by Chinese medicine as 'accumulated heat' (積熱 *jī rè*), 'excessive fire' (實火 *shí huǒ*), and 'heat toxins' (熱毒 *rè dú*), can be treated with Radix et Rhizoma (*dà huáng*).

'Accumulated heat' refers to toxins from waste products that have built up in the intestinal tract and entered the blood. At the same time, these harmful substances cannot be cleared from inside the body, thus harming the organism further. This consequently produces systemic symptoms such as high fever with impaired consciousness, headaches, and bleeding. Using Rhei Radix et Rhizoma (*dà huáng*) for these symptoms flushes out the stomach and intestines, clears out the old to make room for the new, and acts quickly to improve the patient's symptoms.

'Fire excess' manifests in signs of internal fire with such symptoms as headache with red eyes, mouth and tongue sores, vomiting of blood and nosebleeds; these are frequently accompanied by signs of internal excess like constipation, abdominal pain, and an excessive pulse. In these circumstances, Rhei Radix et Rhizoma (*dà huáng*) is able to purge and drain out the excessive fire from below, with the result that "firewood is removed from under the cauldron."

'Heat toxin' refers to patients with such infectious disorders as sores and toxic swellings, or red and swollen throats. In addition to its purgative function, Rhei Radix et Rhizoma (*dà huáng*) has excellent antibacterial properties that, together with its purgative action, enable it to both clear heat and resolve toxicity.

Because it also moves blood and transforms stasis, Rhei Radix et Rhizoma (*dà huáng*) is especially effective for treating those with blood stasis accompanied by abdominal pain and constipation. The blood in this presentation tends to be thick, sticky, and dark purple in color, and these types of patients are often both irritable and restless.

Due to the quick efficacy of Rhei Radix et Rhizoma's (*dà huáng*), it is primarily used in treating serious acute febrile diseases such as acute abdominal problems. The ancients metaphorically referred to Rhei Radix et Rhizoma (*dà huáng*) as the general who has the power to knock down doors and suppress turmoil. Even though infectious diseases are now less prevalent, Rhei Radix et Rhizoma (*dà huáng*) has not lost its important place in the therapeutic armamentarium. On the contrary, its scope of clinical use continues to expand. In November 1990, the Rhubarb Studies Conference took place in Shanghai for the first time in China. According to the proceedings, Rhei Radix et Rhizoma (*dà huáng*) was at that time being used to treat 25 different types of illness, including cardiac and cerebrovascular disease, hyperlipidemina, uremia, acute pancreatitis, and digestive tract bleeding. Pharmacological research provides evidence that Rhei Radix et Rhizoma (*dà huáng*) improves immunity, lowers blood lipid levels, and is hemostatic, antipyretic, antibacterial, and purgative.

Rhei Radix et Rhizoma (*dà huáng*), along with its associated family of formulas, is receiving an increasing amount of serious attention in the modern world and is recorded in the materia medica of 19 different countries. Internationally, many countries are researching Rhei Radix et Rhizoma (*dà huáng*), and the research and development of uses for Rhei Radix et Rhizoma (*dà huáng*) is an urgent task for those in the Chinese medicine field. How to properly use this herb is a challenge that concerns all practitioners as the actions of Rhei Radix et Rhizoma (*dà huáng*) are harsh. Used inappropriately, it will cause side effects. The Ming-dynasty physician Zhang Jing-Yue had this admonition: "When considering the amount to use, accurately assess the [balance of] excess and deficiency within the patient. If used to treat a false excess, it is like serving poisoned wine."

Generally speaking, when using Rhei Radix et Rhizoma (*dà huáng*) to treat an acute febrile disease, attention must be paid to the presence of the rhubarb presentation. When using Rhei Radix et Rhizoma (*dà huáng*) for a complicated chronic illness, the deficiency and excess of the patient's constitution must be carefully differentiated.

Rhubarb Presentation (大黄證 *dà huáng zhèng*)

The rhubarb presentation falls within the categories of interior excess and interior heat. Interior excess manifests with symptoms of constipation along with abdominal pain and bloating, an aversion to pressure on the abdomen as felt by the patient, and an increased sense of resistance as felt by the practitioner. These symptoms indicate a state of fullness and excess in the abdomen. Interior heat refers to signs of fever, irritability, and a red tongue with a dry mouth; these are manifestations of a hyperactive metabolism. Similarly, a red complexion, dark red lips, a red tongue with a yellow coating, thick and sticky sputum and fluids, and a tendency toward constipation are all manifestations of heat, and are tendencies of the rhubarb constitution.

Interior excess and interior heat are important concepts in Chinese medicine for making generalizations about the pathologic state of an organism. They are the exact opposite of the aforementioned conditions of exterior deficiency and exterior excess, which are respectively treated by cinnamon twig and ephedra family formulas. Note the following distinguishing qualities of the rhubarb presentation:

1. Abdominal fullness and pain with resistance when pressed, or a feeling of resistance in the abdominal wall, along with constipation
2. Restless spirit, irritability, easily excited, and fever with sweating
3. Red, tough, firm tongue body with a dry, scorched yellow coating (known as the 'rhubarb tongue')

Generally, in acute illness, as long as the rhubarb presentation is seen, one can consider using a Rhei Radix et Rhizoma (*dà huáng*) family formula. The most distinctive feature of this presentation is the tongue. As opposed to those tongues that are pale red or pale, white, puffy, and tender, the tongue body here is red, tough, and firm. A scorched yellow coating means that there is black within the yellow of the coating, making the tongue appear as though it were burnt. This type of coating is usually found on a tongue body that is dried out and lacks moisture, which I call the 'rhubarb tongue.'

The renowned Ming-dynasty doctor Wu You-Xing was an expert on using Rhei Radix et Rhizoma (*dà huáng*) to treat febrile disease. In his *Discussion of Warm Epidemics* (溫疫論 *Wēn yì lùn*), Wu recorded more than 20 distinctive characteristics of the Rhei Radix et Rhizoma (*dà huáng*) tongue. Within his book are many clinical examples of using Rhei Radix et Rhizoma (*dà huáng*) based on just seeing the tongue.

The older generation of doctors with whom I used to study would often repeatedly examine the nature of the patient's tongue and coating whenever considering the use of a Rhei Radix et Rhizoma (*dà huáng*) formula. The importance they placed on the rhubarb tongue in diagnosis was evident. It should be noted, however, that while many patients who suffer from chronic illness do not have the classic rhubarb tongue, their tongues still tend to have a relatively thick yellow coating and the body of the tongues tends to be red and tough.

The abdominal pain, restlessness, easy excitability, and fever with sweating of the rhubarb presentation may seem to be similar to the cinnamon twig presentation. However, whereas with the cinnamon twig presentation there is an aversion to wind with sweating and abdominal pain that feels better with pressure, in the rhubarb presentation there is fever with a preference for cold and abdominal pain that worsens with pressure. Furthermore, there is a clear difference between the rhubarb tongue, which is red and firm with a dry, burnt yellow coating, and the cinnamon twig tongue, which is moist with a thin, white coating.

Rhubarb Constitution (大黃體質 *dà huáng tǐ zhì*)

The rhubarb constitution is the body type that frequently manifests with presentations matching those of rhubarb family formulas. Manifestations of the rhubarb presentation are not as obvious in chronic illnesses as they are in acute ones, so the use of Rhei Radix et Rhizoma (*dà huáng*) in such cases is based primarily on whether the patient has a rhubarb constitution.

- *External appearance.* A robust physique with strong and firm musculature, a reddish, oily complexion or one that is greasy and dirty looking, thick, darkened red lips, and a tongue with a thick, dry coating
- *Commonly expressed symptoms.* Ordinarily dreads heat and favors coolness, excessive appetite, tendency toward dizziness or vertigo and constipation, only sweats lightly or unevenly, chest stuffiness, a dry mouth with thick and sticky fluids (including sputum and saliva), hyperlipidemia, hypertension, and abdominal tenderness or resistance to pressure

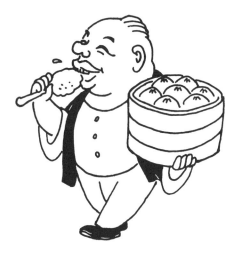

The rhubarb constitution is one of heat and fire. The 'heat' spoken of here primarily manifests as symptoms such as a severe aversion to heat with preference for coolness, a vigorous appetite, dry mouth with a bitter taste, thick and sticky sputum and fluids, as well as constipation. 'Fire' here refers to symptoms such as readily feeling lightheaded and dizzy, frequent headaches, or, in severe cases, a stroke affecting the ability to speak.

The genesis of the rhubarb constitution within a patient is, apart from hereditary factors, primarily due to a long-term inappropriate diet with overconsumption of meats, fats, and sweets and an accompanying lack of physical exercise. In recent years, the number of patients with the rhubarb constitution in China has been increasing in parallel with changes in dietary habits.

4.1 **Major Order the Qi Decoction** (大承氣湯 *dà chéng qì tāng*)

SOURCE: *Discussion of Cold Damage*

Rhei Radix et Rhizoma (*dà huáng*) 5-12g

Magnoliae officinalis Cortex (*hòu pò*) 6-15g

Aurantii Fructus immaturus (*zhǐ shí*) 6-15g

Natrii Sulfas (*máng xiāo*) 6-10g

Just like Cinnamon Twig Decoction (*guì zhī tāng*) of the cinnamon twig formula family and Minor Bupleurum Decoction (*xiǎo chái hú tāng*) of the bupleurum formula family, Major Order the Qi Decoction (*dà chéng qì tāng*) is the representative formula within the rhubarb formula family. It is one of the important traditional prescriptions used to treat acute life-threatening illnesses. Over the past few thousand years, it is unknown how many lives it has saved from an illness of a serious life-threatening nature. This is the extraordinarily effective formula that renowned doctors often prescribed during dangerous junctures of various acute illnesses with high fever, loss of consciousness, cold extremities, abdominal fullness, and pain with extreme agitation, or when the body is burning up with fever and the tongue has a scorched black coating with spiky prickles. With it, all manner of dangerous symptoms can be cured. These types of cases are easily found within old Chinese medicine books and in the case studies of famous doctors. I do not know how many times I have heard old Chinese doctors tell stories about how Rhei Radix et Rhizoma (*dà huáng*) was used to save patients' lives!

While appreciating the miraculous efficacy of Major Order the Qi Decoction (*dà chéng qì tāng*), I admire even more the thinking of the ancients. In the development of many diseases they identified a common pathological condition, namely, the internal excess heat presentation (裡實熱證 *lǐ shí rè zhèng*). In *Discussion of Cold Damage*, what is called 'Stomach excess' (胃家實 *wèi jiā shí*) or 'dried stool in the Stomach' (胃中有燥屎 *wèi zhōng yǒu zào shǐ*) is what later generations have come to call '*yáng míng* organ excess' (陽明腑實 *yáng míng fǔ shí*). This condition manifests with abdominal fullness and pain, constipation, fever with sweating, and a red tongue with a scorched yellow coating. No matter what type of illness, and regardless of its pathogenesis, as long as it manifests with an interior excess heat presentation, the treatment is basically the same. Fever with wheezing from acute pneumonia, abdominal pain from acute pancreatitis, vomiting, irritability and madness due to mental illness, tenesmus from bacterial dysentery, and abdominal fullness with reduced urine from infectious hemorrhagic fevers can all be treated with Major Order the Qi Decoction (*dà chéng qì tāng*). This is precisely what Chinese doctors mean when they say, "The same treatment can be effective for different illnesses" (異病同治 *yì bìng tóng zhì*).

Natrii Sulfas (*máng xiāo*) in Major Order the Qi Decoction (*dà chéng qì tāng*) is the mineral mirabilitum (also known as Glauber's salt) in refined crystalline form. As its ions are not easily assimilated by the mucosa of the large intestine, after ingestion, they remain in the gut, resulting in a hyperosmotic solution, which increases the amount of fluid in the large intestine and stimulates peristalsis. Chinese doctors refer to this function as 'softening hardness and moistening dryness' (軟堅潤燥 *ruǎn jiān rùn zào*).

Magnoliae officinalis Cortex (*hòu pò*) and Aurantii Fructus immaturus (*zhǐ shí*), in this formula, are the herbs traditionally used to treat abdominal distention, and pharmacological research indicates that both of these medicinals stimulate the intestines. Additionally, Aurantii Fructus immaturus (*zhǐ shí*) has been shown to act as a cardiotonic.

Evidence from pharmacological research into Major Order the Qi Decoction (*dà chéng qì tāng*) indicates that this formula markedly stimulates peristalsis; it not only significantly increases motility of the large intestine in laboratory animals, but also increases the volume of contents within the intestinal tract, thus giving it a significant laxative effect. Additionally, it functions to improve the blood circulation of intestinal tissue in cases of histamine-induced circulatory obstruction, has a significant ability to strengthen resistance to pathological microorganisms, and is anti-inflammatory, biliary regulating, antipyretic, and regulates digestive enzymes.

In *Discussion of Cold Damage* and *Essentials from the Golden Cabinet* (金匱要略 *Jīn guì yào lüè*), there are 29 lines of text discussing the ability of Major Order the Qi Decoction (*dà chéng qì tāng*) to treat drizzly sweating of the palms and soles, tidal fever with delirium, wheezing with an inability to lay flat, unclear eyes and pupils that do not work together, abdominal fullness with pain, dry mouth and throat, clear, watery diarrhea, and a pulse that is rapid and slippery. Although the illnesses treated vary greatly from one another, analysis of the signs and symptoms in the original texts shows they all possess signs of fullness, fever, or excess, and that all of the pulses associated with this formula are sinking, excessive, or slippery. The 'fullness' mentioned here indicates the presence of a type of abdominal fullness and distention that ancient people described as "a hard and swollen belly that seems to be made of roof tiles." What is referred to in the texts as 'high fever' indicates a severe fever with agitation to the point that the patient flails their arms and legs, has an aversion to heat, and prefers to be kept cool. 'Excess' simply indicates constipation, with the area around the navel feeling hard, like a smooth stone. The 'sinking pulse' indicates that the illness is in the interior, the 'excessive pulse' means the illness is of an excess type, and the 'slippery pulse' means that there is heat in the interior. Specific details of the Major Order the Qi Decoction (dà chéng qì tāng) presentation are as follows:

1. Intense abdominal pain and distention with fullness and hardness, an aversion to having one's abdomen pressed, and constipation or sticky, thin stools that contain blood and pus
2. Persistent or tidal fever with sweating, and dry tongue and lips
3. Irritability, delirium, and disturbances in consciousness
4. A forceful, excessive pulse, and a dry, scorched yellow tongue coating with red prickles

Compared to the rhubarb presentation, the abdominal distention and pain of the Major Order the Qi Decoction presentation is more severe. These patients often have particularly malodorous flatulence, palpable abdominal fullness and hardness, or an abdomen that feels as though one were pressing on a rubbery pillow. While palpating, the patients often complain that their abdomens feel uncomfortably bloated and painful. The other symptoms of tidal fever—copious sweating, irritability, delirious speech, and abnormal changes in consciousness—are clues to the seriousness of the situation.

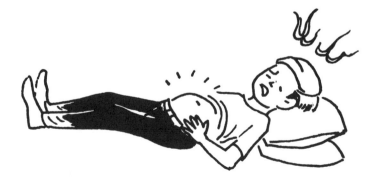

From a glance at modern day clinical reports, the Major Order the Qi Decoction presentation is often seen in the following acute, life-threatening illnesses:

1. Acute Abdomen

- *Acute intestinal obstruction*. The four major distinguishing symptoms—pain, distention, vomiting, and obstruction—are quite similar to the Major Order the Qi Decoction presentation. There is a report of using a modified version of Major Order the Qi Decoction (*dà chéng qì tāng*) where the Aurantii Fructus immaturus (*zhǐ shí*) was replaced with Aurantii Fructus (*zhǐ ké*), and Persicae Semen (*táo rén*), Paeoniae Radix rubra (*chì sháo*), and Raphani Semen (*lái fú zǐ*) were added to treat intestinal obstruction due to adhesions in 1,234 patients. Of these, 828 were successfully treated, and among these, 579 had results after taking only one to four packets of herbs, and, in most of these cases, the obstruction was gone within 24 to 48 hours.[1] It is generally thought that the use of Major Order the Qi Decoction (*dà chéng qì tāng*) is excellent for treating intestinal obstruction from adhesions, roundworms, intestinal calculus, lack of peristaltic force, and tuberculosis of the pelvic cavity.

- *Acute pancreatitis*. Rhei Radix et Rhizoma (*dà huáng*) inhibits digestive enzymes, including pancreatic enzymes, and its strong purgative/laxative function is helpful in flushing out any pancreatic enzymes that have already been activated. Additionally, eliminating retained stool from the intestines helps to reduce the load on the pancreas. There is a report of Rhei Radix et Rhizoma (*dà huáng*) with Natrii Sulfas siccatus (*xuán míng fěn*), a highly refined form of Natrii Sulfas (*máng xiāo*), taken in a liquid form to treat 100 subjects with acute pancreatitis. All of the patients recovered, with symptoms being alleviated in an average of two days. Urinary levels of amylase returned to normal within an average of three days, and fevers were reduced in an average of 3.5 days.[2] For 117 patients where Major Order the Qi Decoction (*dà chéng qì tāng*) was the primary treatment, almost all of them recovered.[3] Clinically, abdominal pain that diminishes with the passing of stool reflects the old Chinese maxim, "When blocked, there is pain, [and] when unblocked, there is no pain" (不通則痛, 通則不痛, *bù tōng zé tòng, tōng zé bù tòng*).

- *Acute appendicitis*. Major Order the Qi Decoction (*dà chéng qì tāng*) can be used alone, or in combination with Rhubarb and Moutan Decoction (*dà huáng mǔ dān tāng*), to treat acute appendicitis. If there is paralytic ileus or acute appendicitis with a perforated appendix, or when there is general peritonitis accompanying paralytic ileus, a modified formulation of Major Order the Qi Decoction (*dà chéng qì tāng*) can be used.

- *Cholecystitis and cholelithiasis*. This formula is often combined with Minor Bupleurum Decoction *(xiǎo chái hú tāng)* or Virgate Wormwood Decoction *(yīn chén hāo tāng)*. There is a report of using three of the Order the Qi Decoctions—Major Order the Qi Decoction *(dà chéng qì tāng)*, Minor Order the Qi Decoction *(xiǎo chéng qì tāng)*, and Regulate the Stomach and Order the Qi Decoction *(tiáo wèi chéng qì tāng)*—to treat 226 patients with biliary infections, with the primary symptoms being pain, vomiting, fever, and jaundice. All of the patients experienced hypochondria and abdominal fullness and pain, 59.7 percent had nausea and vomiting, 53.5 percent had a fever of at least 100.4°F (38°C), 27.9 percent had jaundice, and 27.9 percent had constipation. Fifty-three of the patients were treated with Major Order the Qi Decoction *(dà chéng qì tāng)*, 11 were treated with Minor Order the Qi Decoction *(xiǎo chéng qì tāng)*, and 162 patients were treated with Regulate the Stomach and Order the Qi Decoction *(tiáo wèi chéng qì tāng)*; 93.7 percent of the patients had their hypochondriac, abdominal fullness and pain alleviated within 72 hours, 48.8 percent had their fever resolve, 57.1 percent had their jaundice recede, and 76.2 percent had their constipation relieved. Of the patients in this study, all were either cured or improved; there were no fatalities.[4]

- *Other*. Because this formula increases intestinal peristalsis, it effectively treats paralytic ileus due to a plethora of origins, especially paralysis resulting from abdominal surgery. There is a report of applying a compounded formulation of Major Order the Qi Decoction *(dà chéng qì tāng)* within 20 to 24 hours after abdominal surgery as a retention enema for patients. For the most part, passage of gas and stool and intestinal peristaltic movement returned to normal within 12 to 24 hours.[5]

  There is another report of using a modification of Major Order the Qi Decoction *(dà chéng qì tāng)* infused into the rectum to treat 55 patients with abdominal distention after abdominal surgery. Among these patients, 24 had generalized distention, while 31 had severe distention. Within 10 hours, abdominal distention had completely disappeared in 45 patients; in another nine patients, it took 10 to 24 hours for the distention to disappear; and in the one remaining patient, it took one to two days.[6]

2. Acute Infectious Disease

- *Wide variety*. This formula effectively treats a wide variety of acute infectious diseases as long as they have the Major Order the Qi Decoction presentation. These include epidemic hemorrhagic fevers, influenza, acute pneumonia, epidemic encephalitis B, acute dysentery, symptomatic hepatitis, typhoid, conjunctivitis, keratitis, rhinitis, and pyogenic tonsillitis.

3. ACUTE ILLNESS

- *Shock.* It is reported that this formula, combined with heat-clearing, toxicity-resolving herbs, treats septic shock.[7] A modification of this formula was used to treat 63 cases of septic shock due to bile duct/gallbladder disease; among these patients, 61 recovered from shock within three days.[8] With this kind of shock, despite a hidden pulse and cold extremities, there will be a stiff and painful abdomen, constipation, and the tongue will have either a rough and yellow, or burnt and black coating.

- *Crush syndrome.* This disease is frequently accompanied by a stiff painful abdomen, constipation and urinary retention, and a dry, burnt coating on the tongue. There is a report of using this formula with the addition of blood-invigorating herbs, which, when taken orally, quickly reduced blood potassium levels and nitrogen levels in the urine.[9] This formula also works when it is prescribed as a retention enema.[10]

- *Stroke.* There is a report of using a modification of Major Order the Qi Decoction (*dà chéng qì tāng*) to treat 72 patients who had gone four days without a bowel movement after suffering a stroke. Among these patients, 11 had cerebral hemorrhages and 61 had cerebral thromboses. In these types of cases, this formula is able to alleviate such symptoms and ease the patient's condition. Indeed, it was effective in treating their symptoms of constipation, abdominal fullness and distention, and nausea with vomiting. Additionally, of the 18 patients who were comatose, 10 responded.[11]

- *Other.* Furthermore, there are reports of using this formula with the additions of Polygoni multiflori Radix (*hé shǒu wū*), Gentianae Radix (*lóng dǎn cǎo*), and Polygonati Rhizoma (*huáng jīng*) to treat Cushing's syndrome;[12, 13, 14] combined with Peony and Licorice Decoction (*sháo yào gān cǎo tāng*) to treat lead poisoning;[15] and with the additions of Arnebiae Radix/Lithospermi Radix (*zǐ cǎo*), Salviae miltiorrhizae Radix (*dān shēn*), and Glycyrrhizae Radix (*gān cǎo*) to treat allergic purpura with abdominal pain.[16] In practice, for these presentations, there are usually also signs of abdominal pain that is aggravated by pressure, a yellow, greasy tongue coating, and a strong, excessive pulse.

  Major Order the Qi Decoction (*dà chéng qì tāng*) is a strong purgative. When using this formula, one should be attentive to ensure an accurate differential diagnosis. The herbs used must fit the presentation. Misdiagnosis, overuse, or other misuse of this formula is unacceptable. Extra caution is required, especially for the elderly, pregnant women, children, and those with a weak constitution. Proper diagnosis is vitally important; as long as a patient presents with the rhubarb constitution or presentation, Rhei Radix et Rhizoma (*dà huáng*) formulas can be confidently prescribed. There are even reports where up to 100 packets of Major Order the Qi Decoction (*dà chéng qì tāng*) were prescribed, not only without any side effects, but with good results.[17]

MODIFICATIONS

Two modifications, Minor Order the Qi Decoction (*xiǎo chéng qì tāng*) and Regulate the Stomach and Order the Qi Decoction (*tiáo wèi chéng qì tāng*), are similar to Major Order the Qi Decoction (*dà chéng qì tāng*). However, their purgative effect is not as pronounced. Two other modifications, Increase the Fluids and Order the Qi Decoction (*zēng yè chéng qì tāng*) and Jade Candle Powder (*yù zhú sǎn*), are also described.

- Minor Order the Qi Decoction (*xiǎo chéng qì tāng*) comes from *Discussion of Cold Damage*; it is composed of Rhei Radix et Rhizoma (*dà huáng*) 6-12g, Magnoliae officinalis Cortex (*hòu pò*) 5-10g, and Aurantii Fructus immaturus (*zhǐ shí*) 6-12g. This is Major Order the Qi Decoction (*dà chéng qì tāng*) where Natrii Sulfas (*máng xiāo*) and Glycyrrhizae Radix (*gān cǎo*) were omitted and the dosages of Magnoliae officinalis Cortex (*hòu pò*) and Aurantii Fructus immaturus (*zhǐ shí*) were reduced. This formula has a weaker purging action than Major Order the Qi Decoction (*dà chéng qì tāng*). It is primarily used for rhubarb presentations marked by abdominal fullness and distention.

- Regulate the Stomach and Order the Qi Decoction (*tiáo wèi chéng qì tāng*) is derived from *Discussion of Cold Damage*; it is made up of Rhei Radix et Rhizoma (*dà huáng*) 6-12g, Glycyrrhizae Radix (*gān cǎo*) 3-6g, and Natrii Sulfas (*máng xiāo*) 6-12g. This formula is appropriate for rhubarb presentations where there is a significantly dry, thick, and yellow tongue coating accompanied by constipation, or where there is a rhubarb presentation with significant fever, sweating, and dry stools that come out in small, chestnut-sized balls. Contributing factors to the formation of this formula's presentation are persistent fever and copious sweating leading to dehydration or long-term illness where patients are bedridden, leading to constipation with dry stool. Other than using the interview to confirm this formula's presentation, the key diagnostic points are a dry tongue coating and a firm and full abdomen upon palpation, particularly when accumulation of fecal matter can be palpated around the navel. In practice, this formula's presentation is usually seen in illnesses that manifest with abdominal pain and constipation, such as intestinal obstruction.

• Increase the Fluids and Order the Qi Decoction (*zēng yè chéng qì tāng*) is a modification of Regulate the Stomach and Order the Qi Decoction (*tiáo wèi chéng qì tāng*) where Glycyrrhizae Radix (*gān cǎo*) is removed and Scrophulariae Radix (*xuán shēn*), Rehmanniae Radix (*shēng dì huáng*), and Ophiopogonis Radix (*mài mén dōng*) are added. It can be used to treat those who display the original formula presentation, but who have a red tongue with fever and sweating. Also, it can be used for those patients with chronic illness or whose constitution is relatively weak, but still have the rhubarb presentation.

• Regulate the Stomach and Order the Qi Decoction (*tiáo wèi chéng qì tāng*) can be combined with Four-Substance Decoction (*sì wù tāng*) to make Jade Candle Powder (*yù zhú sǎn*); this also treats women with amenorrhea or those who are thin and suffer from bulimia.

4.2 Peach Pit Decoction to Order the Qi

(桃核承氣湯 *táo hé chéng qì tāng*)

SOURCE: *Discussion of Cold Damage*

Persicae Semen (*táo rén*)..10-25g
Rhei Radix et Rhizoma (*dà huáng*)...................................6-12g
Cinnamomi Ramulus (*guì zhī*)...6
Glycyrrhizae Radix (*gān cǎo*)..3-6
Natrii Sulfas (*máng xiāo*)..6-10g

Peach Pit Decoction to Order the Qi (*táo hé chéng qì tāng*) is the rhubarb formula family prescription for invigorating the blood and transforming stasis, functioning both to purge downward and dispel stasis. From a look at its constituent herbs, it can be seen that Peach Pit Decoction to Order the Qi (*táo hé chéng qì tāng*) is Regulate the Stomach and Order the Qi Decoction (*tiáo wèi chéng qì tāng*) with the addition of Persicae Semen (*táo rén*) and Cinnamomi Ramulus (*guì zhī*). The *Divine Husbandman's Classic of the Materia Medica* says that Persicae Semen (*táo rén*) "masters blood stasis." Pharmacological experimentation provides evidence that Persicae Semen (*táo rén*) both functions as an anticoagulant and prevents the formation of thrombi *in vitro*. Infusing this herb into laboratory mice significantly extends the length of time they bleed before clotting. It also has a relatively strong effect in increasing the volume of blood moving through the femoral artery of dogs. Cinnamomi Ramulus (*guì zhī*) is the herb traditionally used to open the yang and invigorate the blood. Pharmacological research indicates Cinnamomi Ramulus (*guì zhī*), Persicae Semen (*táo rén*), and Rhei Radix et Rhizoma (*dà huáng*) all have a relatively strong inhibitory action on the concentration of platelets in collagen tissue and the adrenal glands.

Peach Pit Decoction to Order the Qi (*táo hé chéng qì tāng*) is the *Discussion of Cold Damage* formula Zhang Zhong-Jing used to treat presentations of "heat clumping in the Bladder, where the patients are manic-like and there is bleeding with defecation" and "acute clumping in the lower abdomen." In this context, the word 'Bladder' is a synonym for the pelvis. 'Clumped heat' (熱結 *rè jié*) is a pattern of interior excess heat. The 'manic-like' behavior of these patients refers to a condition of agitation with an inability to calm down due to overexcitement of the nervous system, delirium, and other similar states of emotional disorder.

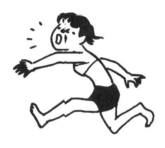 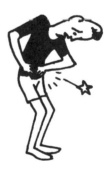

These are the primary signs in presentations of blood stasis and internal heat. When this condition is severe, there are psycho-emotional abnormalities. 'Urgent clumping in the lower abdomen' (少腹急結 *shào fù jí jié*) refers to the lower abdomen being rigid and painful with pain that is aggravated by pressure. The Japanese practitioner Higuchi Kazuko believes that urgent clumping in the lower abdomen refers to severe pain in the lower left portion of the abdomen that, when pressed, causes the patient to flex the left hip in pain. Sometimes when palpating deeply, one can come into contact with a soft, rope-like structure. Some patients will have significant tenderness in the left groin area.[18] In line with the characteristic signs of blood stasis, the blood seen in bleeding with defecation is purplish black in color and readily congeals. Guidelines for the use of Peach Pit Decoction to Order the Qi (*táo hé chéng qì tāng*) are as follows:

1. A rhubarb presentation
2. Rigidity and pain in the lower abdomen that is aggravated by pressure
3. Bleeding of purplish black blood that readily clots and coagulates
4. Irritability with an inability to calm down, as in mania
5. Dark red or purple tongue body, the top of the tongue is dry, dark red lips, and a reddish complexion

The Peach Pit Decoction to Order the Qi presentation is often seen in cases of mental illness, obstetrical and gynecological disease, vascular disease, acute infections, acute abdomens, urinary disorders, and traumatic injuries.

• Schizophrenic patients often present with mania. Zhao reports using this formula to treat 26 patients with schizophrenia, 23 of whom experienced some favorable effect from the treatment. He believes that this formula is effective for mania, schizophrenia, reactive psychosis, and some forms of hysteria with overexcited gesticulation.[19] Niu used this formula with the addition of Carthami Flos (*hóng huā*), Haematitum (*dài zhě shí*), Citri reticulatae viride Pericarpium (*qīng pí*), Chuanxiong Rhizoma (*chuān xiōng*), and Curcumae Radix (*yù jīn*) as the primary treatment to supplement a low dose of a psychoactive pharmaceutical in treating 40 women with schizophrenia. Of these patients, 10 recovered and six had obvious improvement. Those who had fallen ill within the past two years experienced better results from the treatment, while those with chronic illness of five years or more experienced less success with the treatment.[20] Most patients for whom the treatment was effective had signs of blood stasis such as a dark and purple tongue or a rough pulse.

• The Japanese practitioner Arichi Shigeshi used this formula to treat 25 patients who had arteriosclerosis and high blood pressure where the main symptom was acute clumping in the lower abdomen and where the patients tended to be robust or overweight with additional symptoms of constipation, headaches, frozen shoulder, or chills. After using the formula for 12 weeks, significant improvement in the symptoms could be seen in nine patients, some improvement in 11, and in five there was no change.[21]

• There are reports of this formula being effective in treating dysmenorrhea, amenorrhea, spotting, manic behavior during the period, pelvic inflammatory disease, bleeding after miscarriage, lochiorrhea, retention of the placenta, as well as postpartum vaginal bleeding and swelling, abdominal pain during pregnancy, and ectopic pregnancy. These patients often present with purple black menstrual blood with clots and lower abdominal pain that is aggravated by pressure, as well as symptoms such as constipation, a dark tongue, a reddish complexion, and mood swings.

- The presentation for this formula can also be seen in cases of orthopedic and urinary diseases where the primary manifestations are abdominal pain and fullness. There is a report of using this formula with modified amounts of Rhei Radix et Rhizoma (dà huáng) and Natrii Sulfas siccatus (xuán míng fěn) as an enema to treat 20 cases of thoracic-lumbar vertebra fracture with accompanying ileus. Patients were able to defecate after using the herbs and reported a sense of comfort and relief throughout the body, as the abdominal pain disappeared and their oral intake increased.[22] Chen reports using this formula to treat 11 cases of colic from stones in the urinary system. Taking two to three packets of herbs stopped the pain.[23]

- This formula's presentation should be compared and contrasted with that of Cinnamon Twig and Poria Pill (guì zhī fú líng wán) and Drive Out Stasis from the Mansion of Blood Decoction (xuè fǔ zhú yū tāng). All three of these formulas can treat blood stasis with abdominal pain. However, with respect to the location of the pain, the chest and hypochondria are painful in the Drive Out Stasis from the Mansion of Blood Decoction presentation, while in the presentations for Cinnamon Twig and Poria Pill and this formula, the pain is in the lower abdomen. In addition, the presentation here also includes clear signs from the rhubarb presentation, with more severe mental-emotional conditions and constipation.

4.3 Rhubarb and Ground Beetle Pill
(大黃蟅蟲丸 dà huáng zhè chóng wán)

SOURCE: *Essentials from the Golden Cabinet*

Rhei Radix et Rhizoma (dà huáng) 300g

Eupolyphaga/Stelophaga (tǔ biē chóng) 30g

Persicae Semen (táo rén) 60g

Toxicodendri Resina (gān qī) 30g

Holotrichia (qí cáo) 60g

Hirudo (shuǐ zhì) 60g

Tabanus (méng chóng) 60g

Scutellariae Radix (*huáng qín*) 60g
Armeniacae Semen (*xìng rén*) 60g
Rehmanniae Radix (*shēng dì huáng*) 300g
Paeoniae Radix (*sháo yào*) 120g
Glycyrrhizae Radix (*gān cǎo*) 90g

I have never used this formula in decoction form, but always prescribe it as a patent, which is readily available in pharmacies in China.

Rhubarb and Ground Beetle Pill (*dà huáng zhè chóng wán*) is a gentle blood-invigorating, stasis-transforming prescription. *Essentials from the Golden Cabinet* states: "Long-term gazing damages the blood; long-term lying down damages the qi; long-term sitting damages the flesh; long-term standing damages the bones; long-term walking damages the sinews. These are the damages that [lead to] the five consumptions. Rhubarb and Ground Beetle Pill (*dà huáng zhè chóng wán*) masters them by reviving the middle and tonifying deficiency." In China, herb stores carry this formula for sale in prepared form.

Combining Rhei Radix et Rhizoma (*dà huáng*) with insects is the distinctive characteristic of this formula. Eupolyphaga/Stelophaga (*zhè chóng*), also known as 'earth turtle bug' (土鳖蟲 *tǔ biē chóng*), is an earthbound insect with a flat, oval-shaped body that likes to live under walls in rural areas. They are now primarily bred for medicinal use. It functions to invigorate the blood, transform stasis, dispel hardness, and heal trauma. Clinically, it is used for blood stasis congealing into pain, amenorrhea from blood stasis, swellings from blood stasis, back pain, trauma, broken bones and fainting from traumatic injury. In practice, it is common to use 1-2g daily in pill or powder form. If it is cooked as a decoction, each dose should be 6-10g. This medicinal has significant efficacy and is widely used with good effect as a single herb in many folk remedies. For example, Eupolyphaga/Stelophaga (*zhè chóng*) is slowly baked until it turns yellow and then is ground into a powder, with the equivalent of three insects taken once in the evening with either boiled water or sorghum wine. It is effective for both external trauma and chronic back pain. A folk remedy for sciatica that is still used involves pounding 20-30 fresh insects into a white liquid.

There are many reports of using Eupolyphaga/Stelophaga (*zhè chóng*) as the main herb to treat a variety of conditions. When it is combined with Notoginseng Radix (*sān qī*), Hominis Placenta (*zǐ hé chē*), Gigeriae galli Endothelium corneum (*jī nèi jīn*), and Curcumae Radix (*yù jīn*), it treats chronic active hepatitis or cirrhosis. When it is combined with Moschus (*shè xiāng*), Crotonis Semen (*bā dòu*), Olibanum (*rǔ xiāng*), Daemonoropis Resina (*xuè jié*), and Pyritum (*zì rán tōng*), it treats post-traumatic coma. When it is combined with Scorpio (*quán xiē*), Angelicae sinensis Radix (*dāng guī*), Ginseng Radix (*rén shēn*), Strychni Semen (*mǎ qián zǐ*), Chuanxiong Rhizoma (*chuān xiōng*), Hominis Placenta (*zǐ hé chē*), and Lycii Fructus (*gǒu qǐ zǐ*), it treats postconcussion syndrome. The blood-invigorating and stasis-transforming properties of Eupolyphaga/Stelophaga (*zhè chóng*) are relatively mild. It can be used when treating a blood stasis presentation in those with a weak and deficient constitution without causing side effects, and thus the scope of its clinical use is quite expansive.

Hirudo (*shuǐ zhì*), also known as 'water horse locust' (水馬蝗 *shūi mǎ huáng*), is found in warm marshes and rice paddies throughout China. It has a mouth that acts like a sucker, and these creatures frequently attach themselves to people's skin and feed on their blood. The stasis-transforming ability of this medicinal is extremely strong. It is used to treat blood stasis and abdominal pain or blood stasis with fever in patients with a relatively robust and excess constitution, a face that is entirely purple or reddish black, a dark red tongue, and blood with a high degree of viscosity. Generally speaking, this medicinal is used in powdered form, with daily dosages of 1-3g. There are reports of Hirudo (*shuǐ zhì*) powder being used effectively to treat rheumatic heart disease, coronary heart disease, and postsplenectomy thrombocytosis.

The Tabanus (*méng chóng*) within this formula is also an insect, and its blood-invigorating function is also quite strong. It is not commonly used in modern clinical practice and can be omitted from this formula.

Pharmacological experimentation has shown that this formula has the ability to activate the fibrinolytic system and control the formation of thrombi. It also has a mild effect in preventing the formation and development of experimentally induced intestinal adhesions. There are also reports of its use in treating those with chronic active hepatitis, peripheral vascular disease, cerebral thrombosis, sequelae to stroke, pain from external injury to the back or legs, intestinal adhesions, amenorrhea, pelvic inflammatory disease, infertility, and uterine leiomyoma where there are accompanying signs of blood stasis.

The type of blood stasis disease treated by this formula is that of a dry blood (乾血 *gān xuè*) variety, also referred to as 'long-term stasis defeating the blood' (久瘀敗血 *jiǔ yū bài xuè*). This is where there has been a lengthy disease process and the patient's body appears more emaciated with each passing day. There is a dark cast to the complexion, with the area around the eyes being a dark bluish color, dry skin that in extreme cases becomes scaly, and a dark purple tongue body. There is abdominal pain with hard lumps due to the blood stasis in the interior, or frequent episodes of abdominal fullness and distention.

This presentation is quite different from that of Peach Pit Decoction to Order the Qi (*táo hé chéng qì tāng*) in that, with the Peach Pit Decoction to Order the Qi presentation, there is new static blood, the patient is physically strong, and the disease process is relatively short. Therefore, symptoms such as abdominal pain with constipation, mania, fever, and a red tongue would be seen. The treatment method is to use Peach Pit Decoction to Order the Qi (*táo hé chéng qì tāng*) as a decoction so that its purgative action will be relatively strong. However, Rhubarb and Ground Beetle Pill (*dà huáng zhè chóng wán*) is used in pill form; not only is the amount of Rhei Radix et Rhizoma (*dà huáng*) smaller, but it has also been steamed, so its purgative action is milder. As a result, it is relatively rare to see patients have diarrhea after taking this pill. Here, the use of Rhei Radix et Rhizoma (*dà huáng*) is primarily for its ability to invigorate the blood and transform stasis. The Rhubarb and Ground Beetle Pill presentation is as follows:

1. Lower abdominal pain or hard lumps, along with a feeling of abdominal fullness or distention
2. Emaciation with a darkened complexion, dry, scaly skin, and dark circles around the eyes
3. A dark purple tongue body or stasis spots on the tongue, and a thin, rough pulse

The Rhubarb and Ground Beetle Pill presentation can be seen in illnesses such as cerebral thrombosis, thrombocytopenia, aplastic anemia, chronic hepatitis, peritoneal tuberculosis, peripheral vascular disease, and dermatological problems. Liu used this formula to treat 40 cases of chronic active hepatitis, while a control group of 20 was treated with inosine. Both groups were given vitamins C and E and glucurolactone. One 3g Rhubarb and Ground Beetle Pill (*dà huáng zhè chóng wán*) was taken two to three times a day at the beginning. After a week, it was increased to two pills. These were taken for two months to one year. The results for the Rhubarb and Ground Beetle Pill (*dà huáng zhè chóng wán*) group were full recovery in 17 patients, some effect in 19, and no effect in four, while in the inosine group, four recovered completely, there was some effect in 12, and four experienced no effect. Analysis shows a statistically significant difference between the two treatments.[24] There is also a report of this formula being used to treat 19 patients with peripheral vascular disease, which resulted in complete recovery in five, improvement in 12, and no effect in the other two.[25]

There are other similar blood-invigorating and stasis-transforming prescriptions in *Essentials from the Golden Cabinet*. One example is Purge Static Blood Decoction (*xià yū xuè tāng*), which consists of Rhei Radix et Rhizoma (*dà huáng*) 6g, Persicae Semen (*táo rén*) 10g, and Eupolyphaga/Stelophaga (*zhè chóng*) 10g. *Essentials from the Golden Cabinet* states: "For pregnant women with abdominal pain, the method to employ is Unripe Bitter Orange and Peony Powder (*zhǐ shí sháo yaò sǎn*). In the event this does not cure the patient, it is because there is dry blood in the abdomen below the navel; using Purge Static Blood Decoction (*xià yū xuè tāng*) masters it; additionally, it treats menstrual difficulties." Compared with the previously noted Peach Pit Decoction to Order the Qi (*táo hé chéng qì tāng*), this formula contains Eupolyphaga/Stelophaga (*zhè chóng*), but there is no Cinnamomi Ramulus (*guì zhī*), Natrii Sulfas (*máng xiāo*), or Glycyrrhizae Radix (*gān cǎo*), and the amounts used of Rhei Radix et Rhizoma (*dà huáng*) and Persicae Semen (*táo rén*) are smaller by half. Naturally, this formula's purging ability is not as strong as that of Peach Pit Decoction to Order the Qi (*táo hé chéng qì tāng*). However, the use of the Eupolyphaga/Stelophaga (*zhè chóng*) strengthens its ability to treat 'dry blood.' With dry blood below the navel, there are symptoms of lower abdominal pain, lumps, and pain that is aggravated by pressure. Additionally, there are signs of blood stasis such as abdominal fullness and distention, anxiety, and feverishness. This formula can treat postpartum abdominal pain or irregular menstruation and amenorrhea, lower abdominal pain that is aggravated by pressure, or fever, anxiety, difficulty sleeping, and a dark red tongue body.

The method of preparation and consumption of this formula is special in that wine is used to decoct it. Alcohol promotes the circulation of blood and fluids, and increases the blood-invigorating action of the formula. Currently, water decoctions are also used.

4.4 **Virgate Wormwood Decoction** (茵陳蒿湯 *yīn chén hāo tāng*)

SOURCE: *Discussion of Cold Damage*

Artemisiae scopariae Herba (*yīn chén*) 10-30g
Gardeniae Fructus (*zhī zǐ*) 6-12g
Rhei Radix et Rhizoma (*dà huáng*) 6-12g

Virgate Wormwood Decoction (*yīn chén hāo tāng*) is the rhubarb family formula specifically for jaundice. Strictly speaking, it is a formula that treats yang-type jaundice. Chinese medicine generally divides jaundice into the two main categories of yin and yang types. Yang jaundice (陽黃 *yáng huáng*) has signs of heat and excess. This jaundice has a fresh and bright color, and is accompanied by a dry mouth, fever with sweating, constipation, yellow urine, and a red tongue with a yellow coating. Yin jaundice (陰黃 *yīn huáng*) has accompanying signs of cold and deficiency. Here the jaundice is dark in color, the patient has an insipid taste in the mouth and a lack of thirst, the body feels cold, the stools are loose, and the urine is clear. The tongue is pale and with a white coating. Jaundice accompanying the rhubarb presentation falls within the scope of the yang type.

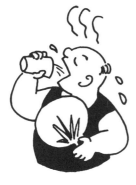

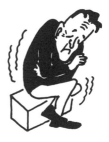

YANG JAUNDICE   YIN JAUNDICE

The Virgate Wormwood Decoction presentation is as follows:

1. Bright colored jaundice with scanty yellow urine
2. Chest stuffiness, irritability, and fever with sweating
3. Signs of the rhubarb presentation

Artemisiae scopariae Herba (*yīn chén*) is specifically used to reduce jaundice. *Divine Husbandman's Classic of the Materia Medica* states: "It masters the pathogenic qi of wind, dampness, cold, heat, and heat clumped jaundice." Other sources state: "It treats whole body jaundice." Modern pharmacological research shows evidence of Artemisiae scopariae Herba's (*yīn chén*) biliary-regulating, hepatic-protective, antipyretic, and diuretic functions. Gardeniae Fructus (*zhī zǐ*) is the fruit of Gardeniae Jasminoidis. It is an herb traditionally used to clear heat and is often employed in the treatment of jaundice, stomach pain, irritability, and bleeding. Pharmacological research shows that Gardeniae Fructus (*zhī zǐ*) has biliary-strengthening, antipyretic, sedative, and antihypertensive functions.

Virgate Wormwood Decoction (*yīn chén hāo tāng*) with its constituent herbs of Rhei Radix et Rhizoma (dà huáng), Artemisiae scopariae Herba (yīn chén), and Gardeniae Fructus (zhī zǐ) possesses a significant ability to clear heat and reduce jaundice. It is now used extensively to treat acute infectious hepatitis, severe cases of hepatitis, cholecystitis, cholelithiasis, jaundice, hemorrhagic leptospinosis, and hyperbilirubinemia.

- This formula is effective in treating jaundice from infectious hepatitis. It reduces the jaundice, lowers the liver enzyme levels, improves the appetite, and restores the digestive function. Chinese reports about these aspects of its effectiveness are numerous. In recent years, statistics were compiled where the formula was used to treat 1,184 cases of acute viral hepatitis; the cure rate was over 95 percent. There are quite a few studies comparing Chinese and Western medicines for this problem, and the reports demonstrate that Virgate Wormwood Decoction (yīn chén hāo tāng) has proven to be a very effective formula.

- This formula is effective in treating severe cases of hepatitis. With the additions of Coptidis Rhizoma (huáng lián), Scutellariae Radix (huáng qín), and Phellodendri Cortex (huáng bǎi), this formula was made into an injectable solution and used to treat 32 cases of severe hepatitis, of which 29 were cured. It both promptly reduced the jaundice and lowered the mortality rate.[26] There are also reports about the effectiveness of this formula when it is combined with modifications of Minor Decoction [for Pathogens] Stuck in the Chest (xiǎo xiàn xiōng tāng), Peach Pit Decoction to Order the Qi (táo hé chéng qì tāng), Coptis Decoction to Resolve Toxicity (huáng lián jiě dú tāng), and Rhinoceros Horn and Rehmannia Decoction (xī jiǎo dì huáng tāng) to treat severe cases of hepatitis.

- This formula is effective in treating hemolytic diseases in newborns. There is a report of the use of this formula where Gardeniae Fructus (zhī zǐ) was removed and Scutellariae Radix (huáng qín) and Glycyrrhizae Radix (gān cǎo) were added to make infusion granules to treat 40 newborns with this kind of blood disease. Among these cases were 16 with ABO-type blood incompatibilities, two with RH-type blood incompatibilities, two with infections, and 20 whose illness was of unknown origin. Other than three cases who underwent blood transfusions, all recovered within three to four days. As confirmed by blood tests, this formula has a definite ability to inhibit anti-A and anti-B antibodies.[27]

- Virgate Wormwood Decoction (yīn chén hāo tāng) is effective in treating acute biliary tract infection. Generally, it is combined with modifications of Minor Bupleurum Decoction (xiǎo chái hú tāng) or Major Bupleurum Decoction (*dà chái hú tāng*). There is a report of using a combination of Chinese and Western medicine to treat 211 cases of acute ascending cholangitis. In the treatment of bile duct infections using this formula, combining Virgate Wormwood Decoction (*yīn chén hāo tāng*) with Major Bupleurum Decoction (*dà chái hú tāng*) and Five-Ingredient Drink to Eliminate Toxin (*wǔ wèi xiāo dú yǐn*)* brought about better treatment results.[28]

• There are also reports of using this formula to treat allergic dermatitis, psoriasis, urticaria, and jaundice from trauma to the liver.

The differentiation of yang-type jaundice is the key to proper use of this formula. As noted above, jaundice that is accompanied by the rhubarb presentation falls within the scope of yang-type jaundice. The differences are generally not difficult to grasp, and the differentiation can simply be made on the basis of color. The color of yang jaundice is a bright orange, like the color of the fruit, whereas the color of yin jaundice is dark, like that of something that has been smoke cured. Additionally, the tongue body and coating, high or low body temperature, and constipation or loose stools are also critical points of differentiation.

The use of Rhei Radix et Rhizoma (*dà huáng*) for illnesses with jaundice is not limited to its facilitation of bowel movements, but also for its ability to clear heat and invigorate the blood. Therefore, the amount used in this formula is less than that used in Order the Qi Decoctions. Aside from changing the amount of time it is cooked, wine-fried Rhei Radix et Rhizoma (*jiǔ dà huáng*) can also be used. Wine-frying Rhei Radix et Rhizoma (*dà huáng*) reduces its purgative effect. If the jaundice has receded, the amount of Rhei Radix et Rhizoma (*dà huáng*) can be reduced, or one can switch to using Virgate Wormwood and Five-Ingredient Powder with Poria (*yīn chén wǔ líng sǎn*).†

4.5 Saposhnikovia Powder that Sagely Unblocks
(防風通聖散 *fáng fēng tōng shèng sǎn*)

SOURCE: *Formulas from the Discussion Illuminating the Yellow Emperor's Basic Questions* (黃帝素問宣明論方 *Huáng dì sù wèn xuán míng lùn fāng*)

---

* Lonicerae Flos (*jīn yín huā*), Chrysanthemi Flos (*jú huā*), Taraxaci Herba (*pú gōng yīng*), Violae Herba (*zǐ huā dì dīng*), and Begoniae fimbristipulatae Herba (*hóng tiān kuí*).

† Artemisiae scopariae Herba (*yīn chén*), Poria (*fú líng*), Polyporus (*zhū líng*), Atractylodis macrocephalae Rhizoma (*bái zhú*), and Alismatis Rhizoma (*zé xiè*).

Rhei Radix et Rhizoma (*dà huáng*) 15g

Natrii Sulfas (*máng xiāo*) 15g

Saposhnikoviae Radix (*fáng fēng*) 15g

Forsythiae Fructus (*lián qiào*) 15g

Ephedrae Herba (*má huáng*) 15g

Menthae haplocalycis Herba (*bò hé*) 15g

Chuanxiong Rhizoma (*chuān xiōng*) 15g

Angelicae sinensis Radix (*dāng guī*) 15g

Paeoniae Radix (*sháo yào*) 15g

Atractylodes macrocephalae Rhizoma (*bái zhú*) 15g

Schizonepetae Herba (*jīng jiè*) 15g

Gardeniae Fructus (*zhī zǐ*) 15g

Scutellariae Radix (*huáng qín*) 30g

Gypsum fibrosum (*shí gāo*) 30g

Platycodi Radix (*jié gěng*) 30g

Glycyrrhizae Radix (*gān cǎo*) 60g

Talcum (*huá shí*) 90g

The rhubarb constitution's distinctive characteristic of interior excess heat has been discussed previously. Generally speaking, people with interior excess have an exterior that is deficient in that they usually sweat easily and have a red, moist, lustrous complexion. However, this is not always the case. If patients with a rhubarb constitution get a cold from being attacked by wind-cold, they can manifest with signs of exterior excess and exterior heat such as fever with a lack of sweating, a yellowish red but dark complexion, headache and dizziness, throat discomfort, red and painful eyes, cough with wheezing, and itchy skin rashes. At the same time, signs of interior heat and interior excess are even more apparent, resulting in manifestations such as constipation, abdominal fullness and distention, focal distention and stuffiness in the chest and diaphragm, thick and viscous nasal discharge and saliva, a greasy feeling with a bitter taste in the mouth, and a thick tongue coating. At this point, use of a strictly purgative formula would not completely address the problem. Saposhnikovia Powder that Sagely Unblocks (*fáng fēng tōng shèng sǎn*) is directed precisely at the above-noted mixed condition and indeed was created for just such a presentation. The Saposhnikovia Powder that Sagely Unblocks presentation is as follows:

1. Fever with sweating, or headache with dizziness, or red, swollen, painful eyes, itchy rashes, or sores and toxic swellings

2. Constipation, abdominal distention, chest and diaphragm fullness and stuffiness
3. A thick tongue coating that could be either greasy or dry

Traditionally, this formula is said to be a prescription that resolves both the exterior and interior, meaning that it can both promote sweating to resolve the exterior while purging to unblock the interior. Additionally, it clears heat and eliminates irritability. In practice, as long as the differential diagnosis is correct, results will be quickly obtained. Clinically, this formula is commonly used for dermatological diseases, flat warts, suppurating infections, and multiple furuncles. It also treats obesity, hyperlipidemia, hypercholesterolemia, headaches, frozen shoulder, constipation, toothache, bloodshot eyes, and inflammatory diseases affecting the face when seen with the above-mentioned presentation. It is especially suitable for treating the headaches and dizziness, common cold with fever, and dermatological illnesses of those with the rhubarb constitution. Additionally, it can be used as a prescription for weight loss.

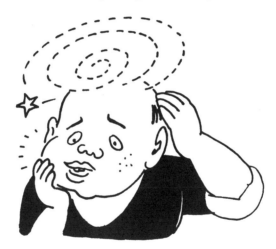

4.6 **Rhubarb and Aconite Accessory Root Decoction**
(大黃附子湯 *dà huáng fù zǐ tāng*)

SOURCE: *Essentials from the Golden Cabinet*

Rhei Radix et Rhizoma (*dà huáng*) 3-10g
Aconiti Radix lateralis preparata (*zhì fù zǐ*) 6-10g
Asari Herba (*xì xīn*) 3-6g

All of the Rhei Radix et Rhizoma (dà huáng) formulas that have been introduced thus far are prescriptions that clear heat and purge. While those with a rhubarb constitution do have a tendency toward heat and excess, this is not to say that they cannot develop illnesses with cold presentations. As a result of being overtired, of long-term use of purgative or heat-clearing herbs, or of excessive intake of food that harms the Stomach and Intestines, those with a rhubarb constitution can also manifest with a cold presentation. Clinically, constipation, abdominal distention accompanied by aversion to cold with fever, cold extremities, and a greasy, white tongue coating are seen. When this occurs, the warming purgative formula Rhubarb and Aconite Accessory Root Decoction (dà huáng fù zǐ tāng) can be used. *Essentials from the Golden Cabinet* states: "Patients with tendency toward pain under the ribs, fever, and a tight and wiry pulse, this is a cold condition. Use warming herbs to purge it; Rhubarb and Aconite Accessory Root Decoction (dà huáng fù zǐ tāng) is appropriate."

This formula consists of Rhei Radix et Rhizoma (dà huáng) combined with Aconiti Radix lateralis preparata (zhì fù zǐ) and Asari Herba (xì xīn). Aconiti Radix lateralis preparata (zhì fù zǐ) and Asari Herba (xì xīn) are both excellent analgesics. In *Discussion of Cold Damage* and *Essentials from the Golden Cabinet*, Aconiti Radix lateralis preparata (zhì fù zǐ) prescriptions are frequently used for aversion to cold, for limbs and joints that are painful, heavy, or numb, or for frigid extremities. They also treat abdominal pain with diarrhea. Asari Herba (xì xīn) prescriptions are often used for chest fullness, cough, edema, counterflow qi leading to chest stuffiness, shortness of breath and an inability to lay flat, and hypochondriac pain. There is evidence from pharmacological research that after Aconiti Radix lateralis preparata (zhì fù zǐ) is absorbed, it has anesthetic effects on the sensory and motor nerves and also functions as an analgesic by first stimulating and then numbing the peripheral nerve endings in the mucous membranes and skin. The volatile oils in Asari Herba (xì xīn) have a significant inhibitory effect on the central nervous system, and decoctions of this herb have sedative, analgesic, and hypnotic effects. Low concentrations of Asari Herba's (xì xīn) volatile oils can reduce smooth muscle tone. Therefore, this formula is typically emphasized for use when there is a tendency toward pain under the ribs with a tight and wiry pulse. 'Under the ribs' (脅下 xié xià) in this context indicates the abdominal area; 'tends to be painful' (偏痛 piān tōng) means there is primarily pain, not distention; and 'a tight and wiry pulse' is a pain pulse. The abdominal pain of this formula's presentation can be quite intense, and it is reasonable to consider that constipation will be part of the presentation. Simply stated, this formula's presentation is the rhubarb presentation with the addition of the presentation of Aconiti Radix lateralis preparata (*zhì fù zǐ*) or Asari Herba (*xì xīn*); or it can be thought of as the rhubarb presentation with signs of interior cold.

Within the ephedra formula family is the prescription Ephedra, Asarum, and Aconite Accessory Root Decoction (*má huáng xì xīn fù zǐ tāng*). This formula is the same, but it uses Rhei Radix et Rhizoma (*dà huáng*) instead of Ephedrae Herba (*má huáng*). Ephedra, Asarum, and Aconite Accessory Root Decoction (*má huáng xì xīn fù zǐ tāng*) treats those with the ephedra presentation who are listless and dispirited, have a dull, lusterless complexion, cold hands and feet, and a sinking pulse. Therefore, this formula's presentation can be understood to be the rhubarb presentation with the appearance of any of the above signs. The Rhubarb and Aconite Accessory Root Decoction presentation is as follows:

1. Intense abdominal pain with an aversion to pressure, and accompanying constipation
2. Listless and dispirited affect with a dark and lusterless complexion, sweating and aversion to cold, cold hands and feet, and a sunken, wiry, and tight pulse
3. A greasy, white tongue coating, a relatively dry tongue surface, and a stiff, hard tongue body

The Rhubarb and Aconite Accessory Root Decoction presentation is often seen in cases of intestinal obstruction, cholecystitis, cholelithiasis, biliary ascariasis, urinary tract stones, appendicitis, or swollen and sore throats in those with a weak constitution. The renowned contemporary Ningbo physician Fan Wen-Hu is adept at using a modification of this formula—Rhei Radix et Rhizoma (*dà huáng*) 9g, Asari Herba (*xì xīn*) 1g, Aconiti Radix lateralis preparata (*zhì fù zǐ*) 3g, Natrii Sulfas siccatus (*xuán míng fěn*) 9g, Pinelliae Rhizoma preparatum (*zhì bàn xià*) 9g, and Glycyrrhizae Radix (*gān cǎo*) 3g—to treat acute tonsillitis. Ordinarily with acute tonsillitis, the tongue coating is white, while the tongue body itself is slightly red, and there are other signs of 'heat wrapped by cold' (寒包熱 *hán bāo rè*). One dose will typically resolve the heat and cure the painful, swollen throat.[29]

The function of this formula is similar to that of the *Important Formulas Worth a Thousand Gold Pieces* (千金要方 *Qiān jīn yào fāng*) formula Warm the Spleen Decoction (*wēn pí tāng*): Rhei Radix et Rhizoma (*dà huáng*) 12g, Aconiti Radix lateralis preparata (*zhì fù zǐ*) 9g, Zingiberis Rhizoma (*gān jiāng*) 6g, Ginseng Radix (*rén shēn*) 6g, and Glycyrrhizae Radix (*gān cǎo*) 6g. It treats those with cold accumulation constipation or long-term dysentery with stools that contain blood and pus, along with accompanying abdominal pain, cold hands and feet, and a pulse that is sinking and wiry.

CHAPTER 5

ASTRAGALUS FORMULA FAMILY

....

黄耆類方 huáng qí lèi fāng

ASTRAGALI RADIX (*huáng qí*) is the stem of the perennial *Astragalus membranaceus* that can be yellow, brown, or mahogany in color and grows to the height of two to three feet. It primarily grows in the Chinese provinces of Gansu, Inner Mongolia, Shanxi, and Dongbei. The first recorded mention of Astragali Radix (*huáng qí*) is found in *Divine Husbandman's Classic of the Materia Medica* (神農本草經 *Shén Nóng běn cǎo jīng*); traditionally, it is used as an important tonic herb. Astragali Radix (*huáng qí*) has a sweet taste and is slightly warming; it can be used to treat various types of symptoms such as debility with spontaneous sweating, edema, urinary difficulty, chronic nonhealing ulcers, diabetes, or poststroke hemiplegia. Astragali Radix (*huáng qí*) is commonly used in combination with Cinnamomi Ramulus (*guì zhī*), Bupleuri Radix (*chái hú*), Atractylodis macrocephalae Rhizoma (*bái zhú*), Aconiti Radix lateralis preparata (*zhì fù zǐ*), Stephaniae tetrandrae Radix (*hàn fáng jǐ*), Angelicae sinensis Radix (*dāng guī*), Glycyrrhizae Radix (*gān cǎo*), or Ginseng Radix (*rén shēn*), and potentiates their function by enabling them to more fully express their therapeutic actions. For example, when it is paired with Cinnamomi Ramulus (*guì zhī*) in the formula Astragalus and Cinnamon Twig Five-Substance Decoction (*huáng qí guì zhī wǔ wù tāng*), it treats exterior deficiency with spontaneous sweating; when it is paired with Bupleuri Radix (*chái hú*) in the prescription Tonify the Middle to Augment the Qi Decoction (*bǔ zhōng yì qì tāng*), it treats weakness of the middle qi leading to an aversion to wind, poor appetite, chest and hypochondriac fullness and discomfort, and anal prolapse; when it is paired with Stephaniae tetrandrae Radix (*hàn fáng jǐ*) in Stephania and Astragalus Decoction (*fáng jǐ huáng qí tāng*), it treats debility with edema and joint pain; when it is paired with Aconiti Radix lateralis preparata (*zhì fù zǐ*), it treats yang deficiency joint pain; and when it is paired with Angelicae sinensis Radix (*dāng guī*) in Tangkuei Decoction to Tonify the

Blood (*dāng guī bǔ xuè tāng*), it treats fever from blood deficiency, thirst, malar flush, and an empty pulse.

In Chinese medicine there is an adage, "Support the normal while dispelling the pathogenic" (扶正祛邪 *fú zhèng qū xié*), and thus when the organism's ability to resist disease is low, the guiding treatment principle is to safeguard and support the normal qi. When the normal qi is full and flourishing, the pathogenic influence is naturally defeated. Illnesses that are treated with Astragali Radix (*huáng qí*) are a subset of those due to an insufficiency of the body's normal qi, that is, those with what is called a qi deficiency presentation. Astragali Radix's (*huáng qí*) is relatively mild, has few side effects, and so is suitable for long-term use. Therefore, it is said that Astragali Radix (*huáng qí*) is an herb that can be used in the "beneficent kingly way" of medicine, versus those methods using harsher medicinals, which are considered to be more like ruling by force. That being said, Astragali Radix (*huáng qí*) is not an herb to be abused. Because it is slightly warm in temperature, it will not only be ineffective, but it can cause adverse reactions if it is used in treating the wrong patients. These include people with an excess or hot constitution, poor digestion, fevers from acute infectious disease, or abdominal fullness, pain, and constipation. Key pointers for the proper use of Astragali Radix (*huáng qí*) are discussed here.

Astragalus Presentation (黃耆證 *huáng qí zhèng*)

Spontaneous sweating or night sweats with edema are the distinctive signs of the astragalus presentation. As previously noted, ancient people said that Astragali Radix (*huáng qí*) primarily treats 'fluids in the outer muscle layer' (肌表之水 *jī biǎo zhī shuǐ*). The spontaneous sweating of the astragalus presentation is relatively severe with the clothes often becoming completely soaked and with sweat stains that sometimes have a yellowish color. For some people, the sweating is worse when they eat, with significantly more sweating from the upper portion of the body. For other people, in addition to spontaneous sweating in the daytime, there are also night sweats, which manifest as waking to find the entire body soaking wet as if having just been immersed in water. The majority of these patients will be seen with accompanying cold limbs, an aversion to wind, susceptibility to the common cold, lower leg edema, and scanty urination. Because of the accompanying edema, there is often a subjective sense of the body feeling heavy and uncoordinated. It should be pointed out that sometimes the astragalus presentation does not manifest with a significant amount of spontaneous sweating. However, the interview process reveals that the patient is usually prone to some type of sweating: readily sweats on minimal exertion or has a history of spontaneous or night sweating.

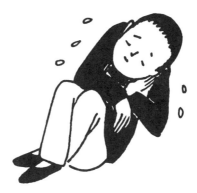

Traditionally, Astragali Radix *(huáng qí)* has been used as a medicinal for various diseases that affect the skin, and it is an indispensable herb in the treatment of nonsupporative ulcers, chronic nonhealing ulcers, or areas of nonregenerating flesh. There are two essential aspects to the diagnosis, the first being local: the skin color of the ulcerated area is dark, the top is flat or sunken, there is not a great amount of pain; or when the problem is a chronic, nonhealing ulcer, there is a thin, clear exudate with the wound itself looking pale and not fresh. The second aspect is that systemically the patient's condition is rather poor. In a similar fashion, Astragali Radix *(huáng qí)* can also be used to treat patients with upper gastrointestinal tract ulcers. The astragalus presentation, therefore, is as follows:

1. Spontaneous sweating, night sweats, aversion to wind, a body that feels heavy, or limbs that are numb and uncomfortable
2. Edema with a heavy feeling in the body, and urinary difficulty
3. Long-term nonhealing ulcers with clear, watery exudate

The cinnamon twig presentation discussed previously is similar to the astragalus presentation, as both are marked by spontaneous sweating with an aversion to wind. However, in the cinnamon twig presentation, spontaneous sweating is accompanied by a fever or feverishness, insomnia, headache, and palpitations; these do not occur in the astragalus presentation. Additionally, the differences in constitution are quite significant. Those with the cinnamon twig constitution, for the most part, are thin and have a tight musculature, while the astragalus body type tends to have soft, relaxed muscles as well as edema.

Astragalus Constitution (黃耆體質 *huáng qí tǐ zhì*)

The astragalus constitution is simply the body type that tends to develop an astragalus presentation. Distinctive characteristics include the following:

- *External distinguishing characteristics.* A lusterless complexion that is yellowish pale, or yellowish and faintly red, or dark yellow; soft and loose musculature that appears edematous; eyes that lack liveliness; and a pale complexion. The abdominal wall is soft, weak, and without strength. The tongue is pale and flabby, and with a wet coating.
- *Predisposition.* Sweats very easily and has an aversion to wind; allergies, coughs, and wheezing, or rhinitis are readily exacerbated by drafts or chills, or there may be a tendency to catch colds. Thin, watery, and unformed stools, or stools that are dry at first and then watery. These people have poor appetites and readily experience abdominal fullness and distention. There is a marked tendency toward edema, especially in the feet, as well as a predilection toward numbness in the hands and feet.

Those with an astragalus constitution appear to have soft and loose musculature with a surplus of water and dampness, very much like that of a leather bag full of water. The edema in these patients can vary in different parts of body. For some, there is swelling in the lower legs that feels stiff and turgid, while the abdomen feels soft; in others, the abdomen feels hard, while the four limbs have a spongy feel when palpated.

This kind of body type, when not due to genetics, develops as a result of long-term lack of physical exercise, poor nutrition, anemia, or chronic illness. The propensity to sweat easily and the aversion to wind associated with this constitutional type resembles that of the cinnamon twig constitution, but without the lower abdominal tightness and pain. The edema and tendency toward wheezing and nasal congestion is similar to that of the ephedra constitution; however, the ephedra constitution's lack of sweating and body aches is lacking. In clinical practice, there are occasions when various constitutional types are blended together, and in these situations, the prescription should conform to this mixed presentation. Examples of such formulas are Cinnamon Twig plus Astragalus Decoction (*guì zhī jiā huáng qí tāng*), Stephania and Astragalus Decoction plus Cinnamon Twig (*fáng jǐ huáng qí jiā guì zhī tāng*), and Ephedra Decoction plus Atractylodes and Astragalus (*má huáng jiā zhú huáng qí tāng*).

Pharmacological research reports that Astragali Radix (*huáng qí*) promotes immune system function, increases the spleen's production of antibodies, and acts as an anti-allergen. It strengthens the contractive ability in healthy hearts; this effect is even more pronounced when there is cardiac insufficiency, either experimentally induced by toxins or from exhaustion. Astragali Radix (*huáng qí*) vasodilates and improves circulation and nutrition to the skin. Additionally, it lowers blood pressure and counteracts adrenaline. Oral and injectable preparations of Astragali Radix (*huáng qí*) both have documented diuretic effects. It also has a certain ability to counteract experimentally induced nephritis, especially with regard to stopping proteinuria. Large dosages of powdered Astragali Radix (*huáng qí*) taken orally impeded the development of serum nephritis in rats, specifically delaying the development of proteinuria and hypercholesterolemia. For rats which already had proteinuria, those who were orally given Astragali Radix (*huáng qí*) powder recovered faster than the control group that did not. Astragali Radix (*huáng qí*) also has hepatoprotective functions, preventing a reduction in liver glycogen levels, and additionally functions to lower blood sugar. These pharmacological research reports help give us a better understanding of the astragalus presentation.

5.1 Jade Windscreen Powder (玉屏風散 *yù píng fēng sǎn*)

SOURCE: *Essential Teachings of [Zhu] Dan-Xi (丹溪心法 Dān Xī xīn fǎ)*

Astragali Radix (*huáng qí*) 30g
Atractylodis macrocephalae Rhizoma (*bái zhú*) 60g
Saposhnikoviae Radix (*fáng fēng*) 30g

Jade Windscreen Powder (*yù píng fēng sǎn*) is the prescription that effectively treats the profuse sweating and susceptibility to the common cold of those with the astragalus constitution. True to its ancient name, it is just like a precious jade screen that blocks out wind; it is clinically effective because it assists in warding off pathogenic wind. The majority of those with the astragalus constitution have signs of edema, urinary difficulty, or musculature that is soft and loose. Therefore, to address these symptoms, this formula contains Atractylodis macrocephalae Rhizoma (*bái zhú*), which functions to promote urination, and Saposhnikoviae Radix (*fáng fēng*), which disperses wind-cold from the exterior, ameliorates aches and pain in the body and head from the common cold, and treats abdominal pain. Chinese medicine holds that Astragali Radix (*huáng qí*) gathers while Saposhnikoviae Radix (*fáng fēng*) scatters. In this way, the exterior is stabilized, but without retaining the pathogens, while the pathogens are dispersed without harming the normal qi. Pharmacological research suggests that this formula and Astragali Radix (*huáng qí*) function to simultaneously regulate both PDE and cAMP in the spleen cells of laboratory mice, thus indicating they have a kind of immune-regulating pharmacological activity.[1] Clinical research also indicates that this formula is useful in treating patients who easily catch cold, which can then lead to recurrent glomerulonephritis. It was further discovered that not only was there an improvement in the clinical symptoms, but additionally their immune function either recovered or improved.[2] In practice, this formula has a relatively good effect in preventing illness in children susceptible to respiratory infections; this could be related to its ability to increase the body's IgA (immunoglobulin A) level.[3]

The Jade Windscreen Powder presentation is as follows:

1. Susceptibility to colds, aversion to wind, spontaneous sweating, sneezing, and body aches or headache
2. Edema or propensity toward edema, scanty urination, or thin, watery stools

This formula's presentation is a synthesis of the presentations of Astragali Radix (*huáng qí*), Atractylodis macrocephalae Rhizoma (*bái zhú*), and Saposhnikoviae Radix (*fáng fēng*). Astragali Radix (*huáng qí*) primarily treats symptoms of edema and sweating, Atractylodis macrocephalae Rhizoma (*bái zhú*) treats edema and urinary difficulty, and Saposhnikoviae Radix (*fáng fēng*) mainly addresses the aversion to wind, body aches, and headache.

The essential differences between the Jade Windscreen and Cinnamon Twig Decoction presentations are:

• *The constitutions are different.* The differences in the external characteristics of the cinnamon twig and astragalus constitutions are relatively easy to discern.

• *The characteristic presentations are different.* The characteristic Jade Windscreen Powder presentation includes symptoms of internal water accumulation such as edema, urinary difficulty, or thin and watery stools, while for the Cinnamon Twig Decoction presentation, it is the tense nature of the abdomen and joint pain that are the defining signs. That being said, in practice, it is common to see patients in whom both presentations occur simultaneously, in which case these formulas can be combined: Cinnamomi Ramulus (*guì zhī*) can be added to Jade Windscreen Powder (*yù píng fēng sǎn*), or Astragali Radix (*huáng qí*) may be added to Cinnamon Twig Decoction (*guì zhī tāng*).

Other than the commonly seen deficient patient who suffers from frequent colds, the Jade Windscreen Powder presentation is commonly seen in cases of sweating due to autonomic dystonia, allergic rhinitis, allergic purpura, dermatological disease, nephritis, chronic enteritis, and pediatric summerheat. Clinically, this formula is usually prescribed in a modified form. There is a report of using Jade Windscreen Powder (*yù píng fēng sǎn*) with the addition of Angelicae sinensis Radix (*dāng guī*), Magnoliae Flos (*xīn yí*), Schisandrae Fructus (*wǔ wèi zǐ*), Acori tatarinowii Rhizoma (*shí chāng pǔ*), Paeoniae Radix alba (*bái sháo*), Cicadae Periostracum (*chán tuì*), Asari Herba (*xì xīn*), and Glycyrrhizae Radix (*gān cǎo*) to treat 34 patients with chronic allergic rhinitis. Treatment resulted in 26 of the patients being completely cured, seven whose condition improved, and one for whom there was no effect.[4] Beijing Xiyuan hospital, which is attached to the China Academy of Traditional Chinese Medicine, has an empirical prescription that consists of this formula with the additions of Six-Gentlemen Decoction (*liù jūn zǐ tāng*), Hominis Placenta (*zǐ hé chē*), and Psoraleae Fructus (*bǔ gǔ zhǐ*) in pill form that is used to treat chronic bronchitis and asthma. There are also reports of this formula with the additions of Artemisiae annuae Herba (*qīng hāo*), Gentianae macrophyllae Radix (*qín jiāo*), Trionycis Carapax (*biē jiǎ*), Lonicerae Flos (*jīn yín huā*), and Lophatheri Herba (*dàn zhú yè*) satisfactorily treating cases of pediatric summerheat.

5.2 Stephania and Astragalus Decoction
(防己黃耆湯 *fáng jǐ huáng qí tāng*)

SOURCE: *Essentials from the Golden Cabinet* (金匱要略 *Jīn guì yào lüè*)

Stephaniae tetrandrae Radix (*fěn fáng jǐ*) 6-12g
Astragali Radix (*huáng qí*) 10-30g
Atractylodis macrocephalae Rhizoma (*bái zhú*) 6-12g
Glycyrrhizae Radix (*gān cǎo*) 3g
Zingiberis Rhizoma recens (*shēng jiāng*) 6g
Jujubae Fructus (*dà zǎo*) 10g

MODIFICATIONS IN THE SOURCE TEXT:

- For those with wheezing, add
  Ephedrae Herba (*má huáng*) 3-6g

- For those with Stomach disharmony, add
  Paeoniae Radix alba (*bái sháo*) 10-20g

- For those with a sensation of upward-surging, add
  Cinnamomi Ramulus (guì zhī)...10-20g
- For those with recalcitrant pain, back and leg pain, or
  abdominal pain, add Asari Herba (xì xīn).........................3-6g

While traditionally a few different herbs have been used as 防己 (fáng jǐ), at present the most commonly used one in China is Stephaniae tetrandrae Radix (fěn fáng jǐ), the root of the perennial vine *Stephania tetrandra* S. Moore. Commonly known as Stephaniae tetrandrae Radix (hàn fáng jǐ), it is round and twisted, brownish grey in color with longitudinal veins, and with a powdery white, grainy interior. Combining Astragali Radix (huáng qí) with Stephaniae tetrandrae Radix (hàn fáng jǐ) and Atractylodis macrocephalae Rhizoma (bái zhú) further strengthens its diuretic function. Therefore, Stephania and Astragalus Decoction (fáng jǐ huáng qí tāng) is the representative prescription traditionally used for reducing edema through diuresis. In *Essentials from the Golden Cabinet* it is said to treat "those with wind-dampness, a floating pulse and heavy body, who sweat and have an aversion to wind." In *Arcane Essentials from the Imperial Library* (外台秘要 Wài tái mì yào), it is used to treat "swelling below the waist reaching to the perineum, with difficulty in flexing and extending." In modern clinical practice, this formula is commonly used to treat edema, various illnesses involving excessive sweating, arthritis, chronic nephritis, obesity, and dermatological disease. The Stephania and Astragalus Decoction presentation is as follows:

1. Edema, especially of the lower extremities, aversion to wind, sweating, and reduced urine
2. Joint pain, especially of the knees, which in addition to being painful are also swollen, or muscle aches

This formula's presentation and that of the ephedra family formula Maidservant from Yue's Decoction plus Atractylodes (Yuè bì jiā zhú tāng) are quite similar. Both formulas share the symptoms of edema, joint pain, profuse sweating, and scanty urination. In clinical practice, it is common to use these two formulas in the treatment of joint pain and edema. The differences between the two are:

- *The constitutions are different.* The physical strength of the ephedra constitution is relatively substantial, while that of the astragalus constitution is less so. The skin of the ephedra type is both thicker and coarser, and has a darkish look about it; these people ordinarily do not sweat very much. The skin of the

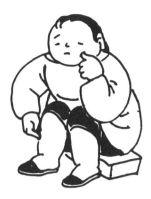

astragalus type is relatively fine and tender, and these patients usually sweat easily.

• *Degree and character of the symptoms are also different.* The course of the illness with the Maidservant from Yue's Decoction plus Atractylodes presentation is relatively short, accompanied by heat signs such as thirst and fever, and its associated edema tends to affect the entire body. By contrast, the course of the illness for this formula's presentation is comparatively long with symptoms that come and go, usually accompanied by an aversion to wind, fatigue, or edema of the lower limbs.

Clinical use of this formula often involves modifications. For example, for patients with wheezing, add Ephedrae Herba *(má huáng)* and Armeniacae Semen *(xìng rén)*; for those with joints of the lower leg feeling cold and painful, add Asari Herba *(xì xīn)*; for those with excessive sweating, thirst, and fever, add Gypsum fibrosum *(shí gāo)*; for those with sweating accompanied by an aversion to cold with coldness and pain in the four limbs, add Aconiti Radix lateralis preparata *(zhì fù zǐ)*; for those with edema, thirst, and scanty urine accompanied by palpitations and dizziness, add Cinnamomi Ramulus *(guì zhī)*, Poria *(fú líng)*, and Alismatis Rhizoma *(zé xiè)*; and for those with headaches and numbness of the four limbs, add Gastrodiae Rhizoma *(tiān má)* and Pinelliae Rhizoma preparatum *(zhì bàn xià)*.

I once treated a patient with temporomandibular joint disorder who came to the clinic because of profuse sweating. Because the patient had a full-figured physique with soft and loose musculature and a pale, purplish tongue, I prescribed this formula with the addition of Puerariae Radix *(gé gēn)*, Carthami Flos *(hóng huā)*, Poria *(fú líng)*, Alismatis Rhizoma *(zé xiè)*, Pinelliae Rhizoma preparatum *(zhì bàn xià)*, and Gastrodiae Rhizoma *(tiān má)*. The sweating stopped after taking five packets. After continuing to take the formula for two months, the temporomandibular joint problem resolved and did not recur. Furthermore, the patient's girth shrunk significantly, the spirit was more vibrant, and there were no recurrences of dizziness.

5.3 Astragalus and Cinnamon Twig Five-Substance Decoction
(黃耆桂枝五物湯 *huáng qí guì zhī wǔ wù tāng*)

SOURCE: *Essentials from the Golden Cabinet*

Astragali Radix (*huáng qí*) 15g
Cinnamomi Ramulus (*guì zhī*) 10g
Paeoniae Radix alba (*bái sháo*) 10g
Zingiberis Rhizoma recens (*shēng jiāng*) 15g
Jujubae Fructus (*dà zǎo*) 12g

Astragalus and Cinnamon Twig Five-Substance Decoction (*huáng qí guì zhī wǔ wù tāng*) is the *Essentials from the Golden Cabinet* formula particularly used for the treatment of painful obstruction of the blood (血痹 *xuè bì*). This type of painful obstruction of the blood manifests as a lack of sensitivity in the body (身體不仁 *shén tǐ bù rén*), resulting in numbness of the limbs and poor coordination. This disease develops, according to *Essentials from the Golden Cabinet*, "in the venerated and honored [i.e., those who do not normally do physical labor] with weak bones and an abundance of flesh who, after working hard to the point of fatigue and sweating, lie down, have frequent tremors, and with the addition of a slight breeze, develop this." The "venerated and honored," those who we might simply call "soft," is one kind of astragalus constitution. They usually are lacking in physical exercise, are overweight with a soft and loose musculature, and have bodies that feel heavy and lethargic, or sweat easily. Additionally, should they get cold after sweating, it results in qi and blood obstruction that in turn gives rise to weakness of the limbs, a lack of coordination, numbness with a lack of sensitivity, extremely achy muscles, or an atrophy of the muscles and flesh. The concept of painful obstruction of the blood does not conform with modern biomedical concepts of disease. Rather than saying this is a disease, perhaps it would be more appropriate to say it is a presentation that can be seen in the course of numerous illnesses because, in practice, many illnesses such as peripheral neuritis, cervical spine disease, diabetes-induced peripheral neuropathy, Raynaud's disease, rheumatoid arthritis, autonomic dystonia, frozen shoulder, sciatica, bone spurs, and the sequelae of stroke can all fall into this category of painful obstruction of the blood. The Astragalus and Cinnamon Twig Five-Substance Decoction presentation is as follows:

1. Weakness of the limbs, clumsiness, numbness with a lack of sensation, achy pain or muscular atrophy
2. Edema, spontaneous sweating, and an aversion to wind
3. Tongue body that is dark and pale

From a look at the common patterns of herb usage as set forth in *Essentials from the Golden Cabinet*, Astragali Radix (*huáng qí*), Cinnamomi Ramulus (*guì zhī*), and Paeoniae Radix alba (*bái sháo*) are often used together to treat sweating with a feeling of heaviness. Examples of this usage are found in Cinnamon Twig plus Astragalus Decoction (*guì zhī jiā huáng qí tāng*)—which treats a patient whose body has a sensation of heaviness, sweating, low back and hip weakness and pain, and urinary difficulty—and in the formula Astragalus, Peony, and Cinnamon Twig in Bitter Wine Decoction (*huáng qí sháo guì kǔ jiǔ tāng*)—which treats those with yellow sweat and a sensation of heaviness. Thus, it follows that in this formula's presentation there must be signs of sweating, a sensation of heaviness, urinary difficulty, or edema. In this case, the patient sweats spontaneously during the daytime even without physical exertion or a warm environment. There are also those who sweat at night to the point of soaking their nightclothes; this sweat often has a yellow color.

This formula is made by taking Cinnamon Twig Decoction (*guì zhī tāng*) and removing the Glycyrrhizae Radix (*gān cǎo*), adding Astragali Radix (*huáng qí*), and increasing the amount of Zingiberis Rhizoma recens (*shēng jiāng*). Even though just one herb has been removed and another added, it causes a rather large change in the formula's presentation. Glycyrrhizae Radix (*gān cǎo*), an herb used primarily to resolve spasms, is commonly paired with Paeoniae Radix (*sháo yào*) to treat abdominal pain with interior tension or hypertonicity. Therefore, formulas such as Minor Construct the Middle Decoction (*xiǎo jiàn zhōng tāng*) and Cinnamon Twig Decoction (*guì zhī tāng*) make use of this particular combination. In this formula, the Glycyrrhizae Radix (*gān cǎo*) presumably has been removed not only because of the lack of any symptoms of abdominal pain or urgency, but because of the presence of abdominal fullness and a sensation of heaviness. Because Glycyrrhizae Radix (*gān cǎo*) contains antidiuretic constituents and because "the sweet taste makes the inside full" (甘能令人中滿 gān néng lìng rén zhōng mǎn), it is removed from this formula. The Astragali Radix (huáng qí) serves to treat sweating, swelling, and numbness; combining it with Cinnamomi Ramulus (guì zhī) and Paeoniae Radix (sháo yào) promotes the circulation of both qi and blood, and unblocks painful obstruction of the blood. Zingiberis Rhizoma recens (shēng jiāng) is acrid, warm, and disperses cold; when a relatively large amount of it is combined with Jujubae Fructus (dà zǎo), this combination also benefits the Stomach. All in all, it is not difficult to distinguish between the presentation of this formula and that of cinnamon twig decoction.

The dark or purple tongue body indicates that the movement of qi and blood is not smooth. Herbs such as Angelicae sinensis Radix (dāng guī) and Carthami Flos (hóng huā) are often added to enhance the therapeutic blood-invigorating and stasis-removing effect of this formula.

It must be emphasized that this formula is primarily prescribed for a lack of sensation in the body. Patients complain of achy and numb limbs, a lack of mobility in the joints, and an aggravation of symptoms when exposed to wind and cold. There may be mild pain, but numbness is the primary complaint. If, for example, there is extreme pain with joints that are swollen and deformed, this is not a presentation that would be treated with this formula; prescriptions from the ephedra and cinnamon twig families are more suitable and should be selected for that type of problem.

Based on many reports, the dosage of Astragali Radix (huáng qí) in this formula should be large. There is a report of this formula with Astragali Radix (huáng qí) 60-120g, Paeoniae Radix (sháo yào) 15g, Cinnamomi Ramulus (guì zhī) 6-10g, Zingiberis Rhizoma recens (shēng jiāng) 10g, and Jujubae Fructus (dà zǎo) 20 pieces being used to treat 35 patients with polyneuritis. For those with more marked decrease in sensation, Angelicae sinensis Radix (dāng guī) 10g was added, and for those with more of a decrease in range of motion, Aconiti Radix lateralis preparata (zhì fù zǐ) 5-15g and Atractylodis macrocephalae Rhizoma (bái zhú) 10g were added along with the application of wine-soaked ginger compresses. Treatment resulted in six patients completely recovering, 10 having significant improvement, 16 showing some effect, and three showing no effect.[5] There is another report of using this formula with a large amount of Astragali Radix (huáng qí), over 60g, that cured two patients with Raynaud's disease.[6] Still another report used a formula where the main ingredients were Astragali Radix (huáng qí) 100g, Paeoniae Radix rubra (chì sháo) 10g, Cinnamomi Ramulus (guì zhī) 3g, and Saposhnikoviae Radix (fáng fēng) 10g to treat 17 patients suffering from frozen shoulder. Twelve were cured, two improved, two patients experienced no effect, and one did not complete the course of treatment. The fewest packets of herbs taken was six and the most was sixteen.[7]

5.4 **Astragalus Decoction to Construct the Middle**
(黃耆建中湯 *huáng qí jiàn zhōng tāng*)

SOURCE: *Essentials from the Golden Cabinet*

Astragali Radix *(huáng qí)* 6-30g
Cinnamomi Ramulus *(guì zhī)* 5-12g
Glycyrrhizae Radix *(gān cǎo)* 3-10g
Jujubae Fructus *(dà zǎo)* 12g
Paeoniae Radix *(sháo yào)* 10-20g
Zingiberis Rhizoma recens *(shēng jiāng)* 5-10g
Maltosum *(yí táng)* 10-15g

Essentials from the Golden Cabinet states: "For deficiency consumption (虛勞 *xū láo*), interior tension (裡急 *lǐ jí*), with all being insufficient (諸不足 *zhū bù zú*), Astragalus Decoction to Construct the Middle *(huáng qí jiàn zhōng tāng)* masters it." Deficiency consumption refers to chronic debilitating illness. Interior tension implies a colicky type of abdominal pain. [All] being insufficient means the exterior and interior are both in a state of deficiency; consequently, there are symptoms of spontaneous sweating with an aversion to wind, a physical sensation of heaviness, mild edema, or loose stools. This formula's presentation can be seen as the chronic abdominal pain of the cinnamon twig constitution accompanied by signs of the astragalus presentation, or someone with the astragalus constitution who has chronic abdominal pain. As this formula is Minor Construct the Middle Decoction *(xiǎo jiàn zhōng tāng)* with the addition of Astragali Radix *(huáng qí)*, it stands to reason that it can be seen as a blending of the cinnamon twig formula family's Minor Construct the Middle Decoction presentation with the symptomology of the astragalus presentation. Its presentation is as follows:

1. Chronic abdominal pain that responds well to warmth and pressure
2. Prone to spontaneous sweating or night sweats, cold with an aversion to wind, a wan complexion, and the body feeling heavy or being slightly edematous

3. The tongue is pale red or dark, and the pulse is large and deficient

The composition of this formula and Astragalus and Cinnamon Twig Five-Substance Decoction *(huáng qí guì zhī wŭ wù tāng)* are almost identical. However, this formula uses a larger amount of Paeoniae Radix *(sháo yào)* and also contains Glycyrrhizae Radix *(gān cǎo)* and Maltosum *(yí táng)*. Paeoniae Radix *(sháo yào)* and Glycyrrhizae Radix *(gān cǎo)* function to resolve spasms and stop pain; Maltosum *(yí táng)* tonifies the Spleen and Stomach, and its sweet taste relaxes tension. Thus, Astragalus Decoction to Construct the Middle *(huáng qí jiàn zhōng tāng)* is used to treat those who have chronic abdominal pain accompanied by the astragalus presentation. On the other hand, Astragalus and Cinnamon Twig Five-Substance Decoction *(huáng qí guì zhī wŭ wù tāng)* uses larger amounts of Astragali Radix *(huáng qí)* and Zingiberis Rhizoma recens *(shēng jiāng)* and has the ability to dispel dampness, scatter cold, and open the channels and collaterals. Therefore, it is most suitable for those patients who have numbness and a lack of sensation in the limbs accompanied by the astragalus presentation.

• The Astragalus Decoction to Construct the Middle presentation is often seen in patients with peptic ulcers where chronic pain is the primary symptom, and in cases of chronic gastritis, gastrointestinal neurosis, and porphyria. Liu reports good results using a modification of Astragalus Decoction to Construct the Middle *(huáng qí jiàn zhōng tāng)* to treat 50 patients with ulcers. He believes that effective treatment is assured when using this formula for ulcers of the deficiency-cold type. The distinctive characteristics of this presentation are long-term upper abdominal pain, tender spots that respond favorably to pressure, or pain that is more pronounced when hungry and alleviated by eating, favoring warmth and an aversion to cold, usually accompanied by a pulse that is deficient and either moderate or wiry, and a pale tongue with a white coating. On the other hand, if the tender spots get worse with pressure, or there is no relation of the pain to eating, or the pain is of an intermittent stabbing nature, and the mouth and tongue are dry with a lack of interest in drinking along with constipation, then this presentation belongs to the category of blood stasis, and this formula will have no effect.[8] Some patients with chronic hepatitis or chronic colitis often have accompanying digestive tract ulcers or a history of such. So long as there is spontaneous sweating, a wan complexion, and a dark, pale tongue, this formula may be used.

• The Astragalus Decoction to Construct the Middle presentation is often seen in cases of anemia, nervous exhaustion, autonomic dystonia, and feverishness where the primary symptoms are a feeling of cold with a slight fever, spontaneous or night sweating, a yellowish complexion or deficiency edema. Yang treated a patient with hemolytic jaundice who had fever, night sweats, diarrhea with watery, bloody stools, dizziness with palpitations, a withered and sallow complexion, and significant whole body fatigue. Based on symptoms of a large pulse, pale tongue, wan complexion, watery stools, and normal urination, Astragalus Decoction to Construct the Middle (*huáng qí jiàn zhōng tāng*) was prescribed. After taking 20 packets, the symptoms improved as did the blood tests. Continuing to take a modified version of this formula for three months resulted in a complete cure.[9]

Maltosum (*yí táng*), being a sugar, is sweet. If patients do not like to eat sweet foods, have abdominal distention, or have a thick tongue coating, Hordei Fructus germinatus (*mài yá*) can be used as a substitute. If patients have constipation, honey can be used instead as it has the multiple functions of tonifying the middle as it moistens the bowels to facilitate the movement of the stool.

5.5 Tonify the Middle to Augment the Qi Decoction
(補中益氣湯 *bǔ zhōng yì qì tāng*)

SOURCE: *Clarifying Doubts about Damage from Internal and External Causes* (內外傷辨惑論 *Nèi wài shāng biàn huò lùn*)

Astragali Radix (*huáng qí*) 10-20g
Ginseng Radix (*rén shēn*) 6-10g
Angelicae sinensis Radix (*dāng guī*) 6-10g
Atractylodis macrocephalae Rhizoma (*bái zhú*) 6-12g
Glycyrrhizae Radix (*gān cǎo*) 3-6g
Citri reticulatae Pericarpium (*chén pí*) 3-6g
Cimicifugae Rhizoma (*shēng má*) 3-6g
Bupleuri Radix (*chái hú*) 6-10g

Li Dong-Yuan, the renowned Jin-dynasty doctor, created the famous prescription Tonify the Middle to Augment the Qi Decoction (*bǔ zhōng yì qì tāng*) to treat a presentation involving internal injury to the Spleen and Stomach. This presentation is accompanied by relatively significant feverishness along with agitation or headache as well as thirst and a large pulse. This is different from the high fever from an infection as here it is a fever produced by heat from deficiency due to weakness of the patient's body. Unfortunately, Li did not write a precise set of indications and guidelines for the use of this formula. From its constituent herbs, we can see that it includes aspects of the astragalus, bupleurum, ginseng, white atractylodes, and tangkuei presentations: the spontaneous sweating with edema, propensity toward catching colds, and limb numbness of the astragalus presentation; the alternating fever and chills and chest and hypochondriac fullness and discomfort of the bupleurum presentation; the epigastric focal distention with firmness and being worn out in both body and spirit of the ginseng presentation; the edema and urinary difficulty of the white atractylodes presentation; and the abdominal and body pain of the tangkuei presentation. Specific aspects of the Tonify the Middle to Augment the Qi Decoction presentation are as follows:

1. Wan or anemic complexion, a relatively tall and thin physique, or thin now after being overweight in the past, a tender, pale red tongue with a thin, white coating
2. Subjective feeling of feverishness, or spontaneous sweating with an aversion to wind, significant whole body lethargy, a slight feeling of chest and hypochondriac fullness and discomfort, or cold hands and feet
3. May have any of the following: prolapse of the internal organs or anus, diarrhea, constipation, abdominal pain, headache, dizziness, edema, or urinary difficulty

I think this type of constitution is primarily a blend of the astragalus and bupleurum constitutions. The symptoms are a blend of the astragalus and bupleurum presentations. Therefore, this formula can be given to those who have either:

• An astragalus presentation with accompanying chest and hypochondriac fullness and discomfort, and alternating fever and chills
• A bupleurum presentation accompanied by spontaneous sweating, aversion to wind, edema, and an anemic complexion
• A Jade Windscreen presentation which at the same time shows chest and hypochondriac fullness and discomfort
• A Minor Bupleurum Decoction presentation and concurrent overall physical weakness

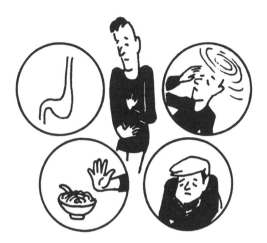

The Tonify the Middle to Augment the Qi Decoction and Bupleurum and Cinnamon Twig Decoction presentations are quite similar, the differences being:

- *Physical strength.* Those with the Tonify the Middle to Augment the Qi Decoction presentation tend to be weaker and appear to be worn out, both mentally and physically.

- *Duration of the illness.* Those with the Tonify the Middle to Augment the Qi Decoction presentation tend to have chronic diseases, while that may or may not be the case for those with the Bupleurum and Cinnamon Twig Decoction presentation.

- *Presentation.* The Bupleurum and Cinnamon Twig Decoction presentation is marked by clear cinnamon twig symptoms, namely, spontaneous sweating, aversion to wind, and abdominal or joint pain. In the Tonify the Middle to Augment the Qi Decoction presentation, it is the astragalus symptoms of edema, scanty urination, anemia, muscle weakness, and whole body fatigue that are relatively more pronounced.

  The presentations for Tonify the Middle to Augment the Qi Decoction (*bǔ zhōng yì qì tāng*) and Astragalus Decoction to Construct the Middle (*huáng qí jiàn zhōng tāng*) are also similar. However, chronic abdominal pain is the key distinguishing symptom of the Astragalus Decoction to Construct the Middle presentation, while edema, spontaneous sweating, a general sense of heaviness with muscular weakness, chronic diarrhea, and a poor appetite are the main markers of the Tonify the Middle to Augment the Qi Decoction presentation.

- Tonify the Middle to Augment the Qi Decoction (*bǔ zhōng yì qì tāng*) originally was used to treat fevers; not surprisingly, the presentation for this formula is often seen in patients with feverishness. Li Dong-Yuan said this sweet, warming formula "has the ability to eliminate severe fevers." This kind of severe feverishness obviously is not that of the White Tiger Decoction or Major Order the Qi Decoction presentations. It is instead a type of fever that is not due to an infectious process, or is of a low-grade, or which over time has become chronic in those with a weak and deficient constitution. Gan reports using this formula with higher dosages of Bupleuri Radix (*chái hú*) and Cimicifugae Rhizoma (*shēng má*) to treat 30 qi deficient patients with influenza. All of their fevers were quickly reduced, and they recovered within three to four days.[10] Li reports that of 77 children suffering from summertime fevers, 13 were treated using Tonify the Middle to Augment the Qi Decoction (*bǔ zhōng yì qì tāng*) with double the amounts of Bupleuri Radix (*chái hú*) and Cimicifugae Rhizoma (*shēng má*); on average, their fevers receded within three days. Two had relapses within a week but were cured by another round of this formula.[11]

- Patients with illnesses marked by reduced muscle tone often have this presentation. They primarily suffer from a lack of tension in the smooth muscles of the digestive tract, striated muscles, or sphincters. Because these symptoms can occur in the course of a variety of illnesses, in practice, modifications must be made to the formula. There is a report of using a version of this formula with the addition of Aurantii Fructus (*zhǐ ké*), Crataegi Fructus (*shān zhā*), Gigeriae galli Endothelium corneum (*jī nèi jīn*), Curcumae Radix (*yù jīn*), Dioscoreae Rhizoma (*shān yào*), and Jujubae Fructus (*dà zǎo*) to treat 108 patients with gastric prolapse. All of the patients had the diagnosis of reduced stomach tone and slowed peristalsis, as confirmed by X-ray imaging. After undergoing 15 to 60 days of treatment, 50.9 percent of the patients had been completely cured, 25 percent had significant improvement, and 21.3 percent experienced some effect from the treatment.[12] Gu reports using this formula to treat 23 cases of uterine prolapse. Patients were divided into those with first-degree (21.7 percent), second-degree (43.5 percent), and third-degree (34.8 percent) prolapse. After receiving treatment, 18 of the cases were cured, two had some improvement, and there was no effect in three.[13] Chen reports using this formula with the addition of Poria (*fú líng*), Coicis Semen (*yì yǐ rén*), and Malvae Fructus (*dōng kuí guǒ*) to treat 24 patients with postpartum urinary retention. Among these, 22 had undergone delivery by forceps, and the remaining two delivered naturally, but after a prolonged labor. All the patients were first treated unsuccessfully with hot compresses and then Western medication. The length of urinary retention ranged between 48 and 144 hours. Urination returned to normal, with the quickest recovery occurring after just one packet and the slowest after three packets.[14] Additionally, Tonify the Middle to Augment the Qi Decoction (*bǔ zhōng yì qì tāng*) can treat illnesses involving severe muscle weakness, renal prolapse, habitual constipation in the elderly, and prolapse of the anus.

- Illnesses such as low blood pressure, nervous exhaustion, and cerebrovascular disease often present with dizziness and headache. Patients with a tall, thin physique often have low blood pressure with accompanying symptoms of dizziness and cold limbs. Dr. He used this formula with the additions of Aurantii Fructus (*zhǐ ké*) and Schisandrae Fructus (*wǔ wèi zǐ*) as the base formula to treat 16 cases of low blood pressure, none of whom had heart disease, and whose blood pressure ranged from 80/50 to 86/56 mmHg. After a course of treatment consisting of six to 24 packets of herbs, six cases had their blood pressure reach 100/70 mmHg, and the remaining 10 cases averaged a blood pressure of 90/60 mmHg.[15] In Japan, there are reports of using this formula to treat men with low sperm counts. These men usually have symptoms of dizziness and fatigue, a thin physique, and show varying degrees of the Tonify the Middle to Augment the Qi Decoction presentation.

- People with chyluria also frequently have a Tonify the Middle to Augment the Qi Decoction presentation. Cao reports using this formula modified in accord with the differential diagnosis to treat 14 patients, with varying degrees of success in 13 of them.[16] Later he also reports treating 30 patients, with 19 being cured, eight showing improvement, and three experienceing no effect. This treatment, besides clearing the urine, also improved their anemic condition and restored their vigor and strength.[17]

- Tonify the Middle to Augment the Qi Decoction (*bǔ zhōng yì qì tāng*) is often used in conjunction with chemotherapy and radiation therapy to ameliorate their side effects. Takada et al. used 2.5 grams of an extract of this formula, which was taken three times daily for two to 21 months, to treat the adverse side effects of anticancer treatment in 15 patients. This resulted in a significant improvement in their appetite and fatigue. Furthermore, their white blood cell count remained within normal levels. Additionally, the time chemotherapy could be tolerated increased from 4.19 ± 0.48 months up to 10.17 ± 2.05 months.[18]

• The Tonify the Middle to Augment the Qi presentation is commonly seen in patients with EENT diseases. Chinese medicine holds that the five senses are the places where the clear qi is abundant. As Li Dong-Yuan stated: "Once the Stomach qi is deficient, the ears, eyes, mouth, and nose become diseased." This formula is used extensively in ophthalmology as it is effective in treating a variety of eye diseases. Effective treatment is assured when this formula's presentation is seen concurrently with diseases such as paralytic strabismus, keratitis, papilledema, optic nerve atrophy, retinitis, detached retina, corneal ulcer, cataracts, night blindness, and dry eyes. When treating eye diseases, not just the eyes should be examined, but the overall condition of the body should be taken into account. Additionally, this formula's presentation is often seen in cases of retracted tympanic membrane, tinnitus, neurogenic deafness, recurrent aphthous ulcers, chronic rhinitis, and chronic pharyngitis.

The range of practical clinical uses of Tonify the Middle to Augment the Qi Decoction (bǔ zhōng yì qì tāng) is unusually wide. Furthermore, the broader a formula's range of indications, the more important it is to be rigorous in grasping when and how it should be used.

5.6 Tonify the Yang to Restore Five-Tenths Decoction
(補陽還五湯 bǔ yáng huán wǔ tāng)

SOURCE: Correction of Errors among Physicians (醫林改錯 Yī lín gǎi cuò)

Astragali Radix (huáng qí) 12-60g
Angelicae sinensis Radix (dāng guī) 6-10g
Paeoniae Radix rubra (chì sháo) 6-12g
Pheretima (dì lóng) 3-6g
Chuanxiong Rhizoma (chuān xiōng) 3-10g
Carthami Flos (hóng huā) 3-10g
Persicae Semen (táo rén) 3-10g

This prescription, created by the famous Qing-dynasty physician Wang Qing-Ren, is directed at the treatment of hemiplegia as the sequelae from cerebrovascular accident. Wang points out: "Hemiplegia comes about when the primal qi (元氣 yuán qì) is exhausted and injured. The primal qi spreads out all over the body; if it is exhausted and injured in over half [the body], the channels and collaterals will of course follow and become empty and deficient … thereby resulting in hemiplegia." Later writers summed this up as "qi deficiency and blood stasis." Chinese medical thought holds that qi is the motive force that moves blood throughout the body. The movement of qi invigorates the blood, and when qi stagnates, the blood in turn becomes static; where there is deficiency of qi, there is also blood stasis. Whenever the qi and blood do not flourish and support the limbs, the result is withering, wasting, and paralysis. Tonify the Yang to Restore Five-Tenths Decoction *(bǔ yáng huán wǔ tāng)* is a formula that addresses this issue as it both tonifies the qi and invigorates the blood. The primary herb in this prescription is a large dose of Astragali Radix *(huáng qí)*, which strongly tonifies the qi. Angelicae sinensis Radix *(dāng guī)*, Paeoniae Radix rubra *(chì sháo)*, Chuanxiong Rhizoma *(chuān xiōng)*, Pheretima *(dì lóng)*, Carthami Flos *(hóng huā)*, and Persicae Semen *(táo rén)* are all medicinals that invigorate the blood and remove stasis. They are suitable for use in presentations involving qi deficiency and blood stasis.

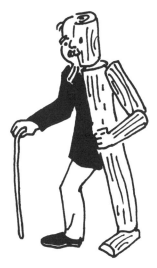

A firm grasp of the dynamics involved in the presentation of qi deficiency and blood stasis is the key to using Tonify the Yang to Restore Five-Tenths Decoction *(bǔ yáng huán wǔ tāng)* well in practice. The symptoms of qi deficiency here are primarily those of the astragalus presentation. Because up to 120g of Astragali Radix *(huáng qí)* can be used in this formula, the astragalus presentation signs of spontaneous sweating and edema, or numbness with a lack of sensation, or deficiency edema must be present. The primary signs of blood stasis will appear on the tongue as the tongue body is usually dark purple or has stasis spots. Of course, if laboratory results show increases in the viscosity of the blood, this also is an important diagnostic indicator of blood stasis. The presentation for this formula is as follows:

1. Hemiplegia, limbs that are numb and lacking sensation, or body pain
2. Edema, especially in the lower limbs, spontaneous sweating, and aversion to wind
3. The tongue is usually pale, puffy, and dark purple in color, or has stasis spots; the pulse is deep and moderate, or thin and rough

Although hemiplegia is the primary symptom addressed by this formula, its clinical applications are not limited only to it. This formula can be used in treating the sequelae of any type of cerebrovascular accident where signs of qi deficiency with blood stasis are seen, for example, ischemic cerebrovascular disease, cerebral arteriosclerosis, coronary heart disease, angina, myocardial infarction, neuritis, sciatica, headache, thromboangiitis obliterans, Takayasu's disease, as well as those with a variety of autoimmune disorders leading to chronic nephritis or systemic lupus erythematosus.

Clinical observation reveals that patients with cardiac and cerebral vascular disease receive excellent results when treated with Tonify the Yang to Restore Five-Tenths Decoction (*bǔ yáng huán wǔ tāng*); not only does it improve the usual clinical symptoms, it also reduces the level of blood viscosity. Wang reports treating 60 patients who suffered a recent (within eight days) acute cerebral thrombosis episode. Within this group, 95 percent had the clot lodged in the carotid vascular system, while five percent had it in the vertebrobasilar system; 91.7 percent of the patients had accompanying high blood pressure, 43.3 percent had coronary disease, and 20 percent suffered from diabetes. A randomized group of 30 were treated with Tonify the Yang to Restore Five-Tenths Decoction (*bǔ yáng huán wǔ tāng*), the remaining 30 subjects by way of comparison were treated with an infusion consisting of a low dose of glucose and Salviae miltiorrhizae Radix (*dān shēn*). Reviewing the results over an extended period of time, at the beginning of the treatment, both groups displayed incremental improvement; however, after two months, the rate of improvement for the group taking Tonify the Yang to Restore Five-Tenths Decoction (*bǔ yáng huán wǔ tāng*) was significantly higher than that of the comparison group. The majority of those taking this formula showed improvement after just three weeks, and achieved the best results after two months. At this juncture, 11 patients could be considered to have a complete recovery, 14 showed significant improvement, one had some improvement, and four showed no effect. Taking the herbs for longer than two months did not, however, result in any further significant improvement. Laboratory testing of the blood revealed a significant lowering of viscosity levels, fibrin content, and other indicators in the second week of the herbal treatment.[19] Zheng used this formula to treat coronary heart disease in 41 subjects. After undergoing two months of treatment, of the 21 patients who had mild angina, five had experienceed a significant effect, 13 had some improvement in their condition, and three experienceed no effect. Within this group were 26 patients whose electrocardiogram displayed chronic coronary artery insufficiency; the treatment had a significant effect for four of these patients and improvement in the condition of another 17. After four months of treatment, one other patient's condition also improved. Laboratory blood tests and impedance differential cardiograms all showed improvement.[20]

This formula is the astragalus formula family's blood-invigorating and sta-sis-transforming prescription. It is similar to Cinnamon Twig and Poria Pill (*guì zhī fú líng wán*) of the cinnamon twig family and the bupleurum family's Drive Out Stasis from the Mansion of Blood Decoction (*xuè fǔ zhú yū tāng*) in that they all treat blood stasis presentations. There are, however, significant differences. The Cinnamon Twig and Poria Pill presentation is a combina-tion of the cinnamon twig presentation with signs of blood stasis, resulting in symptoms of lower leg pain, abdominal pain when palpated, headaches, a red face, and irregular menstruation, with a purple and dark tongue body that is often tough and firm as well. The Drive Out Stasis from the Mansion of Blood Decoction presentation is a combination of the bupleurum presentation with blood stasis signs; therefore, symptoms of chest and hypochondriac fullness and discomfort, or upper abdominal distention and pain are seen. The tongue here is also frequently tough and firm. Aspects of the astragalus presentation are relatively prominent in the Tonify the Yang to Restore Five-Tenths Decoction presentation, commonly with symptoms involving motor and mental changes, simultaneously accompanied by spontaneous sweating, edema, and a dark, pale, but puffy tongue.

The presentations for Tonify the Middle to Augment the Qi Decoction (*bǔ zhōng yì qì tāng*) and for Astragalus and Cinnamon Twig Five-Substance Decoction (*huáng qí guì zhī wǔ wù tāng*) both belong to the category of qi deficiency and blood stasis, however, the degree of blood stasis seen in this formula's presentation is more severe than that of the Astragalus and Cin-namon Twig Five-Substance Decoction presentation. This is reflected in limb numbness that can advance into hemiplegia and a tongue that starts off dark and becomes purple as the condition worsens.

CHAPTER 6

GYPSUM FORMULA FAMILY

石膏類方 *shí gāo lèi fāng*

Gypsum fibrosum (*shí gāo*) is a sedimentary mineral, with a mono-clinic crystal system, and is comprised of calcium sulfate. White in color, heavy in nature, when broken it is possible to see its transparent crystal-line structure that in longitudinal view has a fine, glossy, grain-like, densely packed structure. Gypsum fibrosum (*shí gāo*) is primarily produced in the Chinese provinces of Hubei, Anhui, Henan, Shandong, Sichuan, and Gansu, with Hubei's Yingcheng City and Anwei's Fengyang City being the most famous producers of this medicinal.

Gypsum fibrosum (*shí gāo*) is a medicinal traditionally used to clear heat. *Divine Husbandman's Classic of the Materia Medica* (神農本草經 *Shén Nóng běn cǎo jīng*) states: "[It] primarily treats wind-attack with chills and fever, counterflow qi in the epigastrium, fright asthma, a dry mouth, and burnt tongue." *Miscellaneous Records of Famous Physicians* (名醫別錄 *Míng yī bié lù*) says: "[It] eliminates seasonal disease with headache and fever, intense heat in all the three burners, the skin is hot, blocked up heat in the Stomach and Intestines ... stops thirst, irritability and counterflow." For thousands of years, Chinese doctors have used Gypsum fibrosum (*shí gāo*) and its associated family of formulas to reduce fevers and eliminate irritability. Much like Rhei Radix et Rhizoma (*dà huáng*), Gypsum fibrosum (*shí gāo*) can be lifesaving to those at a critical juncture of a serious illness. Its therapeutic efficacy is thus well praised. Numerous references to the use of Gypsum fibrosum (*shí gāo*) are found within the essays and informal writing of many poets and scholars. For instance, the Qing-dynasty poet Yuan Mei details in his famous *Poems and Talks from Sui's Garden* (隨園詩話 *Suí yuán shī huà*) how he nearly died from summerheat malaria, but thanks to Gypsum fibrosum (*shí gāo*), he was cured. Ji Xiao-Lan (紀曉嵐), another Qing-dynasty literary giant, in the *Fantastic Tales* (閱微草堂筆記 *Yuè wēi cǎo táng bǐ jì*) recorded stories from many survivors of the

1793 epidemic in the nation's capital of a doctor from Tongcheng in Anhui who saved many lives using prescriptions containing large doses of Gypsum fibrosum (shí gāo). The modern medical community also has its share of experts that excel at using Gypsum fibrosum (shí gāo) to treat disease. The famous modern doctor Zhang Xi-Chun (張錫純) liked to use untreated Gypsum fibrosum (shí gāo) along with aspirin to reduce fevers in a formula called Aspirin and Gypsum Decoction (阿斯匹靈石膏湯 ā sī pǐ líng shí gāo tāng). One of Beijing's four most famous doctors in the mid-twentieth century, Kong Bo-Hua (孔伯華), because of his expertise in using Gypsum fibrosum (shí gāo), was nicknamed Gypsum Kong (孔石膏).

Gypsum Presentation (石膏證 shí gāo zhèng)

The heat presentations treated by Gypsum fibrosum (shí gāo) are not what in common parlance is referred to as fever, but rather it is a kind of illness presentation where the main symptoms are thirst, dry mouth, a hot body with profuse sweating, and a flooding and forceful pulse. Chinese doctors call this a dry and hot presentation (燥熱證 zào rè zhèng) or qi-level heat (氣熱證 qì rè zhèng); in this book, it is referred to as a gypsum presentation (石膏證 shí gāo zhèng). Dryness (燥 zào) is indicative of the patient manifesting symptoms of thirst and a dry tongue. The physiological reaction to this condition is similar to the reaction one might have to an intense summer heat wave, which is to say there is profuse sweating, thirst, irritability and restlessness, and a mild headache. This type of dry heat presentation is frequently seen in acute febrile illnesses, but also can be seen in chronic and allergic types of illnesses as well. Its distinguishing symptoms are:

1. Irritability and thirst with a desire to drink
2. Aversion to heat and profuse sweating
3. A very dry tongue
4. Large and flooding pulse, or one that is floating and slippery

Irritability and thirst with a desire to drink is indicative of the patient not only being intensely thirsty, but also being able to drink a large volume of fluids. Chinese doctors of the past used the two words 'big thirst' (大渴 dà kě) as a way of describing this condition. Aversion to heat simply means that the patients have a strong aversion to heat and are drawn toward cold environments and beverages. Heat makes them feel irritable, restless, and uneasy; additionally, they tend to sweat profusely. The profuse sweating cools the skin, which otherwise

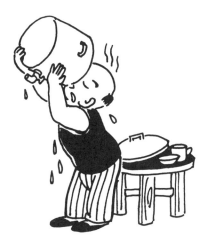

would be hot to the touch. There may be a tongue coating, but the tongue itself will surely be very dry. If the tongue coating is moist, slippery, or greasy, it is not a gypsum presentation. The large and flooding, or floating and slippery, pulse reflects the acceleration in the body's metabolic processes. Patients whose entire body feels hot and who sweat profusely frequently have this type of pulse. The above four symptoms are usually seen together, and their intensity is directly proportional to the severity of the illness.

The gypsum and rhubarb presentations are different. The latter is marked by constipation, abdominal pain and fullness with a tender abdomen, along with a red tongue and a thick, burnt yellow or greasy coating. These indicate the presence of foul, dried-out stool within the digestive tract, which is considered to be a presentation of excess heat with form. Constipation, abdominal pain, and assorted digestive system symptoms are not so prominent in the gypsum presentation; the characteristic signs here are intense thirst, fever, profuse sweating, and a large, flooding pulse. These express within the body due to an unformed, pervasive, scorching dry heat and therefore are considered to be a dry heat or qi-level heat presentation.

The gypsum and cinnamon presentations should also be differentiated as there are obvious differences between them even though there are some apparent similarities, namely, spontaneous sweating, a subjective sense of feverishness, and a large, floating pulse. Spontaneous sweating is accompanied in the cinnamon twig presentation by aversion to wind, while in the gypsum presentation there is aversion to heat with profuse sweating. The cinnamon twig presentation is without thirst, whereas the gypsum presentation has irritability along with extreme thirst. While the pulse is large in both presentations, it is also lax in the cinnamon twig presentation, while it is flooding and slippery in the gypsum presentation. What is more, the cinnamon twig presentation is commonly seen in chronic illness, while the gypsum presentation is more common in acute febrile illnesses.

The gypsum presentation can manifest within the course of many different diseases, therefore Gypsum fibrosum (*shí gāo*) is commonly paired with other medicinals. Gypsum fibrosum (*shí gāo*) used together with Anemarrhenae Rhizoma (*zhī mǔ*), as in the formula White Tiger Decoction (*bái hǔ tāng*), treats the high fever, irritability, thirst, and profuse sweating of acute febrile diseases. Gypsum fibrosum (*shí gāo*) paired with Ephedrae Herba (*má huáng*), as in the ephedra family formulas Ephedra, Apricot Kernel, Gypsum, and Licorice Decoction (*má xìng shí gān tāng*) and Maidservant from Yue's Decoction plus Atractylodes (*Yuè bì jiā zhú tāng*), treats feverishness and sweating when there is coughing and wheezing, or edema. Gypsum fibrosum (*shí gāo*) combined with Ginseng Radix (*rén shēn*), Anemarrhenae Rhizoma (*zhī mǔ*), and Astragali Radix (*huáng qí*) treats thirst from diabetes. When used with Cinnamomi Ramulus (*guì zhī*), as in the formula White Tiger plus Cinnamon Twig Decoction (*bái hǔ jiā guì zhī tāng*), it treats fever with aversion to wind or joint pain. Gypsum fibrosum (*shí gāo*) together with Rhei Radix et Rhizoma (*dà huáng*), as exemplified in the formula Saposhnikovia Powder that Sagely Unblocks (*fáng fēng tōng shèng sǎn*), treats fever, constipation, irritability, and restlessness. Some of these prescriptions have already been discussed in their respective chapters; this chapter primarily explores White Tiger Decoction (*bái hǔ tāng*) as the representative formula of the Gypsum fibrosum (*shí gāo*) formula family.

The main constituent of Gypsum fibrosum (*shí gāo*) is $CaSO_4 \cdot 2H_2O$, which only has a weak antipyretic function. However, by combining Gypsum fibrosum (*shí gāo*) with other medicinals, they synergistically manifest a relatively strong ability to clear heat.

There is a report of a decocted solution of Gypsum fibrosum (*shí gāo*) being able to reduce an animal model of excess-type fevers in rabbits. It was able to bring the fever down quickly but not able to sustain this function. The calcium ions in Gypsum fibrosum (*shí gāo*) can maintain macrophage function. As a result, Gypsum fibrosum (*shí gāo*) strengthens the immune response. Calcium also functions to reduce blood vessel permeability and acts both as an antipyretic and anti-allergen. Still, this modern pharmacological research does not seem to explain the clinical efficacy of this substance. I therefore believe that for clinical use, it is still best to follow the practices and experience of doctors who have preceded us.

6.1 **White Tiger Decoction** (白虎湯 *bái hǔ tāng*)

SOURCE: *Discussion of Cold Damage* (傷寒論 *Shāng hán lùn*)

Gypsum fibrosum (*shí gāo*) 12-30g
Anemarrhenae Rhizoma (*zhī mǔ*) 6-15g
Glycyrrhizae Radix (*gān cǎo*) 3-6g
Nonglutinous rice (*jīng mǐ*) 10g

In speaking of White Tiger Decoction (*bái hǔ tāng*), the story of its use in the treatment of epidemic encephalitis B must be told. Encephalitis B is an extremely dangerous acute infectious disease, which Western medicine also finds to be quite difficult to treat. In 1954, there was a report that drew a lot of attention; some Chinese doctors in Shijiazhuang, Hebei had used, with excellent therapeutic effect, a large dose of White Tiger Decoction (*bái hǔ tāng*) as the primary treatment of epidemic encephalitis B. Not only did this become the standard method of treatment for encephalitis B in many other places, but at the same time, it caused many of those who had doubts about Chinese medicine's methods to change their views about it. Based on domestically published statistical data, Guo compiled a report on 470 cases of epidemic encephalitis B and found that all used White Tiger Decoction (*bái hǔ tāng*) as the primary method of treatment, sometimes in combination with common biomedical emergency or supportive treatments, and that the cure rate was in the range of 80 to 100 percent, with a mortality rate that was dramatically less than normal for this disease.[1] Pharmacological research has shown that White Tiger Decoction (*bái hǔ tāng*) has significant antipyretic effect against endotoxin-induced fevers in rabbits. It also strikingly lowers the mortality rate of laboratory mice infected with the virus that causes encephalitis B.[2]

In fact, before this incident there was already a very long history of using White Tiger Decoction (*bái hǔ tāng*) to treat febrile disease. It is an important formula found in *Discussion of Cold Damage* to treat febrile diseases at their most extreme phase. Most of the prescriptions used by the Ming-dynasty physician Miao Xi-Yong, renowned for his ability in treating febrile epidemic disease, were variations of White Tiger Decoction (*bái hǔ tāng*), Lophatherum and Gypsum Decoction (*zhú yè shí gāo tāng*), and Ophiopogonis Decoction (*mài mén dōng tāng*), with the amount of Gypsum fibrosum (*shí gāo*) used frequently in the area of 30g, with a large single dosage of up to 100g. In an extreme case, a patient could take 50g in a 24-hour period. The dosage of Gypsum fibrosum (*shí gāo*) used by the famous Qing-dynasty doctor Yu Lin are an even bigger surprise. He was an expert in treating febrile epidemic diseases. In his formula Clear Epidemics and Overcome Toxicity Drink (*qīng wēn bài dú yǐn*), a modification of White Tiger Decoction (*bái hǔ tāng*), a large dosage of Gypsum fibrosum (*shí gāo*) was 180-240g and a smaller dosage was 24-36g. Observers at that time were convinced of its efficacy. The modern disease of encephalitis B belongs to the traditional category of warm pathogen epidemics (溫疫 *wēn yì*); as the dry and hot gypsum presentation commonly manifests during this disease, White Tiger Decoction (*bái hǔ tāng*) can be considered a formula with a positive traditional track record in the treatment of this disease.

Other than Gypsum fibrosum (*shí gāo*) in White Tiger Decoction (*bái hǔ tāng*), there is also the heat-clearing herb Anemarrhenae Rhizoma (*zhī mǔ*), which Chinese doctors use to treat symptoms of irritability and restlessness, a hot body, thirst, constipation, and hacking cough. Zhang Zhong-Jing commonly used the combination of Gypsum fibrosum (*shí gāo*) and Anemarrhenae Rhizoma (*zhī mǔ*) to treat (from paragraph 219) "abdominal fullness, a heavy body that is hard to rotate or bend, a lack of sensation in the mouth, a dirty face, incoherent speech, enuresis, … and spontaneous sweating," or to treat (paragraph 350) "cold damage with a slippery but faint pulse," or to treat (paragraph 176) "cold damage with a floating and slippery pulse." These presentations are just another way to describe high fever, stupor, and convulsions. It can be seen that the heat in the White Tiger Decoction presentation, with its primary herbs Gypsum fibrosum (*shí gāo*) and Anemarrhenae Rhizoma (*zhī mǔ*), is more severe than that of the gypsum presentation alone. The White Tiger Decoction presentation can be seen in the following three situations:

1. Gypsum presentation accompanied by a high fever
2. Gypsum presentation accompanied by irritability, restlessness, and muddled consciousness
3. Gypsum presentation accompanied by severe thirst

• A White Tiger Decoction presentation is very commonly seen in patients during the acute phase of viral infections that present with a high fever. In addition to epidemic encephalitis B, there are reports of this formula being used to treat infectious hemorrhagic fevers. In one report, the formula was used to treat 130 subjects, with excellent results. The associated fevers dropped significantly and there was clear improvement in the symptoms from systemic toxicity (especially those related to consciousness). Of the patients with temperatures of 40°C (104°F) and above, 91.5 percent showed temperatures returning to normal within two days. However, not all cases within this group showed improvement: 10 experienced renal failure and shock, and there was one fatality.[3]

There are numerous reports that detail the use of modifying White Tiger Decoction (*bái hǔ tāng*) with heat-clearing, toxcity-resolving, and yin-nourishing medicinals such as Lonicerae Flos (*jīn yín huā*), Forsythiae Fructus (*lián qiào*), Salviae miltiorrhizae Radix (*dān shēn*), Rhei Radix et Rhizoma (*dà huáng*), and Imperatae Rhizoma (*bái máo gēn*) to treat fevers at the qi level of disease. This formula's presentation is often seen in cases of influenza with a high fever, rheumatic fever, as well as high fevers of unknown origin. There is a report of using this formula with the addition of Isatidis/Baphicacanthis Radix (*bǎn lán gēn*) and Peucedani Radix (*qián hú*) to treat 50 patients with high fever from the flu, all of whom had their fevers recede within two days. It is important to note that in the experience of the authors of this report, if the high fever is accompanied by a lack of sweating, chills, and a mouth that is not dry or there is no thirst, then White Tiger Decoction (*bái hǔ tāng*) is not the formula to use.[4]

White Tiger Decoction (*bái hǔ tāng*) with the addition of Atractylodis Rhizoma (*cāng zhú*) is used to treat high fevers with an accompanying feeling of heaviness and fatigue and a greasy tongue coating; this formula is called White Tiger plus Atractylodes Decoction (*bái hǔ jiā cāng zhú tāng*). There is a report of using this formula with chloramphenicol to treat fevers from typhoid and paratyphoid in 173 patients, and it was found to reliably alleviate high fevers of 40°C (104°F) and control other symptoms.[5] For a persistently high fever with a sparsely coated red tongue and constipation, combining it with Increase the Fluids Decoction (*zēng yè tāng*)* strengthens the therapeutic effect. Xia treated a patient with acute transverse myelitis who had a high fever that persisted for 66 days. The biomedical doctors who had been treating him had been unsuccessful. His body temperature was successfully lowered after taking five packets of a modification of this formula.[6]

- In clinical practice, even in the absence of a high fever, the White Tiger Decoction presentation is frequently seen in cases of ophthalmologic disease, nosebleeds, summertime dermatitis, recalcitrant allergic dermatitis, acute stomatitis, or periodontitis where there are signs of aversion to heat with sweating, or irritability and restlessness with thirst. There is a report of using White Tiger Decoction (*bái hǔ tāng*) with the addition of Scutellariae Radix

---

* Rehmanniae Radix (*shēng dì huáng*), Ophiopogonis Radix (*mài mén dōng*), and Glehniae Radix (*běi shā shēn*).

(huáng qín), Forsythiae Fructus (lián qiào), and Lonicerae Flos (jīn yín huā) to treat four patients with sympathetic ophthalmia and seven who suffered from inflammation of the optic disk, all of whom had a significant increase in their visual acuity. A follow-up interview after four years confirmed the stability of the treatment.[7] Yao, a veteran Chinese doctor, had a lot of experience using White Tiger Decoction (bái hǔ tāng) to treat eye diseases. He set out four main points based on his experiences that indicate when this formula is appropriate:

1. The eyes are severely swollen and red, and symptoms of irritation are relatively severe.
2. The tongue is red and lacking moisture, or red with a dry, yellow coating.
3. The pulse is slippery and rapid, flooding and rapid, or large, flooding, and forceful.
4. The physique is robust, with a ruddy complexion, the nose is dry with a burning sensation, the lips and mouth are dry, and there is irritability and thirst with a desire to drink cold beverages.

Various types of eye diseases can be treated with this formula if they present with the above signs and symptoms.[8]

White Tiger Decoction (bái hǔ tāng) combined with Guide Out the Red Powder (dǎo chì sǎn)* was used to treat 100 children with blistering stomatitis. Within three days, 13 were symptom free, and 80 of the children had their symptoms disappear within seven days; the average time to cure was 4.8 days.[9] There is also a reported use of this formula with the addition of Glehniae/Adenophorae Radix (shā shēn), Lophatheri Herba (dàn zhú yè), Cicadae Periostracum (chán tuì), Sophorae flavescentis Radix (kǔ shēn), and Rehmanniae Radix (shēng dì huáng) to treat 40 subjects with summertime dermatitis, resulting in 24 being cured and 16 improving. It also cured drug rashes in another 13 children.[10]

The types of illnesses treated by White Tiger Decoction (bái hǔ tāng) are not limited to those discussed above. It can be used also for various types of conditions involving inflammation, infection, digestive illness, allergic disease, heat stroke, feverishness, headache and tooth pain, manic episodes, unusually strong appetite, and abnormal sweating when these are accompanied by a White Tiger Decoction presentation. However, to use this formula effectively, it is vitally important to have a good command of the White Tiger Decoction

---

* Rehmanniae Radix (shēng dì huáng), Lophatheri Herba (dàn zhú yè), Akebiae Caulis (mù tōng), and Glycyrrhizae Radix (gān cǎo).

presentation. *Systematic Differentiation of Warm Pathogen Diseases* (溫病條辨 *Wēn bìng tiáo biàn*) points out four contraindications for White Tiger Decoction (*bái hǔ tāng*):

1. A pulse that is floating or wiry and thin
2. A pulse that is sinking
3. Lack of thirst
4. Lack of sweating

A sinking pulse, lack of thirst, or the absence of sweating is usually part of an ephedra or aconite presentation; they belong to the categories of cold and/or deficiency. Their nature and that of the gypsum presentation are exactly the opposite; thus, when they appear, the use of White Tiger Decoction (*bái hǔ tāng*) is prohibited.

I believe that in differentiating the White Tiger Decoction presentation it is especially important to pay attention to the tongue and pulse. The tongue coating must be dry and without any moisture. If the tongue coating is greasy, or glossy and moist, another formula would be appropriate. In addition, the White Tiger Decoction presentation pulse feels slippery, fast, and forceful, in addition to being flooding and large.

Yue reports treating a patient who had a high fever of 41.9°C (107.4°F) and diarrhea; two packets of White Tiger Decoction (*bái hǔ tāng*) were taken in succession, but the illness was unchanged. Careful inspection of the tongue revealed that although the coating was yellow, it was not dry. Furthermore, the patient had nausea and loose stools; this is not a White Tiger Decoction presentation. Switching to the use of Kudzu, Scutellaria, and Coptis Decoction (*gé gēn huáng qín huáng lián tāng*) brought about a cure.[11]

As there are similarities, the White Tiger Decoction presentation should be clearly differentiated from that of collapse from exhaustion, as profuse sweating and a relatively large pulse are also seen during a period of collapse. Furthermore, collapse frequently manifests during a high fever, so it is easy to confuse it with the White Tiger Decoction presentation. There are quite distinct differences between the two. The sweat of a collapse syndrome is a cold sweat; the four limbs are usually cold due to counterflow; the pulse is large but empty or slightly weak; and there is low blood pressure. If White Tiger Decoction (*bái hǔ tāng*) is prescribed erroneously in these cases, the side effects will be severe, so due care must be taken

The White Tiger Decoction presentation should also be differentiated from the Cinnamon Twig Decoction presentation. Both of these formula presentations include sweating and a large, floating pulse. However, the fever of the White Tiger Decoction presentation is either a feeling of the body being hot or one with a very high temperature, and there is an intense feeling of thirst. These signs are not part of the Cinnamon Twig Decoction presentation.

6.2 White Tiger plus Ginseng Decoction
(白虎加人參湯 *bái hǔ jiā rén shēn tāng*)

SOURCE: *Discussion of Cold Damage*

Gypsum fibrosum (*shí gāo*)...12-30g
Anemarrhenae Rhizoma (*zhī mǔ*)....................................6-15g
Glycyrrhizae Radix (*gān cǎo*)..3-6g
Nonglutinous rice (*jīng mǐ*)..10g
Ginseng Radix (*rén shēn*) 6-10g

This formula's pulse presentation is clearly stated in *Discussion of Cold Damage* (paragraph 26): "If after profuse sweating from taking Cinnamon Twig Decoction (*guì zhī tāng*) there is severe irritability and unquenchable thirst along with a large, flooding pulse, White Tiger plus Ginseng Decoction (*bái hǔ jiā rén shēn tāng*) masters it"; in paragraph 168: "For those where the exterior and interior both have heat, an occasional aversion to wind, and severe thirst with a dry tongue coating, irritability, and a desire to drink large amounts of fluids, White Tiger plus Ginseng Decoction (*bái hǔ jiā rén shēn tāng*) masters it"; and in paragraph 169: "Cold damage without a high fever, dry mouth with thirst, irritability, and the back has a slight aversion to cold, White Tiger plus Ginseng Decoction (*bái hǔ jiā rén shēn tāng*) masters it." The passages found in the original text—"after profuse sweating" (大汗出後 *dà hàn chū hòu*) and "desire to drink large amounts of fluids" (欲飲水數升 *yù yǐn shuǐ shù shēng*)—both express the patient's severe sense of thirst and the relatively severe depletion of body fluids that occurs after losing a large amount of fluids from profuse sweating. This condition and that of the high fever usually associated with the White Tiger Decoction presentation discussed above are not the same. From these passages, it can also be seen that the symptoms for which Zhang Zhong-Jing would use Ginseng Radix (*rén shēn*) were depletion of fluids after sweating and a dry mouth with thirst. Other than these signs, the patients themselves feel fidgety, have chest stuffiness, shortness of breath, poor appetite, epigastric focal distention with firmness, or have lost weight.

An analysis of the formulas in *Discussion of Cold Damage* that include Ginseng Radix *(rén shēn)* shows that it is mostly used for symptoms concerning epigastric focal distention with firmness or difficulty in swallowing food. Here, *Discussion of Cold Damage* has only emphasized the particular situation that arises after severe sweating depletes the fluids, but it is a brief outline, and not very detailed.

All of the above symptoms are a reflection of the patient's severe depletion of fluids, which occurs in the aftermath of profuse sweating, severe diarrhea, or large amount of vomiting. When the body fluids have been severely depleted, the ability of the body to homeostatically regulate its internal environment is weakened, thereby falling into a state of what Chinese doctors call damage to both the qi and yin. When this occurs, Chinese medicine emphasizes the treatment principle of supporting the normal while dispelling the pathogenic (扶正驅邪 *fú zhèng qū xié*), often utilizing qi-tonifying and qi-benefiting herbs such as Ginseng Radix *(rén shēn)* that strongly tonify the primal qi to increase physical strength. Modern pharmacology has provided evidence of Ginseng Radix *(rén shēn)* being able to markedly strengthen the body's ability to regulate the neuro-endocrine systems, strengthen the immune system, and improve the function of the cardiovascular, respiratory, and digestive systems, thereby improving specific and nonspecific immunity and strengthening the body's adaptogenic abilities.

White Tiger plus Ginseng Decoction *(bái hǔ jiā rén shēn tāng)* can be used in the following three contexts:

1. Repeated episodes of sweating, feeling listless and dispirited, White Tiger Decoction presentation accompanied by severe thirst
2. The absence of a high temperature or profuse sweating, but the presence of a chronic illness with thirst as the chief complaint
3. Presence of the White Tiger Decoction presentation, but without a strong pulse, as the patient's physical condition is compromised

• White Tiger plus Ginseng Decoction *(bái hǔ jiā rén shēn tāng)* significantly reduces blood sugar levels.[12] Therefore, this formula is primarily used to treat diabetes. There are reports of such an application from both Japan and China. Dong reports using this formula to treat eight diabetes patients, resulting in the resolution of all their clinical symptoms. Fasting blood sugar levels dropped to 120mg/dl or lower, and urine glucose tests showed negative results three times in a row. There were no relapses after more than six months.[13] There is pharmacological evidence that Atractylodis Rhizoma (*cāng zhú*) can function to reduce blood sugar. This plus the fact that diabetes patients often have symptoms of irritably, thirst, a heavy feeling in their bodies, and edema can help explain why this formula is modified by the addition of Atractylodis Rhizoma (*cāng zhú*) when treating diabetics.

• The primary use of White Tiger plus Ginseng Decoction (*bái hǔ jiā rén shēn tāng*) is still the treatment of febrile diseases that manifest with irritability and thirst. Guo reports on pediatric summerheat and how its primary characteristics of fever, thirst, and copious urination coincide with this formula's presentation, which he used with satisfying results to treat 50 children.[14] There is also a report of using White Tiger plus Ginseng Decoction (*bái hǔ jiā rén shēn tāng*) with the addition of Lonicerae Flos (*jīn yín huā*), Forsythiae Fructus (*lián qiào*), Trichosanthis Radix (*tiān huā fěn*), Dioscoreae Rhizoma (*shān yào*), and Isatidis/Baphicacanthis Radix (*bǎn lán gēn*) to treat with good effect a variety of tumors with fever in 11 patients.[15] Additionally, this formula's presentation is seen in cases of sunstroke, pneumonia, tuberculous meningitis, rheumatic fever, and acute febrile illnesses where the patients are weak and debilitated.

Based on the prescribing habits of Chinese medicine doctors in my home province of Jiangsu, there are four different herbs used as 'ginseng' in White Tiger plus Ginseng Decoction (*bái hǔ jiā rén shēn tāng*). They are divided into four types: Ginseng Radix (*rén shēn*), preferably from Jilin province, Panacis quinquefolii Radix (*xī yáng shēn*), Codonopsis Radix (*dǎng shēn*), and Glehniae Radix (*běi shā shēn*). When there is an extreme amount of sweating, listless spirit, and a deficient, forceless pulse, use Ginseng Radix (*rén shēn*); when there is a dry mouth and tongue, use Panacis quinquefolii Radix (*xī yáng shēn*); when there is epigastric focal distention and a poor appetite, use Codonopsis Radix (*dǎng shēn*); and when there is accompanying hacking cough or constipation, Glehniae Radix (*běi shā shēn*) is the herb of choice.

6.3 White Tiger plus Cinnamon Twig Decoction
(白虎加桂枝湯 *bái hǔ jiā guì zhī tāng*)

SOURCE: *Essentials from the Golden Cabinet* (金匱要略 *Jīn guì yào lüè*)

Gypsum fibrosum (*shí gāo*) 12-30g

Anemarrhenae Rhizoma (*zhī mǔ*) 6-12g

Glycyrrhizae Radix (*gān cǎo*) 3-6g

Nonglutinous rice (*jīng mǐ*) 15g

Cinnamomi Ramulus (*guì zhī*) 6-10g

This formula is White Tiger Decoction (*bái hǔ tāng*) with the addition of Cinnamomi Ramulus (*guì zhī*). *Essentials from the Golden Cabinet* states: "For warm malarial diseases, with a pulse that seems normal, fever without chills, achy and bothersome joints, and occasional vomiting, White Tiger plus Cinnamon Twig Decoction (*bái hǔ jiā guì zhī tāng*) masters it." Fever without any chills (身無寒但熱 *shēn wú hán dàn rè*) is the White Tiger plus Cinnamon Twig Decoction presentation's primary symptom. At the same time, there are symptoms of irritability and restlessness, thirst or a high fever. Achy and bothersome joints belong to the cinnamon twig presentation as do the simultaneous symptoms of aversion to wind and mild sweating. The White Tiger plus Cinnamon Twig Decoction presentation is as follows:

1. Fever without chills, and thirst
2. Joint pain, aversion to wind, and sweat that comes out in patches but is ineffective in resolving the problem
3. Dark red tongue body

The White Tiger plus Cinnamon Twig Decoction presentation is often seen in cases of rheumatic fever, rheumatoid arthritis, and acute febrile illnesses. Cheng reports using a modification of this formula to treat 11 cases of rheumatic fever, resulting in the fevers receding after an average of seven days; joint swelling and pain disappeared after an average of 10.7 days.[16] Li used White Tiger plus Cinnamon Twig Decoction (*bái hǔ jiā guì zhī tāng*) with the addition of Atractylodis Rhizoma (*cāng zhú*) to treat 12 cases of rheumatic fever, resulting in a reduction of the fever within seven to 18 days.[17]

6.4 Lophatherum and Gypsum Decoction
(竹葉石膏湯 *zhú yè shí gāo tāng*)

SOURCE: *Discussion of Cold Damage*

Lophatheri Herba (*dàn zhú yè*) 10-15g

Gypsum fibrosum (*shí gāo*) 12-30g

Pinelliae Rhizoma preparatum (*zhì bàn xià*) 6-10g

Ginseng Radix (*rén shēn*) 6-10g

Ophiopogonis Radix (*mài mén dōng*) 10-12g

Glycyrrhizae Radix (*gān cǎo*) 3-6g

Nonglutinous rice (*jīng mǐ*) 15g

Discussion of Cold Damage states: "After the resolution of cold damage when there is deficiency and emaciation with shortness of breath and counterflow qi with a desire to vomit, Lophatherum and Gypsum Decoction (*zhú yè shí gāo tāng*) masters it." This formula is made by removing the Anemarrhenae Rhizoma (*zhī mǔ*) from White Tiger plus Ginseng Decoction (*bái hǔ jiā rén shēn tāng*) and then adding Lophatheri Herba (*dàn zhú yè*), Pinelliae Rhizoma preparatum (*zhì bàn xià*), and Ophiopogonis Radix (*mài mén dōng*). Based on what is recorded in *Discussion of Cold Damage*, this formula is clearly a prescription used to regulate and adjust the system during the recovery period after an acute febrile disease. Compared with the White Tiger Decoction presentation, the fever of this formula's presentation has already been weakened, and because, generally, there are neither signs of a high temperature nor of muddled consciousness, the use of Anemarrhenae Rhizoma (*zhī mǔ*) is not required. In comparison with White Tiger plus Ginseng Decoction (*bái hǔ jiā rén shēn tāng*), the degree of fluid depletion in this formula's presentation is more severe, thereby manifesting in physical emaciation, a red and sparsely coated tongue, with a dry mouth and tongue, or hacking cough. Ophiopogonis Radix (*mài mén dōng*), as stated in *Divine Husbandman's Classic of the Materia Medica*, primarily treats "emaciation and shortness of breath," and as noted in *Miscellaneous Records of Famous Physicians*, it treats "deficiency consumption from externally-contracted heat, with a parched mouth and thirst." Ginseng Radix (*rén shēn*) works synergistically with Ophiopogonis Radix (*mài mén dōng*) to promote the recovery of physical strength and restore the depleted fluids. Pinelliae Rhizoma preparatum (*zhì bàn xià*) is an anti-emetic herb; its use is aimed at "rebellious qi with a desire to vomit." Its inclusion in this formula's presentation is indicative of there being symptoms of nausea and dry heaves.

The Lophatherum and Gypsum Decoction presentation is as follows:

1. Feverish body, profuse sweating, thirst, and perhaps coughing or dry heaves

2. Listless and dispirited, emaciated, and haggard

3. Red tongue with sparse coating, the tongue body itself is dry,
    and the pulse is deficient and fast

    ....

The Lophatherum and Gypsum Decoction presentation is often seen in the
recovery period following a febrile illness or in the course of illnesses such as
sunstroke, diabetes, stomaticitis, nervous exhaustion, or bronchitis. There is a
report of treating 17 patients suffering from a low-grade fever in the aftermath
of a febrile illness. Among these, five had scarlet fever, seven were recovering
from upper respiratory tract infections, one suffered from a *Salmonella* infection, another was recovering from acute nephritis, and the source of the illness
for three patients was unknown. Using a modification of this formula resulted
in 16 patients experiencing a full recovery, with the fastest recovery occurring
after taking two packets of herb (three patients) and the slowest requiring 15
packets (one patient). On average, the fever receded after taking five packets.[18]
This formula taken internally, and the external application of a patent formula,
were used to treat 120 children with mouth ulcers. Treatment resulted in 55
children being cured within three days, 46 children were cured within four to
seven days, 12 children recovered after eight to 15 days, six children took 15 or
more days, and one child did not continue with the treatment for a sufficient
time and was not cured.[19]

After undergoing chemotherapy or radiation treatment for cancer, patients
often manifest with a dry mouth and tongue, are listless and dispirited, and
have a poor appetite and excessive sweating with a red, sparsely coated tongue.
Use of this formula will most assuredly have a therapeutic effect for these
patients. There is also a report of a modification of this formula being cooked
into a concentrated 100ml decoction—the nonglutinous rice (*jīng mǐ*) of this
formula was not part of the decoction but boiled separately—and ingested
frequently throughout the day in small amounts like tea as a preventive measure
in reducing the toxic side effects from chemotherapy in the treatment of 18
patients with malignant bone cancer. Treatment resulted in significant effect
for five patients, and some effect for another 10 patients.[w]

I once treated a case of Legionnaires' Disease where the patient had a low-
grade fever that had not receded after a month's time. Seeing that he was listless
and dispirited, and had thirst, a poor appetite, coughing, and constipation as
well as a peeled tongue coating, I prescribed this formula with the additions
of Anemarrhenae Rhizoma (*zhī mǔ*), Phragmitis Rhizoma (*lú gēn*), Dendro-
bii Herba (*shí hú*), and Glehniae/Adenophorae Radix (*shā shēn*). There was
improvement after taking five packets, and continuing to take the herbs for half
a month brought his temperature back to normal.

6.5 **Eliminate Wind Powder** (消風散 *xiāo fēng sǎn*)

SOURCE: *Orthodox Lineage of External Medicine*
(外科正宗 *Wài kē zhèng zōng*)

Gypsum fibrosum (*shí gāo*) 12g
Anemarrhenae Rhizoma (*zhī mǔ*) 6g
Atractylodis Rhizoma (*cāng zhú*) 10g
Angelicae sinensis Radix (*dāng guī*) 10g
Rehmanniae Radix (*shēng dì huáng*) 15g
Schizonepetae Herba (*jīng jiè*) 10g
Saposhnikoviae Radix (*fáng fēng*) 10g
Sophorae flavescentis Radix (*kǔ shēn*) 6g
Cicadae Periostracum (*chán tuì*) 5g
Sesami Semen nigrum (*hēi zhī má*) 12g
Arctii Fructus (*niú bàng zǐ*) 10g
Glycyrrhizae Radix (*gān cǎo*) 5g
Akebiae Caulis (*mù tōng*) 5g

Eliminate Wind Powder (*xiāo fēng sǎn*) is a well-known prescription used for treating skin diseases. A look at its constituent herbs shows it to be an augmented version of White Tiger plus Atractylodes Decoction (*bái hǔ jiā cāng zhú tāng*), which treats the White Tiger Decoction presentation when accompanied by a feeling of heaviness and fatigue, or a greasy tongue coating and an inclination toward edema. Schizonepetae Herba (*jīng jiè*), Saposhnikoviae Radix (*fáng fēng*), Arctii Fructus (*niú bàng zǐ*), and Cicadae Periostracum (*chán tuì*) all are Chinese medicine's exterior-releasing and wind-dispersing medicinals, which are frequently used to treat itching, rashes, and fever. Sophorae flavescentis Radix (*kǔ shēn*) and Akebiae Caulis (*mù tōng*) function to promote urination and clear heat, and are commonly used for urinary difficulty or edema accompanied by itchy skin, feverishness, or the oozing of yellow exudate. Angelicae sinensis Radix (*dāng guī*), Rehmanniae Radix (*shēng dì huáng*), and Sesami Semen nigrum (*hēi zhī má*) function to nourish the blood and moisten dryness; they treat itching from chronic sores and dry skin. Altogether, the herbs in this formula give it anti-allergy, antipyretic, and sedative effects. They also dilate the blood vessels and improve blood circulation in the skin, and regulate internal immunological function. In practice, the formula is frequently used to treat urticaria, acute and chronic eczema, itching disorders in the elderly, allergic dermatitis, neurodermatitis, and acute nephritis when accompanied by the following formula presentation:

1. Itchy skin with wheals or weeps when scratched that is chronic and does not improve
2. Feeling of feverishness, irritability and restlessness, and thirst
3. Tendency toward edema, or urinary difficulty

CHAPTER 7

COPTIS FORMULA FAMILY

....

黃連類方 *huáng lián lèi fāng*

Coptidis Rhizoma (*huáng lián*) has an extremely bitter taste, and chewing on it will turn the saliva a red-yellow color. There is hardly a Chinese person who is not familiar with Coptidis Rhizoma (*huáng lián*). Folk sayings like "the mute eat coptis, but cannot speak of its bitterness" and "bitter as coptis" are expressions that reflect the Chinese way of thinking that Coptidis Rhizoma (*huáng lián*) is the foremost representative of the bitter class of medicinals; they are completely clear on the idea that "bitter medicine is good for what ails you" (良藥苦口 *liáng yào kǔ kǒu*).

This medicinal has been used in China for at least two-thousand years. *Divine Husbandman's Classic of the Materia Medica* (神農本草經 *Shén Nóng běn cǎo jīng*) records that Coptidis Rhizoma (*huáng lián*), which it placed in the upper class of medicinals, "masters hot qi leading to eye pain, tearing from injury to the corners of the eyes, it can brighten the eyes, treat Intestinal flow [where food and drink run right through] with abdominal pain and dysentery, as well as swelling and pain in women's privates. With long-term use, people no longer forget." *Discussion of Cold Damage* (傷寒論 *Shāng hán lùn*) contains 12 formulas with Coptidis Rhizoma (*huáng lián*), including:

- Pinellia Decoction to Drain the Epigastrium (*bàn xià xiè xīn tāng*), which combines it with Scutellariae Radix (*huáng qín*) and Pinelliae Rhizoma preparatum (*zhì bàn xià*) to treat the focal distention presentation (痞證 *pǐ zhèng*), which is marked by epigastric focal distention, dry heaves, irritability, and a sense of unease.

- Minor Decoction [for Pathogens] Stuck in the Chest (*xiǎo xiàn xiōng tāng*), which combines it with Pinelliae Rhizoma preparatum (*zhì bàn xià*) and Trichosanthis Fructus (*guā lóu*) to treat clumping in the chest disorder (結胸 *jié xiōng*), which is marked by symptoms of epigastric pain with pressure

183

and a floating, slippery pulse.

- Coptis and Ass-Hide Gelatin Decoction (*huáng lián ē jiāo tāng*), which combines it with Scutellariae Radix (*huáng qín*) and Asini Corii Colla (*ē jiāo*) to treat *shào yīn* disease with irritability and an inability to lie down.

- Coptis Decoction (*huáng lián tāng*), which combines it with Cinnamomi Ramulus (*guì zhī*) to treat abdominal pain with a desire, but inability, to vomit.

- It is also used with Pulsatillae Radix (*bái tóu wēng*) for dysentery, and with Rhei Radix et Rhizoma (*dà huáng*) and Scutellariae Radix (*huáng qín*) to stop nosebleeds.

In the Tang dynasty *Arcane Essentials from the Imperial Library* (外台秘要 *Wài tái mì yào*) are a large number of proven formulas such as Coptis Decoction to Resolve Toxicity (*huáng lián jiě dú tāng*) where Coptidis Rhizoma (*huáng lián*) is combined with Scutellariae Radix (*huáng qín*), Phellodendri Cortex (*huáng bǎi*), and Gardeniae Fructus (*zhī zǐ*) to treat overabundant heat leading to delirium, vomiting of blood, or nosebleeds. When Coptidis Rhizoma (*huáng lián*) is combined with Rehmanniae Radix (*shēng dì huáng*) and Gypsum fibrosum (*shí gāo*), it treats wasting and thirsting disorders (diabetes). Later generations of doctors used Coptidis Rhizoma (*huáng lián*) in such formulas as Aucklandia and Coptis Pill (*xiāng lián wán*) to treat dysentery, Coptis and Perilla Drink (*lián sū yǐn*)* to stop vomiting, Restore the Left [Kidney] Pill (*zǔo guī wán*) to treat lower rib pain, and Grand Communication Pill (*jiāo tài wán*) to treat irritability and insomnia.

The scope of use for Coptidis Rhizoma (*huáng lián*) is quite extensive. Traditionally, Coptidis Rhizoma (*huáng lián*) is said to have the ability to clear and reduce the following types of fire and heat:

- *Heart fire.* The ancient Chinese believed that the human thought process and psycho-emotional activity are primarily related to the function of the Heart. Joy (or happiness) is described as 'happiness in the Heart' (心裡高 興 *xīn lǐ gāo xìng*), grief is described as 'feeling sad in the Heart' (心裡難過 *xīn lǐ nán guò*), and irritability, insomnia, muddled consciousness, delirious speech, forgetfulness, and madness are described as 'Heart fire.' Therefore, when irritability and restlessness accompany high fever, vomiting of blood, subcutaneous bleeding, hematuria, or ulcerations and erosions of the tongue and oral cavity, Coptidis Rhizoma (*huáng lián*) can be used.

---

* Coptidis Rhizoma (*huáng lián*) and Perillae Folium (*zǐ sū yè*).

- *Stomach fire.* Chinese medicine views irritability with thirst and a desire for cold beverages, bad breath, toothache and bleeding gums, or epigastric focal distention with pain as manifestations of Stomach fire.

- *Liver fire.* Chinese medicine holds that the eyes are the openings of the Liver; it then follows that when the Liver has fire, the eyes will be red, swollen, and painful, or there will be irritability, restlessness and irascibility, or headaches with dizziness.

- *Damp-heat.* This is indicated by heat symptoms involving the digestive tract such as epigastric focal distention, nausea and vomiting, stomachache, abdominal distention, dysentery, diarrhea, or bad breath, mouth sores, and hemorrhoids with accompanying feverishness in those who have a red tongue with a greasy, yellow coating.

- *Heat toxin.* This refers to bacterial infections either on or below the skin, as in sores or boils, erysipelas, or as a result of burns. These usually manifest with localized redness, swelling, heat, and pain.

Coptis Presentation (黃連證 *huáng lián zhèng*)

Are there any particularly distinctive symptoms for which the use of Coptidis Rhizoma (*huáng lián*) is indicated? Indeed there are. Guided by the usage of this herb in *Discussion of Cold Damage* and my own clinical experience, the coptis presentation is composed of the following three aspects:

1. Irritability and restlessness, or palpitations, insomnia, unclear consciousness, or a subjective feeling of feverishness
2. Digestive tract symptoms such as epigastric focal distention, stomach ache, abdominal pain, diarrhea, or nausea and vomiting
3. Red or dark red tongue body that is tough and firm, with a greasy, yellow coating that could be either thick or thin, and a somewhat dry tongue surface (also known as the 'coptis tongue')

Irritability and restlessness are the most significant symptoms in the coptis presentation. In *Discussion of Cold Damage*, Coptis and Ass-Hide Gelatin Decoction (*huáng lián ē jiāo tāng*) is the formula that has the largest dosage of Coptidis Rhizoma (*huáng lián*), using up to 12g. It treats irritability in the chest with an inability to lie down. Second to that is Coptis Decoction (*huáng lián tāng)* where up to 9g is used for heat in the chest; this is where there is a subjective oppressive feeling of stuffiness, irritability, and heat in the chest. Coptis Decoction to Resolve Toxicity *(huáng lián jiě dú tāng)*, from *Arcane Essentials from the Imperial Library*, also uses 9g of Coptidis Rhizoma *(huáng lián)* to treat heat diseases involving "extreme feelings of irritability and anxiety accompanied by a physical feeling of oppression in the chest, dry heaves, dry mouth, moaning and groaning, or an inability to lie down." Clinical experience shows that prescriptions containing Coptidis Rhizoma *(huáng lián)* have a significantly positive effect on the symptoms of anxiety and irritability. Therefore, in Chinese medicine, Coptidis Rhizoma *(huáng lián)* is said to eliminate irritability. Additionally, there can be accompanying symptoms of palpitations and nervousness, or light and easily disturbed sleep, which when severe, causes one to toss and turn without a moment of peaceful sleep. In extreme situations, it can manifest with severe psychological symptoms.

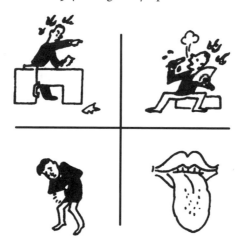

Generally in *Discussion of Cold Damage*, for cases of epigastric focal distention, Coptidis Rhizoma *(huáng lián)* and Scutellariae Radix *(huáng qín)* must be used together. What is referred to as 'epigastric focal distention' is indicative of a subjective feeling on the part of the patient of a distended and stuffy feeling in the area of the upper abdomen, the musculature of which, when palpated by the practitioner, has no feeling whatsoever of being guarded. Some patients will have a mild degree of distending pain, which is aggravated by pressure. While there are some patients who will on their own mention this kind of abdominal symptom, others whose symptoms are not primarily of a digestive nature will frequently neglect to mention this. When this occurs, the practitioner can either inquire about such symptoms or palpate the area around the solar plexus. This will usually cause some discomfort to the patient or trigger a feeling of fullness and distention; there may also be pain.

There is a certain peculiarity about the character of the tongue and tongue coating in the coptis presentation, which I refer to as the 'coptis tongue.' From my experience, the appearance of the coptis tongue, which was already discussed above, is of significant assistance in determining whether to use Coptidis Rhizoma (*huáng lián*) and its associated prescriptions. Generally speaking, a tongue that is pale, whitish, and flabby, or tender with a white, glossy or white, greasy coating is a sign of a cold presentation; these are the exact opposite of the qualities seen in the coptis presentation. Furthermore, even if the tongue body is red, but is also flabby and tender, this would fall into the category of qi or yang deficiency; Coptidis Rhizoma (*huáng lián*) also cannot be used here. To effectively use Coptidis Rhizoma (*huáng lián*), signs of the coptis tongue must be present.

There is a plethora of modern pharmacological reports concerning Coptidis Rhizoma (*huáng lián*) based on its chemical constituents, especially berberine. Here is a summary of its pharmacological activity:

- *Central nervous system effects.* Water decoctions of Coptidis Rhizoma (*huáng lián*) have the ability to reduce voluntary motor function in laboratory animals and can lengthen the hypnotic effects of pentobarbital. While small amounts of berberine can strengthen the excitatory processes in the cerebral cortex of laboratory mice, large amounts will weaken these and simultaneously strengthen inhibitory processes.

- *Antibacterial effects.* Coptidis Rhizoma (*huáng lián*) and berberine have powerful bactericidal and antibacterial effects against a variety of microbes, especially those within the digestive tract.

- *Digestive tract effects.* It stops diarrhea; promotes the secretion of saliva, gastric and pancreatic juices, and bile; and promotes peristalsis in the stomach and intestines. Water decoctions of Coptidis Rhizoma (*huáng lián*) significantly inhibit the generation of stress-related peptic ulcers in laboratory mice regardless of whether it is administered subcutaneously or orally.

- *Anti-inflammatory effects.* Using the experimental device of inducing granulomas in ova, crude preparations of Coptidis Rhizoma (*huáng lián*) as well as berberine have been shown to have clear anti-inflammatory effects.

- *Antihypertensive effects.* Both intravenous and oral administration of Coptidis Rhizoma (*huáng lián*) have antihypertensive effects. It is generally believed that its mechanism for lowering blood pressure and its direct effect on the blood vessels are related to its enhancement of acetylcholine activity.

7.1 Coptis Decoction to Resolve Toxicity
(黃連解毒湯 *huáng lián jiě dú tāng*)

SOURCE: *Arcane Essentials from the Imperial Library*

Coptidis Rhizoma (*huáng lián*)..3-6g
Scutellariae Radix (*huáng qín*)...6-10g
Phellodendri Cortex (*huáng bǎi*) 6-10g
Gardeniae Fructus (*zhī zǐ*)...6-12g

This is a well-known prescription that effectively treats acute febrile diseases. The symptomatology according to the original text reads: "illness that has lasted three days with sweating that has resolved, due to drinking alcohol there is a relapse with extreme feelings of irritability and anxiety accompanied by a physical feeling of oppression in the chest, dry heaves, dry mouth, moaning and groaning, with an inability to lay down." In *Practical Established Formulas* (成方切用 *Chéng fāng qiē yòng*), the Qing-dynasty doctor Wu Yi-Luo stated that this formula "treats all kinds of fire and heat, where there is overabundance in both the exterior and interior with mania and irritability, dry mouth and throat, severe fever and dry heaves, disordered speech, insomnia, vomiting of blood or nosebleeds. When the heat is severe enough, maculae will develop." In the past, during times of epidemic febrile disease, Coptis Decoction to Resolve Toxicity (*huáng lián jiě dú tāng*) was a formula that effectively helped to save lives. This formula can be used to treat acute infectious disease of an excess nature such as epidemic meningitis, encephalitis B, leptospirosis, septicemia, and supporative skin disease. Additionally, it treats damp-heat illnesses such as acute hepatitis, acute gastroenteritis, bacterial dysentery, and urinary tract infections. These days, even though dangerous infectious epidemics don't run rampant, Coptis Decoction to Resolve Toxicity (*huáng lián jiě dú tāng*) is still a favored formula of Chinese doctors. This is because, for some modern illnesses of middle or old age that doctors find difficult to treat, Coptis Decoction to Resolve Toxicity (*huáng lián jiě dú tāng*) demonstrates some exciting results. Japanese reports of these kinds of treatments are especially numerous. Tohkai University's Araki Goro and co-workers used Coptis Decoction to Resolve Toxicity (*huáng lián jiě dú tāng*) over a course of 12 weeks to treat 32 patients who had suffered for three months with cerebrovascular dementia. Using Hasegawa's simple consciousness inventory as a measure to judge the effectiveness of treatment, four patients had significant improvement, there was some improvement in the condition of five patients, a mild degree of improvement for another five, no change for 13, and four patients experienced a deterioration in their condition.[1] In another study, Hasegawa orally administered Coptis Decoction to Resolve Toxicity *(huáng lián jiě dú tāng)*, in granulated form, to treat the sequelae of stroke in 96 patients, resulting in a relatively good effect in the treatment of cognitive symptoms.[2]

There is evidence from pharmacological research that shows Coptis Decoction to Resolve Toxicity *(huáng lián jiě dú tāng)* lowers blood pressure, stops bleeding, increases cerebral blood flow, improves lipid metabolism, inhibits agglutination of platelets, and defends against atherosclerosis. There has already been successful experience with these new clinical usages of Coptis Decoction to Resolve Toxicity *(huáng lián jiě dú tāng)*.

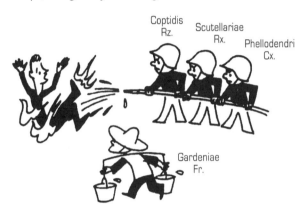

All the ingredients in Coptis Decoction to Resolve Toxicity *(huáng lián jiě dú tāng)* are important medicinals that clear heat and relieve toxicity. Coptidis Rhizoma *(huáng lián)* needs no further introduction. Scutellariae Radix *(huáng qín)*, working synergistically with Coptidis Rhizoma *(huáng lián)*, is particularly good at treating epigastric focal distention and pain, headache, abdominal pain, and bleeding. Phellodendri Cortex *(huáng bǎi)* excels at treating joint swelling and pain, jaundice, and vaginal discharge. Gardeniae Fructus *(zhī zǐ)* is also an important heat-clearing, fire-draining herb that reduces irritability, stops bleeding, and eliminates jaundice. Used together with the other three ingredients, which are known as the 'three yellows' (三黃 *sān huáng*), it gives this formula a remarkable ability to clear heat and drain fire.

In the past, Chinese doctors often used Coptis Decoction to Resolve Toxicity *(huáng lián jiě dú tāng)* to treat acute infectious disease with high fevers, changes in consciousness and disordered speech, irritability, mania, bleeding disorders and macules, and dryness of the mouth and tongue. Chinese doctors refer to this type of condition as one of 'fire, heat, and toxin.' The body, in reaction to the stimulus of toxins produced by bacteria, responds by pushing a variety of functions into a state of hyperactivity: the body temperature rises, the blood thickens, the heart rate and blood pressure both rise, and there is increased activity in the cerebral cortex. Coptis Decoction to Resolve Toxicity (*huáng lián jiě dú tāng*) is effective in eliminating the source of the illness and acting against bacterial toxins; it is also effective as it has antipyretic and anti-inflammatory activity and can promote immune function, acting as a sedative, anticoagulant, and haemostatic. While of course chronic illnesses such as hypertension, cerebral infarction, and senile dementia are not acute contagious diseases, some of these patients also manifest with 'fire or heat' syndromes such as restlessness, fretfulness, and insomnia or emotional disturbances, and have a red, congested face, dry mouth and tongue, and heaviness in the head or headache. In these situations, Coptis Decoction to Resolve Toxicity (*huáng lián jiě dú tāng*) can be used. The Chinese medicine adage that "The same treatment can be effective for different illnesses" (異病同證, 異病同治 *yì bìng tóng zhèng, yì bìng tóng zhì*) is, in principle, the same idea as the previously noted adage, "Prescribe herbs to match the presentation" (有是證便用是方 *yǒu shì zhèng biàn yòng shì fāng*).

The following four items sum up the presentation of Coptis Decoction to Resolve Toxicity (*huáng lián jiě dú tāng*):

1. Irritability, restlessness, anxiety or depression
2. Red face, fire rising upward, dark red lips, tendency toward bleeding
3. Coptis tongue
4. Epigastric focal distention with a feeling of stuffiness and discomfort or dull pain in the upper abdomen when palpated

The above list of symptoms gives insight into the range of use for Coptis Decoction to Resolve Toxicity (*huáng lián jiě dú tāng*). Item number 1 points out the neurological and psychological issues it treats, numbers 2 and 3 reflect pathologic changes in the circulatory system, and number 4 lists the digestive symptoms. In practice, it is not uncommon for patients with digestive symptoms to rarely speak of these as their main complaint; it is only from the interview or palpation of the abdomen that they are discovered.

Patients with the Coptis Decoction to Resolve Toxicity presentation for the most part are strong and robust men who have a red or purplish complexion, whose lips and mouth are dark red, and have a dry, dark red, firm, and tough tongue with a greasy, yellow coating. The interview can be used to discover if the patient has psycho-emotional symptoms such as irritability, restlessness, insomnia, anxiety or depression, headaches with dizziness, loss of memory or problems with concentration. Palpation can reveal epigastric focal distention and stuffiness with discomfort, or increase in resistance of the tissues and tenderness.

This feeling of stuffiness and discomfort (悶不適感 *mēn bù shì gǎn*) is indicative of a kind of discomfort that is like pain, but not particularly painful, or like a feeling of bloating, but there is no visible distention. In practice, patients come in with all kinds of different main complaints when they have this problem. Some say they feel uncomfortable, that their stomach hurts, or that they feel bloated.

A biomedical examination may reveal hypertension, slight tachycardia, or polycythaemia (elevated levels of hemoglobin). The Japanese practitioner Maruyama Ikuro put forth the idea that there are similarities between the Coptis Decoction to Resolve Toxicity presentation and biomedicine's Gaisböck syndrome (also known as polycythemia hypertonica or pseudopolycythaemia). He discovered that in Gaisböck syndrome patients, 40 to 50 percent of their platelet agglutination mechanism, as found in cases of hyperfibrinogenemia, was hyperfunctioning. This is to say that patients with a Coptis Decoction to Resolve Toxicity presentation and those with Gaisböck syndrome are both in a state where there is hyperfunctioning of the agglutinating process, resulting in an increase in the viscosity of the blood.[3] While in practice it is not common to use biomedical test data, as we have our traditional methods of observation and diagnosis, this can nonetheless serve as a microscopic indicator of the Coptis Decoction to Resolve Toxicity presentation and provide the reader with something to consider in their clinical work should they have access to these kinds of test results.

There are reports that Coptis Decoction to Resolve Toxicity (*huáng lián jiě dú tāng*) has been effective in treating hypertension, Behcet's disease, favism, allergic purpura, various skin problems, and trigeminal nerve pain; topically applied, it is also effective in treating cervical erosion.

Coptis Decoction to Resolve Toxicity (*huáng lián jiě dú tāng*) with the addition of Four-Substance Decoction (*sì wù tāng*)* is called Warming and Clearing Drink (*wēn qīng yǐn*), which is a well-known prescription commonly used in the Japanese Kampō tradition. Due to the addition of the blood-nourishing

---

* Rehmanniae Radix preparata (*shú dì huáng*), Angelicae sinensis Radix (*dāng guī*), Paeoniae Radix (*sháo yào*), and Chuanxiong Rhizoma (*chuān xiōng*).

and blood-invigorating Four-Substance Decoction (*sì wù tāng*), this formula's scope of usage is broader than that of Coptis Decoction to Resolve Toxicity (*huáng lián jiě dú tāng*). It is especially applicable for the Coptis Decoction to Resolve Toxicity presentation where there is a tendency toward bleeding or for women with irregular periods.

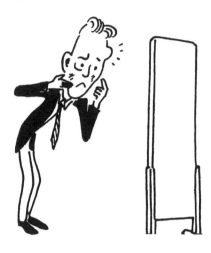

Warming and Clearing Drink (*wēn qīng yǐn*), with the addition of Schizonepetae Herba (*jīng jiè*), Forsythiae Fructus (*lián qiào*), Menthae haplocalycis Herba (*bò hé*), Bupleuri Radix (*chái hú*), Platycodi Radix (*jié gěng*), Angelicae dahuricae Radix (*bái zhǐ*), and Glycyrrhizae Radix (*gān cǎo*), becomes Schizonepeta and Forsythia Decoction (*jīng jiè lián qiào tāng*). It is primarily used for inflammation involving the head and can treat chronic and acute tonsillitis, sinus infections, folliculitis, conjunctivitis, otitis media, and acne with headache, a red face, and fever. From the perspective of Chinese medicine, these symptoms of inflammation involving the head and face all fall within the category of fire and heat. Use of heat-clearing herbs is indispensable; at the same time, they are generally paired with herbs that clear the head and benefit the eyes. Schizonepetae Herba (*jīng jiè*) is fragrant and aromatic; it has a light and subtle ability to resolve heat and induce sweating. It is often used to treat common colds with headache, fever, red eyes, swollen, painful throat, and itchy skin conditions. Forsythiae Fructus (*lián qiào*) is bitter and has been used throughout history as a principal herb in the treatment of sores. Menthae haplocalycis Herba (*bò hé*) is cool and acrid, and treats headache, fever, and EENT diseases. According to *Comprehensive Outline of the Materia Medica* (本草綱目 *Běn cǎo gāng mù*), not only does Bupleuri Radix (*chái hú*) treat alternating fever and chills or chest and hypochondriac fullness and discomfort, it also treats "headaches with vertigo, and cloudy vision; red and painful eyes, weak eyesight with superficial visual obstructions; and loss of aural acuity and tinnitus." Platycodi Radix (*jié gěng*) is an important medicinal for sore throats, and Angelicae dahuricae Radix (*bái zhǐ*) treats all kinds of illnesses involving the head and face; it is an especially important herb in the treatment of headache and nasal problems. These above-mentioned herbs, which clear the head and benefit the eyes, when paired with the heat-clearing, fire-draining Warming and Clearing Drink (*wēn qīng yǐn*), focus its effect even more on the head and face.

The medicinals in Coptis Decoction to Resolve Toxicity (*huáng lián jiě dú tāng*) and other members of its formula family are all of a bitter and cold or acrid and cool nature. Therefore, they should not be used with those who do not have a yang-heat constitution. The salient points of the 'yang-heat constitution' (陽熱體質 *yáng rè tǐ zhì*) are as follows:

- *Distinguishing external characteristics.* Relatively strong and robust physique, flushed or blackish red complexion with an oily sheen, bloodshot eyes with a copious, gummy discharge, dark red or purple red lips, a red or dark red tongue body that is firm, tough and inflexible with a thin and yellow or greasy and yellow coating; and abdominal musculature that is relatively tight with a resistance to palpation or that causes the patient some discomfort when pressure is applied. The coptis tongue is distinguished by being dark and firm due to the presence of old congested blood that is the result of heat impairing the circulation of blood; when extended, it is stiff like a piece of wood as well as tight and contracted, so it does not protrude very far.

- *Predisposition.* Usually favors cold and is averse to heat, enjoys cold beverage, is easily agitated, anxious and physically restless, with a propensity toward insomnia and excessive dreaming; frequent sores and boils, upper abdominal focal distention with a feeling of stuffiness and discomfort, dry mouth with a bitter taste, frequent mouth and tongue sores, sore throat, and scanty, yellow urine.

7.2 **Coptis Decoction** (黃連湯 *huáng lián tāng*)

Source: *Discussion of Cold Damage*

Coptidis Rhizoma (*huáng lián*) 3-6g
Cinnamomi Ramulus (*guì zhī*) 5-10g

Zingiberis Rhizoma (*gān jiāng*) 3-6g
Glycyrrhizae Radix (*gān cǎo*) 3-6g
Ginseng Radix (*rén shēn*) 5-10g
Pinelliae Rhizoma preparatum (*zhì bàn xià*) 6-10g
Jujubae Fructus (*dà zǎo*) 10g

The *Discussion of Cold Damage's* description (paragraph 173) of the presentation for Coptis Decoction (*huáng lián tāng*) is fairly simple: "Cold damage, with heat in the chest and pathogenic qi in the Stomach, abdominal pain and a desire to vomit, Coptis Decoction (*huáng lián tāng*) masters it." Over time, the range of practical clinical applications for this formula grew to become quite extensive. For those with gastrointestinal symptoms that accompany cardiovascular and febrile diseases as well as stomatitis, drunkenness, or insomnia, this formula is rather effective.

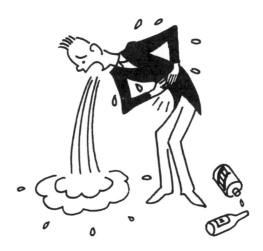

Because of the absence of Scutellariae Radix (*huáng qín*), Phellodendri Cortex (*huáng bǎi*), and Gardeniae Fructus (*zhī zǐ*), the heat-clearing and fire-draining effect of this formula is not as strong as that of Coptis Decoction to Resolve Toxicity (*huáng lián jiě dú tāng*). Because it does contain Cinnamomi Ramulus (*guì zhī*) and Zingiberis Rhizoma (*gān jiāng*), Coptis Decoction (*huáng lián tāng*) can be seen as a conglomeration of the coptis, cinnamon twig, and dried ginger presentations. Its use is appropriate when treating patients of the cinnamon twig constitution who exhibit concurrent coptis and dried ginger presentations, or for those with a coptis presentation who also have aversion to wind, spontaneous sweating, abdominal pain with diarrhea, and a thick tongue coating. The Coptis Decoction presentation is as follows:

1. Aversion to wind, feverishness, and sweating
2. Irritability and restlessness, palpitations
3. Epigastric focal distention as well as perhaps vomiting, abdominal pain, or diarrhea
4. Red or dark red tongue with either a relatively thick, greasy coating or one that is thin on the front and becomes thick and white on the back of the tongue

Aversion to wind, feverishness, and sweating are aspects of the cinnamon twig presentation. The distinctive signs of the Coptis Decoction presentation are sweating accompanied by unremitting fever or having a fever that does not clear; in more severe cases, the sweating is accompanied by irritability and restlessness. The sweating here can be either of a spontaneous nature or that of night sweats. In some cases, there is no measurable fever, however, these patients have a subjective sense of feverishness. Irritability and restlessness are part of the Coptis Decoction presentation; palpitations are part of the Cinnamon Twig Decoction presentation. It follows then that this formula's presentation would include irritability and restlessness along with palpitations. Apart from those with the aforementioned signs, there are also those whose irritability and restlessness are accompanied by an upward-rushing sensation in the chest; other patients will present with irritability and restlessness, a hot body, sweating, and a stifling feeling in the chest. In clinical practice, there are many patients whose main complaint does not concern irritability or restlessness; in order to understand whether a similar process is occurring, the practitioner should inquire about their mood, ability to concentrate, and sleep.

Symptoms of epigastric focal distention with vomiting, abdominal pain, or diarrhea occur in both the coptis and dried ginger presentations. Patients with a Coptis Decoction *(huáng lián tāng)* presentation usually have a thick tongue coating, or one that is both white and yellow, or white underneath but covered by a yellow coating, or one that is thick, dry, and a little sticky. One particular characteristic of the tongue coating is that the back part is thicker and white in color. The tongue body itself, or at least its sides and tip, tends to be red. People who overindulge in food and drink, as well as alcoholics, often have this type of tongue. Chinese medicine regards this as a situation of retained dampness and lurking heat (濕過熱伏 *shī è rè fú*). In these circumstances, the bitter flavor of Coptidis Rhizoma *(huáng lián)* and the acrid flavor of Zingiberis Rhizoma *(gān jiāng)* must be used together, as acrid herbs open up areas of dampness and bitter herbs drain away the heat.

I once treated a man who had a fever for over a week and for whom a variety of herbs used to treat colds had all been ineffective. Before his fever, he had chills throughout the body, which was followed by a fever with sweating. Although the fever would decrease with the sweating, it never completely went away. Additionally, the skin was usually moist from very slight sweating; there was a stifling feeling in the chest, epigastric focal distention with firmness, and occasional watery diarrhea with gurgling sounds from the intestines. He had a red tongue with a thick, greasy coating at the center and rear. After taking Coptis Decoction (*huáng lián tāng*), he experienced a whole body therapeutic sweat and was cured.

7.3 Minor Decoction [for Pathogens] Stuck in the Chest
(小陷胸湯 *xiǎo xiàn xiōng tāng*)

SOURCE: *Discussion of Cold Damage*

Coptidis Rhizoma (*huáng lián*)..3-6g
Trichosanthis Fructus (*guā lóu*) 12-20g
Pinelliae Rhizoma preparatum (*zhì bàn xià*) 6-10g

When the coptis presentation is accompanied by epigastric focal distention and pain that is aggravated by pressure along with constipation, or is accompanied by chest and hypochondriac fullness and discomfort, coughing and wheezing with sticky, sometimes yellow, sputum, merely using Coptidis Rhizoma (*huáng lián*) is not going to solve the problem. In this situation, it is generally recognized that Minor Decoction [for Pathogens] Stuck in the Chest (*xiǎo xiàn xiōng tāng*) should be used.

This formula is made by combining Trichosanthis Fructus (*guā lóu*) and Pinelliae Rhizoma preparatum (*zhì bàn xià*) with Coptidis Rhizoma (*huáng lián*). Trichosanthis Fructus (*guā lóu*) is a gourd that is the mature fruit of the trichosanthes plant. Its peel, Trichosanthis Pericarpium (*guā lóu pí*), and seeds, Trichosanthis Semen (*guā lóu rén*), are both used as medicine, however they have different functions. Trichosanthis Pericarpium (*guā lóu pí*) is mostly used for coughs with sticky phlegm, while the seeds are used to treat constipation. In this formula, both the skin and seeds are used together. Pinelliae Rhizoma preparatum (*zhì bàn xià*) is a commonly used medicinal in Chinese medicine, as noted in *Divine Husbandman's Classic of the Materia Medica*: "It [treats] cold damage with fever and chills, firmness in the epigastrium, a distended feeling in the chest, coughing, dizziness, swollen and painful throat, borborygmus and flatulence, and stops sweating." Furthermore, *Miscellaneous Records of Famous Physicians* (名醫別錄 *Míng yī bié lù*) states that it "eliminates fullness and hot clumped phlegm from the Heart, abdomen, chest and diaphragm; treats coughing with ascending qi, urgency and pain in the epigastrium, focal distention with firmness, and vomiting from seasonal diseases." In this formula, Pinelliae Rhizoma preparatum *(zhì bàn xià)* is primarily used to treat symptoms of chest and hypochondriac fullness and swelling, focal distention with pain, and coughing.

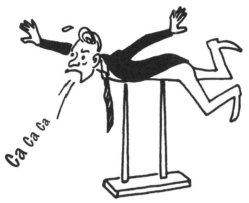

Discussion of Cold Damage says that Minor Decoction [for Pathogens] Stuck in the Chest *(xiǎo xiàn xiōng tāng)* is used to treat a type of disease presentation called "minor clumping in the chest" (小結胸 *xiǎo jié xiōng*). Its primary symptoms are focal distention with a stifling feeling in the chest, hypochondriac, and epigastrium, all of which are made worse when pressed. To confirm the Minor Decoction [for Pathogens] Stuck in the Chest presentation, there must be symptoms of pain in the chest and epigastrium. The specific presentation is as follows:

1. Focal distention and pain in the upper abdomen, chest, and hypochondriac that is aggravated when pressed
2. Red tongue body with a greasy, yellow coating
3. Constipation, or nausea, or coughing with wheezing, and sticky or viscous, yellow sputum

In practice, there is a marked tendency to see the Minor Decoction [for Pathogens] Stuck in the Chest presentation in illnesses of the respiratory, digestive, and neurological systems. This would include bronchitis, pneumonia, pleuritis, chronic and acute gastritis, biliary tract disease, autonomic dystonia, intercostal neuralgia, and hypertension or coronary heart disease.

- This formula treats digestive tract disorders where there are symptoms of pain in the upper abdomen upon palpation, or distending oppressive pain, nausea with vomiting, epigastric discomfort with acid regurgitation, or constipation, with a yellow, greasy coating at the root of the tongue and a wiry or slippery pulse. Commonly for this purpose, Aurantii Fructus immaturus (zhǐ shí) or Gardeniae Fructus (zhī zǐ) is added. There is a report of treating 83 cases of stomach ache; among these cases, 36 had acute or chronic gastritis, 30 had peptic ulcers, and 17 had gastric neurosis. Treatment resulted in a complete cure for 52 cases, improvement in the condition of 29, and no effect for two. The treatment proved most effective for the patients with acute or chronic gastritis.[4] This formula with the addition of Aurantii Fructus immaturus (zhǐ shí) and Paeoniae Radix rubra (chì sháo) was used to treat 26 patients with phlegm-heat type epigastric pain. Patients were given from three to 30 packets of herbs, with the average being 14 packets; all the patients were cured. One to two months after discontinuing the herbs, four patients experienced a relapse; after taking between another nine to 15 packets of herbs, they were cured.[5] This formula is also effective in treating biliary tract disease. It is reported that a modification of this formula was used with satisfactory results to treat 11 cases of biliary ascariasis.[6] The *Revised Popular Guide to the Discussion of Cold Damage* (通俗傷寒論 *Tōng sú shāng hán lùn*) formula Bupleurum Decoction [for Pathogens] Stuck in the Chest (*chái hú xiàn xiōng tāng*), which is composed of this formula with the addition of Bupleuri Radix (*chái hú*), Scutellariae Radix (*huáng qín*), Aurantii Fructus immaturus (*zhǐ shí*), Platycodi Radix (*jié gěng*), and Zingiberis Rhizoma recens (*shēng jiāng*), can also be used in the treatment of cholecystitis.

- Minor Decoction [for Pathogens] Stuck in the Chest (*xiǎo xiàn xiōng tāng*) can be used for respiratory illness where there are symptoms of chest pain, coughing with sticky, yellow phlegm, and a thick, yellow, greasy coating on the tongue. *Comprehensive Medicine According to Master Zhang* (張氏醫通 *Zhāng shì yī tōng*) observes: "Coughing that causes the face to turn red, heat commonly in the chest, abdomen, and hypochondria such that only the hands and feet at times feel cold, along with a flooding pulse, is hot phlegm above the diaphragm, and this formula masters it."

I have treated many patients with cases of bronchitis whose coughs either did not respond to or were not helped much by conventional treatment methods.

Based clinically on coughing with viscous, yellow sputum, chest and hypochondriac pain, epigastric focal distention, a yellow, greasy tongue coating, and constipation, the use of this formula brings quick relief with an effect usually being seen after taking three to seven packets of herbs.

There is a report of using Minor Decoction [for Pathogens] Stuck in the Chest (*xiǎo xiàn xiōng tāng*) together with Ephedra, Apricot Kernel, Gypsum, and Licorice Decoction (*má xìng shí gān tāng*) to treat 50 cases of pediatric bronchitis, resulting in 37 being cured, seven showing improvement in their condition, and six being unchanged. By comparison, another 50 cases were treated with only Ephedra, Apricot Kernel, Gypsum, and Licorice Decoction (*má xìng shí gān tāng*), resulting in 26 cases being cured, five experiencing some improvement, and 19 experiencing no effect. Fevers receded in an average of 2.4 days for the first group and 3.5 days for the second. The average time it took for the coughing and wheezing to resolve, and for other signs such as the complete blood count (CBC) and chest X-rays to return to normal, were better when both formulas were used together.[7] In practice, this formula is commonly modified to treat respiratory illness, or it is combined with Three-Unbinding Decoction (*sān ǎo tāng*),* Honeysuckle and Forsythia Powder (*yín qiào sǎn*),† Trichosanthes Fruit and Chinese Chive Decoction (*guā lǒu xiè bái tāng*),‡ or Ephedra, Apricot Kernel, Gypsum, and Licorice Decoction (*má xìng shí gān tāng*).§

- This formula combined with Frigid Extremities Powder (*sì nì sǎn*) is effective in treating coronary heart disease with angina.

The differences between the presentation for this formula and that of Pinellia Decoction to Drain the Epigastrium (*bàn xià xiè xīn tāng*), discussed in Chapter 10, are as follows:

- *Level of discomfort.* In the Pinellia Decoction to Drain the Epigastrium presentation, focal distention and discomfort are the primary symptoms, whereas with this formula, there is focal distention with pain.

- *Location.* The focal distention and stuffiness in the Pinellia Decoction to Drain the Epigastrium presentation is centered in the epigastrium, while the

---

* Ephedrae Herba (*má huáng*), Armeniacae Semen (*xìng rén*), and Glycyrrhizae Radix (*gān cǎo*).

† Lonicerae Flos (*jīn yín huā*), Forsythiae Fructus (*lián qiào*), Schizonepetae Herba (*jīng jiè*), Platycodi Radix (*jié gěng*), Glycyrrhizae Radix (*gān cǎo*), Menthae haplocalycis Herba (*bò hé*), Arctii Fructus (*niú bàng zǐ*), Lophatheri Herba (*dàn zhú yè*), and Sojae Semen preparatum (*dàn dòu chǐ*).

‡ Trichosanthis Fructus (*guā lóu*) and Allii macrostemi Bulbus (*xiè bái*).

§ Ephedrae Herba (*má huáng*), Armeniacae Semen (*xìng rén*), Gypsum fibrosum (*shí gāo*), and Glycyrrhizae Radix (*gān cǎo*).

focal distention and pain of the Minor Decoction [for Pathogens] Stuck in the Chest presentation is more spread out in the upper abdomen, chest, and hypochondria.

• *Bowel movements.* There can be loose stools, boborygmus, and poor appetite with the Pinellia Decoction to Drain the Epigastrium presentation, while for this formula's presentation, there is constipation with sticky, yellow mucus in the stool.

7.4 **Drain the Epigastrium Decoction** (瀉心湯 *xiè xīn tāng*)

SOURCE: *Essentials from the Golden Cabinet* (金匱要略 *Jīn guì yào lüè*)

Coptidis Rhizoma (*huáng lián*)..3g
Scutellariae Radix (*huáng qín*)..6g
Rhei Radix et Rhizoma (*dà huáng*)...6g

Drain the Epigastrium Decoction (*xiè xīn tāng*), also known as Three-Yellow Drain the Epigastrium Decoction (*sān huáng xiè xīn tāng*), is a powerful prescription that clears heat and drains fire. In *Essentials from the Golden Cabinet* it is used to treat vomiting of blood and nosebleeds. The original text states: "For insufficiency of Heart qi (心氣不足 *xīn qì bù zú*) with vomiting and nosebleeds, Drain the Epigastrium Decoction (*xiè xīn tāng*) masters it." How are we to understand this concept of "insufficiency of Heart qi"? *Important Formulas Worth a Thousand Gold Pieces* (千金要方 *Qiān jīn yào fāng*) uses the often misunderstood phrase "instability of Heart qi" (心氣不定 *xīn qì bù dìng*). Many doctors from later generations believe this is mistake that has been passed down over the years through erroneous copied manuscripts and that instability of Heart qi is in fact exuberant Heart fire (心火旺盛 *xīn huǒ wàng shèng*). I believe that something similar has occurred in *Essentials from the Golden Cabinet*. Accordingly, this formula's presentation should include the heat symptoms of irritability, restlessness, and an inability to calm down. Extrapolating from the herbs that comprise this prescription, this formula's presentation can be seen as a synthesis of the coptis and rhubarb presentations, or it could be said to be a prescription for those with a rhubarb constitution where signs of the coptis presentation are also found. Specifically, the presentation for Drain the Epigastrium Decoction (*xiè xīn tāng*) is as follows:

1. Irritability, restlessness, inability to calm down, a flushed, red face, or signs of the rhubarb constitution

2. Epigastric focal distention, and constipation
3. A dark red, tough, and firm tongue, with a greasy, yellow, or dry coating (coptis tongue)
4. An excessive, forceful, rapid, slippery pulse
5. Vomiting of blood, nosebleeds, or a tendency to easily bleed

This is to say that if a patient is ordinarily listless and dispirited, with a desire for warmth and aversion to cold, is anemic and debilitated, has watery stools and edema, with a whitish yellow complexion, loose musculature, a puffy, pale tongue with a white, slippery, wet coating, it is inappropriate to use Drain the Epigastrium Decoction (xiè xīn tāng). The reader should pay close attention to this point as the nature of the above-mentioned presentation is one of cold and deficiency, and quite different from the hot excess of the (Three-Yellow) Drain the Epigastrium Decoction presentation; care must be taken that it is not mistakenly prescribed for these patients.

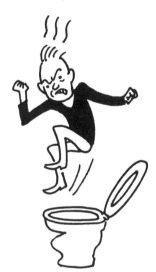

• Pyogenic infections, especially furuncles, swellings on the head and face, conjunctivitis, or pustulated and swollen tonsils that manifest with redness, swelling, heat and pain are often seen with the Drain the Epigastrium Decoction presentation. Surveying the results of 350 cases which were treated with this formula for various types of inflammation due to infections showed that, for most ordinary types of inflammation, the formula does have an effect. Furthermore, it is relatively effective at treating bacterial dysentery, chronic gastroenteritis, tonsillitis, and pleuritis. It is also effective in treating cystitis, urethritis, and pelvic inflammatory disease, especially for chronic gastroenteritis and tonsillitis.[8] In one report, this formula with the addition of Chuanxiong Rhizoma (chuān xiōng), Angelicae sinensis Radix (dāng guī), Lonicerae Flos (jīn yín huā), Forsythiae Fructus (lián qiào), Taraxaci Herba (pú gōng yīng), Olibanum (rǔ xiāng), Myrrha (mò yào), and Glycyrrhizae Radix (gān cǎo) was used to treat 75 patients with suppurative inflammations. Among these were 14 cases of appendicitis (either acute or an acute flare-up in patients with chronic appendicitis), seven cases of acute mastitis or breast abscess, 16 cases of recurrent furuncles, 11 cases of furuncles complicated by lymphadenitis, eight cases of infection due to trauma, and 11 cases of acute abscesses. Good results occurred in both the 33 cases for which only Drain the Epigastrium Decoction (xiè xīn tāng) was used as well as the 42 cases for which it was used in combination with antibiotics (sometimes having the antibiotics used first).[9]

- Bleeding disorders with vomiting of blood, coughing up of blood, or nosebleeds are often seen with this formula's presentation. In a comparative standard-of-care study, the Chengdu College of Traditional Chinese Medicine made a granulated form of this formula that was used to treat 103 patients with upper digestive tract bleeding due to either ulcers or inflammation. Treatment resulted in a complete recovery for 86 patients, significant improvement for 10, some effect for two, and no effect for five. The control group of 72 patients in this study was treated with either orally administered norepinephrine or an injection of etamsylate, resulting in a cure for 38 patients, significant effect for 18, some improvement for another 12, and no effect for four.[10] Gao used a modification of this formula to treat 105 cases of acute pulmonary bleeding. Of these, there were 60 cases of X-ray diagnosed pulmonary tuberculosis, 34 cases of bronchiectasis, six cases of lung cancer, and five cases of coronary heart disease. In addition, the blood lost by these patients was 60 to 500ml in a 24-hour period. Treatment resulted in the cessation of bleeding within two to three days after taking the herbs in 53 cases, and within four days in another 44 cases. The remaining eight cases, in which the bleeding had not stopped after four days, were switched to Western medication.[11] There is also a report of the use of this formula in treating nosebleeds, spitting up of blood due to endometriosis, as well as bleeding from disseminated intravascular coagulation.

- The presentation for this formula can be seen in people with cardiovascular and cerebrovascular diseases. In Japan, Drain the Epigastrium Decoction (xiè xīn tāng) is extensively used for hypertension, arteriosclerosis, stroke, cerebral infarction, hypercholesterolemia, and hyperlipidemia when accompanied by symptoms of a red face, constipation, headache, chest stuffiness, and a feeling of unease.

- Psycho-emotional illness often falls into the category of instability of Heart qi and is often seen with this formula's presentation in cases of everything from insomnia to schizophrenia.

7.5 Coptis and Ass-Hide Gelatin Decoction
(黃連阿膠湯 *huáng lián ē jiāo tāng*)

Source: *Discussion of Cold Damage*

Coptidis Rhizoma (*huáng lián*)......................................3-6g
Scutellariae Radix (*huáng qín*).....................................6-10g
Paeoniae Radix (*sháo yào*)...6-10g
Asini Corii Colla (*ē jiāo*)...10g
Egg yolk (*jī zǐ huáng*)...2 yolks

This is the coptis formula family's prescription for clearing heat, draining fire, and stopping bleeding. It is suitable to use in the treatment of all types of bleeding illnesses accompanied by irritability in the chest with an inability to get to sleep. Irritability is fundamental to the coptis presentation, and the inability to get to sleep shows that the patient's condition is more serious. Asini Corii Colla (*ē jiāo*) traditionally has been used to tonify blood and stop bleeding. It treats all kinds of bleeding presentations such as vomiting of blood, nosebleeds, hematuria, blood in the stool, and metrorrhagia. Almost all of the formulas found in *Discussion of Cold Damage* and *Essentials from the Golden Cabinet* that contain Asini Corii Colla (*ē jiāo*) have to do with conditions involving blood loss. Although the text in *Discussion of Cold Damage* concerning Coptis and Ass-Hide Gelatin Decoction (*huáng lián ē jiāo tāng*) does not mention bleeding or loss of blood, it can be inferred from the formulas' composition that it can treat the presentation of blood loss and irritability with an inability to get to sleep. The Coptis and Ass-Hide Gelatin Decoction presentation is as follows:

1. Irritability with an inability to get to sleep
2. Tendency toward bleeding disorders or any type of bleeding
3. Ashen pallor, listless and dispirited, dry mouth and throat, heat in the palms and soles, tinnitus, dizziness, scanty, yellow urine, and macerated tongue and oral cavity

4. Epigastric focal distention or abdominal pain
5. Red or deep-red colored tongue, with a thin, yellow, or peeled coating, cracks, and a thin, rapid pulse

Irritability with an inability to get to sleep are the primary signs of the Coptis and Ass-Hide Gelatin Decoction presentation. The reasons for insomnia are numerous, and many different formulas can be used to treat it. Therefore, in practice, one cannot use this formula based simply on the presence of irritability and insomnia; clear differentiation based on the presence or absence of several other symptoms from the above list is a must. Special attention must be paid both to the patient's psycho-emotional condition and the pulse. The irritability and insomnia of this formula's presentation and that of Coptis Decoction to Resolve Toxicity (*huáng lián jiě dú tāng*), Drive Out Stasis from the Mansion of Blood Decoction (*xuè fǔ zhú yū tāng*), and Peach Pit Decoction to Order the Qi (*táo hé chéng qì tāng*) are different in that this formula's presentation emphasizes a feeling of being listless and dispirited, a thin, rapid pulse, and a red, sparsely coated tongue. Furthermore, characteristically, they become more irritable when evening falls, while in the daytime, they are relatively calmer. Zheng introduces the experience of how the old Chinese doctor Chen Zi-Guo used this formula with very satisfactory results to treat insomnia in patients who are lightheaded and have vertigo, tinnitus with irritability, dry mouth and red lips, achy calves and feel sluggish, and find themselves either nodding off or suddenly waking up or unable to sleep at all; they have scanty, dark yellow urine, a red, sparsely-coated tongue, and a thin, rapid pulse.[12] Furthermore, patients with irritability often have palpitations, and thus clinically, Coptis and Ass-Hide Gelatin Decoction (*huáng lián ē jiāo tāng*) can also be used to treat tachycardia.

Bleeding is also a distinctive sign of the Coptis and Ass-Hide Gelatin Decoction presentation. This bleeding often involves blood in the stool or urine, coughing of blood, metrorrhagia, or ecchymosis. The color of this blood is usually bright red, and the ecchymosis appears as stasis spots. Chinese doctors of the past frequently used this formula to treat damp-warmth (濕溫 *shī wēn*), which is an emergency condition of an epidemic fever with bloody stools (this corresponds to enteric typhoid with intestinal perforation).

I once treated a patient with a chronic case of bacterial dysentery. He had recalcitrant bloody stools with mucus, accompanied by irritability and restlessness, difficulty sleeping, and a macerated oral cavity and tongue; he also was emaciated and fatigued. Coptis and Ass-Hide Gelatin Decoction (*huáng lián ē jiāo tāng)* with the egg yolk *(jī zǐ huáng)* removed but with the addition of Glycyrrhizae Radix *(gān cǎo)* was prescribed. After taking five packets, the bleeding with the bowel movements stopped; afterward, the treatment consisted of modifications of the original formula for half a month, after which he was all better.

There are clinical reports of this formula effectively treating the coughing blood from pulmonary tuberculosis, hematuria, and dysfunctional uterine bleeding. In practice, the main complaint of patients with this formula's presentation usually concerns either bleeding or insomnia.

Even if there have not been any recent episodes of significant bleeding, utilizing the interview process often leads to the discovery that these patients have a tendency toward problems involving bleeding. Examples are women with menorraghia or postpartum bleeding, or skin that is prone to purpura. Since this is a bleeding disorder, perhaps there are some readers who want to ask why Coptis Decoction to Resolve Toxicity *(huáng lián jiě dú tāng)* or Rhubarb and Coptis Decoction to Drain the Epigastrium *(dà huáng huáng lián xiè xīn tāng)* are not used instead? From Chinese medicine's perspective, while all of these are presentations of bleeding from heat, the issue is whether the condition is of one excess or deficiency. With excess, there must be accompanying signs of irritability and irascibility, a red face with thirst, constipation with a bitter taste in the mouth, abdominal distention or pain, and an excessive, forceful pulse with a stiff and tough tongue. Rhubarb and Coptis Decoction to Drain the Epigastrium *(dà huáng huáng lián xiè xīn tāng)* or Coptis Decoction to Resolve Toxicity *(huáng lián jiě dú tāng)* treat this kind of bleeding from excess presentation. By contrast, the presentation associated with bleeding due to heat from deficiency is indicated by a patient with an ashen complexion who is thin and pallid, speaks with a low voice, is short of breath, dispirited and listless, and has a thin, rapid, forceless pulse and a thin, red tongue with a shiny coating. The bleeding of the Coptis and Ass-Hide Gelatin Decoction presentation is exactly this type of deficiency-heat presentation bleeding.

In *Discussion of Cold Damage*, Coptidis Rhizoma *(huáng lián)* and Scutellariae Radix *(huáng qín)* are frequently prescribed together to treat various presentations involving epigastric focal distention. It can be inferred from looking at the composition of this formula that there should be symptoms of epigastric focal distention and abdominal pain. This is confirmed by reports of this formula being effective in the treatment of atrophic gastritis. The patient herself may only have mild symptoms or even be unaware of any significant symptoms; however, by utilizing palpation, areas with a feeling of localized distention are often found.

The tongue in the Coptis and Ass-Hide Gelatin Decoction presentation has some obvious characteristics: the tongue body itself is red or deep red, what Chinese doctors call a 'deeply red tongue'; the coating could be thin and yellow, or peeled, or there may be cracks on the surface of the tongue; often there are fissures in the mucous membranes of the mouth. Not surprisingly, in clinical practice, this formula's presentation is often seen in cases of recurrent mouth ulcers or other diseases of the oral mucosa.

The Coptis and Ass-Hide Gelatin Decoction presentation is what Chinese doctors refer to as 'yin deficiency with exuberant fire' (陰虛火旺 yīn xū huǒ wàng). This is when the yin and fluids of the body are insufficient, which in turn leads to a pathologic condition where the yang qi becomes relatively overly exuberant. In modern medical terms, this corresponds to illnesses that resemble autonomic dystonia, hypertonus of the sympathetic nervous system, or hyperactive metabolism. In practice, it is common to see infectious diseases of a chronic nature, chronic consumptive illness, nervous exhaustion, and disorders of the endocrine system with this presentation.

7.6 Aucklandia and Coptis Pill (香連丸 xiāng lián wán)

SOURCE: *Materia Medica of the Zhenghe Era*
(政和本草 Zhèng hé běn cǎo)

Coptidis Rhizoma (*huáng lián*) 10g
Aucklandiae Radix (*mù xiāng*) 6g

Dry-fry the Coptidis Rhizoma (*huáng lián*) with Evodiae Fructus (*wú zhū yú*) and then remove the Evodiae Fructus (*wú zhū yú*).

This prescription is a traditional empirical formula for treating dysentery. Coptidis Rhizoma (*huáng lián*) is particularly useful in the treatment of dysentery; modern pharmacological research has already confirmed its powerful antibacterial function. Aucklandiae Radix (*mù xiāng*) is aromatic and relieves pain through its strong qi-moving action; clinically, it is used for treating abdominal pain and distention. Additionally, pharmacological experimentation has evidence of powdered Aucklandiae Radix (*mù xiāng*) functioning as a rather potent antibacterial agent against *Staphylococcus aureus*, *Bacillus subtilis*, *Escherichia coli*, and *Salmonella enterica serovar Typhi*. Water decoctions of Aucklandiae Radix (*mù xiāng*) have a very strong antibacterial effect against *Shigella flexneri*; they also have a stimulating effect on the large intestine that both promotes peristalsis and the release of intestinal secretions, thus alleviating pain and bloating from intestinal gas. This combination of Coptidis Rhizoma (*huáng lián*) and Aucklandiae Radix (*mù xiāng*) is very effective in treating abdominal pain and bloating, diarrhea, and dysenteric stool with blood or pus resulting from gastrocolonic inflammation, dysentery, enteritis, or typhoid fever.

The Aucklandia and Coptis Pill presentation is as follows:

1. Abdominal distention and pain, tenesmus, sticky and malodorous or blood- and pus-streaked dysenteric stool
2. Dark red tongue with a greasy, yellow coating

The Aucklandia and Coptis Pill presentation symptoms of tenesmus, sticky and malodorous or blood- and pus-streaked dysenteric stool, and a dark red tongue with a greasy, yellow coating are indicative of a coptis presentation. Clinically, these patients are usually seen with accompanying symptoms of feverishness and sweating or irritability and restlessness. If the patient has a deficient, cold presentation with watery or semiliquid stool like that of a duck, a feeling of being cold and desirous of warmth, with a pale, flabby, white-coated tongue, the use of Aucklandia and Coptis Pill (*xiāng lián wán*) would be completely inappropriate.

If there is intense abdominal pain, tenesmus, and a burnt, greasy, yellow tongue coating, Rhei Radix et Rhizoma (*dà huáng*) can be added to this formula. After being steamed in alcohol, its purgative function is weakened, while its ability to clear heat and resolve toxicity is retained; it can assist Coptidis Rhizoma (*huáng lián*) in eliminating the above clinical symptoms. Four-Miracle Pill (*sì shén wán*) from the Ming-dynasty work *Introduction to Medicine* (醫學入門 *Yī xué rù mén*) is exactly this combination of Aucklandia and Coptis Pill (*xiāng lián wán*) with the addition of Rhei Radix et Rhizoma (*dà huáng*) plus the qi-regulating Arecae Semen (*bīng láng*).

7.7 **Left Metal Pill** (左金丸 *zuǒ jīn wán*)

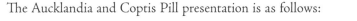

SOURCE: *Essential Teachings of [Zhu] Dan-Xi* (丹溪心法 *Dān Xī xīn fǎ*)

Coptidis Rhizoma (*huáng lián*)...5g
Evodiae Fructus (*wú zhū yú*) 1g

This formula was originally used to treat the presentation of "constrained heat in the Liver channel, acid regurgitation, left costal pain, and hypertense muscles in the lower abdomen, with hernia-like conditions." Today it is commonly used to treat those with bile reflux-induced gastritis, cholecystitis, gastric ulcers, and functional stomach problems where there is upper abdominal pain and vomiting of sour fluids.

This formula has excellent sedative, stomachic, and anti-inflammatory effects. The Evodiae Fructus (*wú zhū yú*) in this formula has a relatively strong analgesic and anti-emetic effect. The *Discussion of Cold Damage* prescription Evodia Decoction (*wú zhū yú tāng*)* is quite good at treating dry heaves, vomiting of saliva, and headaches. Left Metal Pill's (*zuǒ jīn wán*) combining of Coptidis Rhizoma (*huáng lián*) with Evodiae Fructus (*wú zhū yú*) not only clears heat and gets rid of inflammation, but can also stop pain and vomiting; it is most suitable for gastric pain and vomiting that is accompanied by the coptis presentation. The Left Metal Pill presentation is as follows:

1. Upper abdominal pain, hypochondriac distention and pain, a bitter taste in the mouth, intense feeling of hunger and emptiness in the stomach, or vomiting of bitter, sour fluids
2. Red tongue with a yellow coating

Abdominal pain and vomiting of sour, bitter fluids are the characteristic symptoms of the Left Metal Pill presentation. In practice, some patients who also have chronic and continuous stomachache and often vomit sour fluids are seen. This condition seems similar to the Left Metal Pill presentation, however, careful interviewing of the patients reveals that the level of pain is not at all intense and usually occurs when the stomach is empty. The fluids vomited are sour, not bitter, and are copious in amount and of a clear, thin nature; these patients also have a subjective feeling of cold in the upper abdomen and stomach. Additionally, there is an absence of taste, and the tongue usually is pale red with a white, glossy coating. This type of abdominal pain is that of the Minor Construct the Middle Decoction presentation. Please refer to Chapter 1 on the Cinnamon Twig formula family for more details.

Left Metal Pill (*zuǒ jīn wán*) and Aucklandia and Coptis Pill (*xiāng lián wán*) both utilize Coptidis Rhizoma (*huáng lián*) as the primary ingredient. The difference between the two is that Left Metal Pill (*zuǒ jīn wán*) primarily treats upper abdominal pain accompanied by the vomiting of sour, bitter fluids, while Aucklandia and Coptis Pill (*xiāng lián wán*) primarily treats lower abdominal distention and pain accompanied by diarrhea.

---

* Evodiae Fructus (*wú zhū yú*), Ginseng Radix (*rén shēn*), Jujubae Fructus (*dà zǎo*), and Zingiberis Rhizoma recens (*shēng jiāng*).

CHAPTER 8

DRIED GINGER FORMULA FAMILY

:::

乾薑類方 gān jiāng lèi fāng

Mention ginger, and there is not anyone who has not heard of it. Ginger has an intimate connection with the daily lives of the Chinese, Japanese, Indians, and other Asian peoples. It is regarded as an acrid, fragrant spice that gets rid of fishy smells, eliminates greasiness, improves the flavor of food, and strengthens the stomach. Regardless of whether it is used to cook fish, roast meat, flavor a pickling sauce, season a stir-fry, spice up steamed foods, or in the stewing of a soup, Zingiberis Rhizoma recens (*shēng jiāng*) absolutely cannot be done without. Zingiberis Rhizoma recens (*shēng jiāng*) scatters cold, promotes sweating, and warms the Stomach. If a bowl of steaming hot ginger and brown sugar soup is drunk after catching a cold, it will regulate the body, causing a slight sweat that makes one feel comfortably warm and cozy. Fresh ginger when harvested in the winter and then left to dry in the sun or

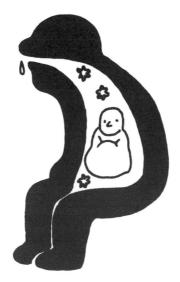

baked in an oven becomes the commonly used middle-warming, cold-scattering medicinal used in Chinese medicine: Zingiberis Rhizoma (*gān jiāng*).

Hot in nature and with an acrid taste, Zingiberis Rhizoma (*gān jiāng*) is an important medicinal that treats nausea and vomiting, abdominal pain and diarrhea, frigid extremities with cold sweating, cold and painful joints, coughing and wheezing with copious phlegm, poor appetite, and coughing of blood or blood in the stool. *Important Formulas Worth a Thousand Gold Pieces* (千金 要方 *Qiān jīn yào fāng*) says to treat cold attack with watery diarrhea (中寒水 瀉 *zhòng hán shuǐ xiè*) by ingesting ground-up Zingiberis Rhizoma preparata (*páo jiāng*). Repeated incessant vomiting can be treated by using a mixture of powdered Zingiberis Rhizoma (*gān jiāng*) and Infantis Urina (*tóng biàn*). In *Emergency Formulas to Keep up One's Sleeve* (肘後備急方 *Zhǒu hòu bèi jí fāng*), Zingiberis Rhizoma (*gān jiāng*) is used alone to treat sudden heart pain (卒心 痛 *cù xīn tòng*) and cold-type dysenteric disorder with dark-colored stools (寒 痢青色 *hán lì qīng sè*). The renowned Qing-dynasty physician Wang Meng-Ying used Zingiberis Rhizoma (*gān jiāng*) to save the lives of those suffering collapse due to loss of yang (虛脫亡陽 *xū tuō wáng yáng*). When combined with medicinals such as Glycyrrhizae Radix (*gān cǎo*), Aconiti Radix lateralis preparata (*zhì fù zǐ*), and Atractylodis macrocephalae Rhizoma (*bái zhú*), its scope of treatment is further expanded.

According to modern pharmacologic research, there is evidence of Zingiberis Rhizoma (*gān jiāng*) having a bidirectional regulating effect on the secretion of stomach acid and gastric juices, a mildly stimulating effect on the digestive tract, and a bidirectional regulating effect on intestinal tract tonus, rhythm, and peristaltic movement. Furthermore, by stimulating the mucous membranes of the intestinal tract, ginger can excite both the vasomotor and respiratory central nervous system centers; it also directly stimulates the heart.

Dried Ginger Presentation (乾薑證 *gān jiāng zhèng*)

The dried ginger presentation falls within the category of internal cold. Internal is reflected primarily in the clinical manifestations of stomach and intestinal symptoms such as vomiting, abdominal distention and pain, and diarrhea; there can also be respiratory tract symptoms such as coughing. Cold is indicated by sluggish or diminished metabolic functions, increased parasympathetic nervous system tone, low blood pressure, and delayed physiologic responses. Clinical manifestations include vomitus or diarrhea that is of a thin, clear, odorless, or watery consistency. These patients have an aversion to cold and favor warmth, have a sallow complexion, cold limbs and body, a soft or weak voice, and a pale white tongue with a white, greasy coating. The ability of Zingiberis Rhizoma (*gān jiāng*) to warm the center and scatter cold is aimed squarely at the above-mentioned symptoms. In practice, the dried ginger presentation is frequently seen in those who are fundamentally yang deficient or who have issues of cold, thin mucus after exposure to cold, are exhausted from overwork, suffer from chronic illness, overindulge in cold beverages, or have been overprescribed cold medicines. The dried ginger presentation is as follows:

1. Clear, thin, and odorless vomitus, saliva, sputum, stool, or urine
2. Abdominal distention, abdominal pain, nausea and vomiting, and perhaps coughing
3. Excess saliva in the mouth and lack of thirst, aversion to cold and desire for warmth, listless and dispirited
4. Pale or pale red tongue, with a greasy coating that is usually white and greasy, but may be dark gray and greasy, or white and slimy (the 'dried ginger tongue')

This presentation is the exact opposite of the rhubarb presentation with its excess interior heat. Even though the dried ginger presentation also includes signs of abdominal distention and pain, the stool is thin and watery like that of a duck. Unlike the dry constipation of the rhubarb presentation, the stool is usually clear, watery, and odorless. The rhubarb presentation includes a dry mouth and burnt tongue coating along with an aversion to heat and desire for cold, while in the dried ginger presentation, there is excess saliva in the mouth, a lack of thirst, and an aversion to cold and desire for warmth. The tongue of the rhubarb presentation is red with a burnt yellow coating, whereas that of the dried ginger presentation is pale with a white, greasy coating. Clearly, these two presentations are the opposite of each other. In my experience, the appearance of the dried ginger presentation tongue has significant diagnostic meaning, so I call this the 'dried ginger tongue.'

The white tongue coating of the dried ginger presentation is indicative of cold, and the greasiness means there is dampness. Clinical use of Zingiberis Rhizoma (*gān jiāng*) based prescriptions, when seeing this type of white and greasy tongue coating, not only can reduce the thickness of the tongue coating, but, as the tongue coating becomes thinner, can also reduce or eliminate the accompanying symptoms. Should the tongue be red or dark red with a sparse coating, or if it is red, shiny, and lacking a coating, these symptoms indicate heat and yin deficiency, which are the opposite of the characteristics associated with the dried ginger presentation. As Zingiberis Rhizoma (*gān jiāng*) is a hot and acrid medicinal, misuse can cause patients to have a dry mouth and tongue, and will aggravate any underlying heat or yin deficiency conditions.

Therefore, before deciding to use a Zingiberis Rhizoma (*gān jiāng*) based prescription, I most assuredly would have a look at the tongue. The surface of the dried ginger tongue usually has a white, slimy coating, and these patients are not thirsty or may have excessive cold saliva in the mouth. Should patients have thirst and a desire to drink, along with a dry tongue surface, even though they may display signs of being listless and dispirited, they cannot be treated as if they have a dried ginger presentation.

The dried ginger presentation is commonly seen in clinical practice and frequently manifests along with the ephedra, cinnamon, bupleurum, aconite, coptis, and pinellia presentations. Consequently, not only is Zingiberis Rhizoma (*gān jiāng*) used alone, but it is often combined with other medicinals. Examples include the ephedra family formula Minor Bluegreen Dragon Decoction (*xiǎo qīng lóng tāng*), the bupleurum family formula Bupleurum, Cinnamon Twig, and Ginger Decoction (*chái hú guì zhī gān jiāng tāng*), and the coptis family formula Pinellia Decoction to Drain the Epigastrium (*bàn xià xiè xīn tāng*).

The following formulas are the representative prescriptions of the dried ginger formula family, as Zingiberis Rhizoma (*gān jiāng*) is the primary medicinal within each of them.

8.1 Regulate the Middle Pill (理中丸 *lǐ zhōng wán*)

SOURCE: *Discussion of Cold Damage* (傷寒論 *Shāng hán lùn*)

Ginseng Radix (*rén shēn*).. 6-10g
Atractylodis macrocephalae Rhizoma (*bái zhú*).................... 6-12g
Zingiberis Rhizoma (*gān jiāng*) 3-10g
Glycyrrhizae Radix (*gān cǎo*).. 3-10g

Zingiberis Rhizoma (*gān jiāng*) combined with Ginseng Radix (*rén shēn*), Atractylodis macrocephalae Rhizoma (*bái zhú*), and Glycyrrhizae Radix (*gān cǎo*) is the well-known formula Regulate the Middle Pill (*lǐ zhōng wán*). This is an indispensable formula used by Chinese doctors to treat abdominal illness of a cold and deficient nature. In *Discussion of Cold Damage*, Regulate the Middle Pill (*lǐ zhōng wán*) is used to treat fever with headache, body aches, aversion to cold, and vomiting and diarrhea, and also to promote recovery after a major illness or for drooling. In *Important Formulas Worth a Thousand Gold Pieces*, this formula is used to treat sudden turmoil disease with vomiting and diarrhea, abdominal fullness, inability to digest food, and epigastric and abdominal pain. There is a use recorded in *Red Water and Dark Pearls* (赤水玄珠 *Chì shuǐ xuán zhū*) for children with Spleen and Stomach weakness after they have been ill with vomiting and diarrhea, with gradual onset of coldness in the limbs; or superficial facial edema and deficiency swelling in the four limbs; or to treat patients who like to keep their eyes closed. In *Discussion of Illnesses, Patterns, and Formulas Related to the Unification of the Three Etiologies* (三因極一病證方論 *Sān yīn jí yī bìng zhèng fāng lùn*) it is used to treat damage to the Stomach with vomiting of blood. Legend has it that Emperor Hui-Zong of the Song dynasty suffered from Spleen illness after eating too much cold food. None of the court physicians was able to cure this disease, so the famous doctor Yang Jie was summoned to the palace. Regulate the Middle Pill (*lǐ zhōng wán*) boiled in ice water cured the problem.

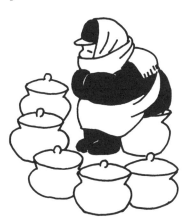

Regulate the Middle Pill (*lǐ zhōng wán*) is the primary prescription used to treat digestive tract diseases that have interior deficiency-cold presentations. The Zingiberis Rhizoma (*gān jiāng*) and Glycyrrhizae Radix (*gān cǎo*) within this formula constitutes the *Discussion of Cold Damage* prescription Licorice and Ginger Decoction (*gān cǎo gān jiāng tāng*). It is used to treat interior cold presentations with irritability and restlessness, vomiting, as well as cold in the Lungs, dizziness, and excessive salivation. Ginseng Radix (*rén shēn*) and Atractylodis macrocephalae Rhizoma (*bái zhú*) are presumably included because of the injury to the gastrointestinal system after illnesses involving vomiting and diarrhea. This injury manifests as reduction in digestive function and being undernourished with symptoms of poor appetite, epigastric focal distention with firmness, thin, watery stools, soft and loose musculature, being listless and dispirited, and a low, fatigued-sounding voice. This type of condition is what Chinese doctors refer to as an 'interior deficiency-cold presentation.' The 'interior' here primarily refers to the Spleen and Stomach, which is to say, the absorptive functions of the digestive system. The physical condition of these patients is relatively poor, as they have either been ill for a long time or are debilitated due to old age. The Regulate the Middle Pill presentation is as follows:

1. Abdominal fullness and distention, vomiting and diarrhea, thin and watery stools, poor appetite, epigastric focal distention with firmness, and perhaps excessive, clear, thin saliva

2. Aversion to cold and attraction to warmth, feeling listless and dispirited, a lack of thirst, or a dry mouth but without a desire to drink

3. Pale red tongue with a white coating that can be thick and greasy, or slimy

- This formula's presentation is often seen in illnesses of the digestive tract. There are clinical reports of the efficacy of this formula and its modifications in treating chronic bacterial dysentery, chronic enteritis, allergic colitis, and acute vomiting and diarrhea in those with deficiency-cold, infantile diarrhea, indigestion, chronic atrophic gastritis, chronic superficial gastritis, gastric ulcers, pyloric spasms, morning sickness, biliary ascariasis, excessive bile secretion after bile duct surgery, chronic hepatitis, recalcitrant abdominal distention, colic, upper digestive tract bleeding, and blood in the stool. For example, chronic gastritis commonly manifests with indistinct stomach pain, a lack of taste, and a poor appetite; it responds well to local application of warmth and pressure and has a tendency to worsen after being chilled, eating raw or cold foods, or becoming exhausted; the tongue coating is thin and white or white and greasy, and the pulse is sinking, thin, and lacks force. The internal medicine department at a Chinese Air Force hospital took this to be a deficiency-cold presentation and used a modification of Regulate the Middle Pill (lǐ zhōng wán) to treat chronic gastritis in 40 patients. Treatment resulted in stomach acid levels returning to normal along with a disappearance of symptoms for 21 patients; another 16 patients experienced a significant improvement as their symptoms basically disappeared and their level of stomach acid showed varying degrees of improvement.[1]

There is also a report of treating a patient who, during gallbladder duct surgery, had a T-duct implanted. After the surgery, there was excessive bile secretion with 5000 to 6000ml of bile being collected in a 24-hour period. Antibiotic treatment did not reduce the flow. The patient had a sallow complexion, was fatigued, emaciated, had cold limbs, watery stools, a lack of taste along with a poor appetite, chest and epigastric focal distention and fullness, a dark tongue with a white coating, and a sinking, slow, and thin pulse. This was diagnosed as a Regulate the Middle Pill presentation, and the patient was given Regulate the Middle Pill (*lǐ zhōng wán*) with the addition of Amomi Fructus (*shā rén*). After taking two packets of herbs, the amount of bile produced within a 24-hour period was reduced to 500ml, and the patient's spirits and appetite both improved significantly.[2]

- Acute infectious illnesses usually manifest with symptoms of heat and excess, however, there are also cases that can manifest with symptoms of deficiency and cold. There is a report of a patient with a case of measles complicated by pneumonia with a persistent fever, a strong desire for sleep, restlessness, neck rigidity and opisthotonos, as well as trembling of the entire body, especially marked in the arms and legs. The patient was given repeated courses of antibiotics, both orally and via an IV drip, but in the end, this failed to produce results as the temperature continued to fluctuate around 38°C (100.4°F). Even though there was a persistent fever, the doctors on the basis of the breath coming out of the nose and mouth feeling cold, watery stools, clear urine, and a deficient and lax pulse, judged this to be a case of true cold with false heat. After taking several packets of Regulate the Middle Pill (*lǐ zhōng wán*) together with Six-Ingredient Pill with Rehmannia (*liù wèi dì huáng wán*) the patient was cured.[3]

- Some patients with bleeding disorders, as in cases of dysfunctional uterine bleeding, nosebleeds, allergic or thrombocytopenic purpura, and digestive tract bleeding, also have a Regulate the Middle Pill presentation. These patients rarely have marked blood loss, but do have a dark, pale complexion. In these circumstances, Zingiberis Rhizoma preparata (*páo jiāng*) is usually substituted for Zingiberis Rhizoma (*gān jiāng*).

- Pediatric patients are often seen with this formula's presentation with such problems as persistent fevers from deficiency, chronic childhood convulsions (慢驚風 *màn jīng fēng*), pediatric pneumonia, dyspepsia, or mouth sores that are accompanied by digestive tract symptoms. I once treated a child who had suffered for two weeks with blistering stomatitis. The illness began with a fever, and afterward many ulcers appeared on the mucosal lining of the mouth, causing the inconsolable child to cry, scream, and continually drool throughout the day. Because the face was edematous and with a yellowish cast, the tongue was pale red with a white coating, and there was a history of loose, unformed stool that contained undigested food particles, Regulate the Middle Pill (lǐ zhōng wán) with the addition of Aconiti Radix lateralis preparata (zhì fù zǐ) and Coptidis Rhizoma (huáng lián) was prescribed. After taking five packets, the problem was resolved.

MODIFICATIONS

In clinical practice, Regulate the Middle Pill (lǐ zhōng wán) is often modified with other herbs:

- For those with vomiting, add Pinelliae Rhizoma preparatum (zhì bàn xià).
- For jaundice, add Artemisiae scopariae Herba (yīn chén).
- For pulsation below the navel, add Cinnamomi Ramulus (guì zhī).
- For palpitations and dizziness, add Poria (fú líng).
- For abdominal pain, add Aucklandiae Radix (mù xiāng).

This formula with the addition of Aconiti Radix lateralis preparata (zhì fù zǐ) is Aconite Accessory Root Pill to Regulate the Middle (fù zǐ lǐ zhōng wán); this is used to treat those with the Regulate the Middle Pill presentation who also present with frigid extremities, a thin, weak pulse, and who feel dispirited and listless. There is a report of treating an infant who spit up lumpy vomitus after feeding and whose stools were greenish black in color. Two to three times a day, about 45 minutes before feeding, the mother would ingest 200 to 300ml of the following decoction: Aconiti Radix lateralis preparata (zhì fù zǐ) 10-12g (which was first decocted for 30 minutes), Codonopsis Radix (dǎng shēn) 20g, Atractylodis macrocephalae Rhizoma (bái zhú) 10g, Zingiberis Rhizoma (gān jiāng) 6g, and Glycyrrhizae Radix (gān cǎo) 6g. After one to two days, the baby recovered completely.[4] There are yet other reports of a modification of this formula being used to treat those suffering allergic purpura who have a deficiency-cold presentation.[5]

This formula modified with Coptidis Rhizoma (huáng lián) is Regulating Decoction with Coptis (lián lǐ tāng), which treats patients with the Regulate the Middle Pill presentation where there is also irritability, epigastric focal distention with pain, a red tongue with a greasy, yellow coating, and dark red lips. Chronic gastritis, chronic colitis, and ulcers in the oral cavity are frequently seen with this formula's presentation.

This formula modified with Cinnamomi Ramulus (*guì zhī*) is Cinnamon Twig and Ginseng Decoction (*guì zhī rén shēn tāng*), which is the formula that will be discussed next. This formula treats those with the Regulate the Middle Pill presentation when accompanied by spontaneous sweating, body aches, and an aversion to drafts.

Regulate the Middle Pill (*lǐ zhōng wán*) with the addition of Aurantii Fructus immaturus (*zhǐ shí*) and Poria (*fú líng*) becomes Unripe Bitter Orange Pill to Regulate the Middle (*zhǐ shí lǐ zhōng wán*). It treats those with the Regulate the Middle Pill presentation with abdominal fullness and distention who dislike having pressure put on the abdomen.

This formula modified by adding Citri reticulatae viride Pericarpium (*qīng pí*) and Citri reticulatae Pericarpium (*chén pí*) is Treat the Middle Pill (*zhì zhōng wán*), which is suitable for treating a Regulate the Middle presentation accompanied by upper abdominal distention.

Regulate the Middle Pill (*lǐ zhōng wán*) with Poria (*fú líng*) substituted for Zingiberis Rhizoma (*gān jiāng*) is Four-Gentlemen Decoction (*sì jūn zǐ tāng*), which is suitable for treating presentations that include symptoms of poor appetite, a sallow complexion, and loose stools due to Spleen and Stomach weakness. Because it lacks Zingiberis Rhizoma (*gān jiāng*), it is appropriate for presentations where there are no significant signs of cold in the middle such as marked aversion to cold, vomiting of clear, watery fluids, diarrhea, or a greasy, white tongue coating.

The nature of these modifications, whether they lean toward warming the interior, clearing heat, tonifying and augmenting the qi, resolving the exterior, or regulating the qi, are more closely related to the complexity of actual clinical reality than is the use of Regulate the Middle Pill (*lǐ zhōng wán*) by itself.

8.2 Cinnamon Twig and Ginseng Decoction

(桂枝入參湯 *guì zhī rén shēn tāng*)

SOURCE: *Discussion of Cold Damage*

Cinnamomi Ramulus (*guì zhī*) 5-10g
Glycyrrhizae Radix (*gān cǎo*) 3-6g
Atractylodis macrocephalae Rhizoma (*bái zhú*) 6-10g
Ginseng Radix (*rén shēn*) 6-10g
Zingiberis Rhizoma (*gān jiāng*) 6-10g

Regulate the Middle Pill (*lǐ zhōng wán*) is also called Ginseng Decoction (*rén shēn tāng*) in *Discussion of Cold Damage*; with the addition of Cinnamomi Ramulus (*guì zhī*), it is known as Cinnamon Twig and Ginseng Decoction (*guì zhī rén shēn tāng*). While the Regulate the Middle Pill presentation treats interior presentations, cinnamon twig treats exterior presentations; it is not uncommon to see illnesses that simultaneously express with both interior and exterior symptoms. *Discussion of Cold Damage* (paragraph 163) states: "When a *tài yáng* disease is purged repeatedly, although the external pattern has not yet been eliminated, comingled heat with diarrhea will follow. For those where the diarrhea is incessant, there is focal distention and firmness below the Heart, and [both] the exterior and interior are unresolved, Cinnamon Twig and Ginseng Decoction (*guì zhī rén shēn tāng*) masters it." This is to say that, if purging herbs are erroneously given while the exterior has not been resolved, the result will be continuous diarrhea, epigastric focal distention with firmness, and a situation in which both the exterior and interior are deficient. In practice, this presentation does not usually arise from erroneous purging; those with constitutional yang deficiency who contract a wind-cold type cold or those with a cold and fever who overwork can both manifest with this presentation. It is especially common in patients with a cinnamon twig constitution who have chronic gastrointestinal diseases. The Cinnamon Twig and Ginseng Decoction presentation is as follows:

1. Regulate the Middle Pill presentation
2. Feverishness with spontaneous sweating; perhaps also with abdominal pain or epigastric focal distention with firmness
3. A pale red tongue, or one that is tender looking and tends toward being dark; and a large, floating pulse

The distinctive aspect of this formula is that it is a blending of the Regulate the Middle Pill and cinnamon twig presentations; there is not just one clinical manifestation of this condition. Patients may have feverishness, joint pain, spontaneous sweating, aversion to drafts, palpitations, periumbilical pulsations, or insomnia. They may also have epigastric focal distention with firmness, abdominal pain, headaches, and stiff necks. Spontaneous sweating and aversion to drafts are the most commonly seen symptoms. Within the symptomology of spontaneous sweating are those who sweat from even very slight physical exertion, those who sweat at night, and also those who do not sweat significantly but whose skin is moist. Most of those with spontaneous sweating have an aversion to drafts and are sensitive to both wind and cold. This formula's presentation can be seen in illnesses that manifest with peptic ulcers, chronic colitis, allergic colitis, as well as abdominal pain, diarrhea, low-grade fever, and spontaneous sweating.

I once treated an elderly woman whose main complaint was that she had been constipated for five days. Her previous doctor had prescribed a formula with Rhei Radix et Rhizoma (*dà huáng*), which proved to be ineffective. This patient was extremely listless and dispirited, her entire body was cold; however, at night, she would get hot and sweat, after which she again felt cold. She would only eat a little congee every day as her appetite was poor. Observation showed her to have a small and thin build, sallow complexion, and a pale red tongue with a thick, white coating. Abdominal diagnosis revealed that her abdomen was flat and the musculature taut and overly tense. The patient herself had an uncomfortable feeling of epigastric distention with firmness. She was diagnosed with a cinnamon twig constitution with a Regulate the Middle Pill presentation; three packets of Cinnamon Twig and Ginseng Decoction (*guì zhī rén shēn tāng*) were prescribed. After taking just one packet, her entire body felt more comfortable, and she passed some soft stool. After three packets, her sweating stopped and she no longer felt cold. I treated another patient with cirrhosis who often experienced diarrhea and abdominal pain, and frequently had bouts of ascites. Furthermore, during the night, he would often have spasms of the calf muscles accompanied by sweating. After taking 30 packets of Cinnamon Twig and Ginseng Decoction (*guì zhī rén shēn tāng*) with the addition of Paeoniae Radix (*sháo yào*), Dioscoreae Rhizoma (*shān yào*), Jujubae Fructus (*dà zǎo*), and Angelicae sinensis Radix (*dāng guī*), his stools became formed, his appetite improved, his complexion became ruddy, and he had no more bouts of ascites.

This formula's presentation should be differentiated from that of Coptis Decoction (*huáng lián tāng*). Both presentations include spontaneous sweating, diarrhea, and epigastric focal distention with firmness. They do, however, differ in that one treats a presentation of cold and deficiency, while the other is for heat and excess. The presentation for Cinnamon Twig and Ginseng Decoction (*guì zhī rén shēn tāng*) falls into the category of deficiency and cold, consequently, there is thin, clear, and odorless diarrhea, and while there is sweating, it is accompanied by an aversion to drafts and cold limbs. These patients are listless, dispirited, and have a despondent sound to their voice. The Coptis Decoction presentation falls into the category of mixed heat and cold with abdominal pain and distention, a hot body with profuse sweating, and irritability with an inability to calm down. More important is the rather clear difference in the tongues of these two formula presentations. Generally, the tongue in a heat presentation is red with a yellow coating, while that of the cold presentation is pale with a white coating; the excess presentation tongue is stiff and inflexible, while the tongue of the deficiency presentation is puffy and tender. It follows, then, that the Coptis Decoction presentation tongue is red, whereas for this formula's presentation, it is pale red. Additionally, the Cinnamon Twig and Ginseng Decoction presentation tongue usually is completely covered with a white coating, but with the Coptis Decoction presentation generally, it is the back half of the tongue that has a thick, white coating.

8.3 Major Construct the Middle Decoction
(大建中湯 *dà jiàn zhōng tāng*)

SOURCE: *Essentials from the Golden Cabinet* (金匱要略 *Jīn guì yào lüè*)

Zingiberis Rhizoma (*gān jiāng*) 5-12g
Zanthoxyli Pericarpium (*huā jiāo*) 2-6g
Ginseng Radix (*rén shēn*) 6-10g

Major Construct the Middle Decoction (*dà jiàn zhōng tāng*) is the ginger formula family's analgesic prescription applicable for treating presentations with cold and pain throughout the abdomen. In *Essentials from the Golden Cabinet*, it is used to treat a specific presentation that includes "severe cold and pain in the Heart and chest, vomiting and an inability to eat or drink, cold in the abdomen, pain due to obstruction of the Intestines where in extreme cases the shape of the [Intestines] pops up [like an animal] that has a head and feet, or the entire abdomen from top to bottom is so painful that [the patient] cannot stand it even close to being touched." In the modern way of looking at this, it is much like a sudden reversal peristalsis in the stomach or intestines. Major Construct the Middle Decoction (*dà jiàn zhōng tāng*) can be used for chronic gastritis, gastric ulcers, functional stomach problems, stomach prolapse, biliary ascariasis, gastric adhesions, and obstructions of the intestines when seen with this formula's presentation. The Major Construct the Middle Decoction presentation is as follows:

1. Relatively intense paroxysmal abdominal pain and distention, functional obstruction of the intestines that leads to visible changes in the abdomen, or borborygmus, often accompanied by vomiting

2. Extremely cold hands and feet, or cold sweats, and excessive clear saliva in the mouth
3. 'Dried ginger tongue'

....

Should there be relatively intense abdominal pain, but with constipation, fever with sweating, and a burnt yellow tongue coating, this would be the exact opposite of this formula's presentation. It falls into the category of pain from heat; therefore, the use of a rhubarb family formula would be the correct choice for that presentation.

8.4 Licorice, Ginger, Poria, and White Atractrylodes Decoction
(甘草乾薑茯苓白朮湯 *gān cǎo gān jiāng fú líng bái zhú tāng*)

SOURCE: *Essentials from the Golden Cabinet*

Zingiberis Rhizoma (*gān jiāng*) 12g
Poria (*fú líng*) 12g
Atractylodis macrocephalae Rhizoma (*bái zhú*) 10g
Glycyrrhizae Radix (*gān cǎo*) 6g

When the Ginseng Radix (*rén shēn*) in Regulate the Middle Pill (*lǐ zhōng wán*) is replaced with Poria (*fú líng*), it becomes Licorice, Ginger, Poria, and White Atractylodes Decoction (*gān cǎo gān jiāng fú líng bái zhú tāng*), which treats lower back pain from cold and dampness. Ginseng Radix (*rén shēn*) is not used in this situation as there are no signs of emaciation, epigastric focal distention with firmness, or poor appetite. Poria (*fú líng*) and Atractylodis macrocephalae Rhizoma (*bái zhú*) are used together here as they treat a sense of heaviness and lethargy, urinary difficulty, and superficial edema.

The lower back should feel warm after taking this prescription. *Essentials from the Golden Cabinet* has the following description of this formula's actions in treating lower back pain: "These people's bodies feel heavy; there is a clear demarcation to the pain, much like they were sitting in a tub of cold water and there is accompanying whole body edema, ... from the waist on down, it feels cold and painful, the back feels heavy, as if carrying 5,000 coins." The distinctive characteristics of this type of lower back pain are cold pain (冷痛 *lěng tòng*) and heavy pain (重痛 *zhōng tòng*); cold indicates that there is pathogenic cold, and heaviness indicates that there is dampness. The Licorice, Ginger, Poria, and White Atractylodes Decoction presentation is as follows:

1. A cold feeling from the waist down, with a feeling of heaviness
   and pressure, or achy pain
2. Edema or predisposition to edema, the entire body feels
   fatigued and sluggish
3. 'Dried ginger tongue'

There is a report of using this formula to treat an elderly patient with joint pain. Because the back had got soaked and felt cold after fatiguing labor, it caused all of the joints both large and small throughout the body to feel painful; there was also a sense of pain and distention in the lower back, along with heaviness and an aversion to cold in the legs. After using six packets of this formula, the pain disappeared.[6]

I once treated an overweight middle-aged woman whose lower back felt cold and painful. She had had this back pain for two weeks; neither acupuncture nor *tuina* had proven effective. Because she had a white, greasy tongue coating and lower leg edema, I used this formula, modified with the addition of Atractylodis Rhizoma (*cāng zhú*) and Coicis Semen (*yì yǐ rén*). After taking five packets, the symptoms were alleviated.

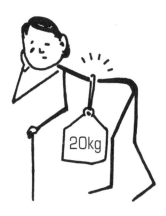

This formula's presentation is often seen in patients who are overweight and have lived for a long time in a cold, damp environment. Their bodies usually feel heavy and tired, the joints and muscles often feel heavy and achy, they are predisposed to edema or watery stools, and the tongue has a white coating. This is a 'damp' body type, much like those of the previously introduced ephedra and astragalus constitutions. When these types of people fall ill, they often experience dizziness, lower back and body aches, diarrhea, abdominal fullness, edema, or palpitations. Therefore, in practice, this formula, other than treating wind-damp lower back pain, also can be used to treat symptoms of edema, joint pain, and diarrhea.

MODIFICATIONS

Licorice, Ginger, Poria, and White Atractylodes Decoction *(gān cǎo gān jiāng fù líng bái zhú tāng)* is commonly used in combination with ephedra, astragalus, and aconite family formulas. When combined with Stephania and Astragalus Decoction *(fáng jǐ huáng qí tāng)*, it treats edema; with Ephedra Decoction plus Atractylodes *(má huáng jiā zhú tāng)*, it treats chills without sweating and joint pain; paired with Frigid Extremities Powder *(sì nì sǎn)*, it treats chills, diarrhea, and frigid extremities. The *Arcane Essentials from the Imperial Library* (外台 秘要 *Wài tái mì yào*) prescription Fixed Kidneys Powder (腎著散 *shèn zhuó sǎn*) is a modification of this formula with the addition of Eucommiae Cortex *(dù zhòng)*, Cinnamomi Ramulus *(guì zhī)*, Achyranthis bidentatae Radix *(niú xī)*, and Alismatis Rhizoma *(zé xiè)*; it treats the same type of presentation discussed here, with excellent results.

CHAPTER 9

ACONITE FORMULA FAMILY

附子類方 *fù zǐ lèi fāng*

Aconiti Radix lateralis preparata *(zhì fù zǐ)* and Rhei Radix et Rhizoma *(dà huáng)* are both considered to be high-ranking generals among Chinese herbs. Aconiti Radix lateralis preparata *(zhì fù zǐ)* has a powerful, virile nature and is like the fierce general that takes pass after pass to lead his army onward; it causes qi-tonifying herbs to circulate through the twelve channels, and it is used to pursue and restore lost or dispersed primal yang (元陽 *yuán yáng*). While the character of these two herbs is completely different, both of them are frequently used to save lives in critical situations. Because Rhei Radix et Rhizoma *(dà huáng)* is cold in nature and purges downward, it is appropriate for excess and heat presentations, and because the nature of Aconiti Radix lateralis preparata *(zhì fù zǐ)* is warm, it returns yang and expels cold and is suitable for use with deficiency and cold presentations.

For centuries, Aconiti Radix lateralis preparata *(zhì fù zǐ)* has been used by Chinese doctors as a yang-warming, cold-dispelling medicinal for the treatment of all types of deep or intractable cold illnesses such as profuse sweating that depletes the yang, heart failure, vomiting and diarrhea with frigidly cold extremities, pain and cold in the chest and abdomen, headache, painful joints, sinew and muscle spasms, lower limb edema, nonhealing sores, and chronic diarrhea or cold-type dysentery. In these kinds of serious or chronic cold-type illnesses, the body's internal organs or the function of the various organ systems have been severely diminished or manifest some type of abnormality, or the metabolic processes have become dysfunctional. Chinese medicine often uses the concept of yang deficiency to describe these conditions. This type of yang deficient presentation can appear within the disease process of all sorts of illnesses. Symptoms of biomedically-defined diseases such as circulatory collapse, heart failure, adrenal insufficiency, or hypothyroidism can all fall within the category of yang deficiency.

The aconite family of formulas, in which Aconiti Radix lateralis preparata (zhì fù zǐ) plays a primary role, all treat presentations of yang deficiency. These are referred to as yang-restoring or yang-warming, cold-expelling prescriptions. By restoring and warming the yang, they stimulate and strengthen debilitated body functions, thus bringing back into play the organism's innate ability to resist disease, resulting in the recovery of health. This way of thinking about treatment is based on Chinese medicine's wholism and theory of internal causes; it is one of the distinctive aspects of Chinese medicine.

Aconiti Radix lateralis preparata (zhì fù zǐ) contains a number of different kinds of alkaloids, including hipaconitine, aconitine, mesaconitine, talatisamine, chuan-wu-base A, and chuan-wu-base B. Pharmacological research has evidence of hydrolyzed aconoitine functioning as a cardiotonic. Water decoctions of Aconiti Radix lateralis preparata (zhì fù zǐ) have a significant cardiotonic effect on *in vitro* experimental animal hearts; cooking it longer increases its efficacy and reduces its toxicity. There is also experimental evidence that decoctions of Aconiti Radix lateralis preparata (zhì fù zǐ) expand the blood vessels of the lower limbs and coronary blood vessels (without being related to blood pressure or heart rate). Aconiti Radix lateralis preparata (zhì fù zǐ) also has significant anti-inflammatory functions and stimulates the pituitary–adrenal axis. Decoctions of Aconiti Radix lateralis preparata (zhì fù zǐ) administered either orally or by abdominal injection have a significant anti-inflammatory effect in laboratory animals with formaldehyde- or albumen-induced ankle swelling. Additionally, it can increase the excretion of 17-ketosteriods in laboratory rats and reduce the eosinophil count in peripheral blood. There is evidence from histochemical analysis of laboratory mice that decoctions of Aconiti Radix lateralis preparata (zhì fù zǐ) cause a reduction in cholesterol levels in the adrenal cortex, increased phosphatase activity, and promote glycogen production. There is also documentation of Aconiti Radix lateralis preparata (zhì fù zǐ) having analgesic effects in experiments that involved the application of electrical shocks to the tails of rats.

Aconiti Radix lateralis preparata (zhì fù zǐ) contains toxins. Symptoms of aconite poisoning include drooling, nausea, vomiting, diarrhea, dizziness, blurry vision, numbness of the mouth, tongue, limbs, or whole body, breathing difficulties, reduced heart rate, twitching of the hands and feet, or muddled consciousness. Other side effects influence the body's regulatory mechanisms such as causing reductions in both blood pressure and body temperature, arrhythmias, as well as incontinence. While caution should be exercised in the clinical use of

Aconiti Radix lateralis preparata *(zhì fù zi)*, in reality, as long as the differential diagnosis is correct, the dosage is not too large, it is appropriately combined to use with other medicinals, and it is decocted for an extended period of time, the toxicity and other side effects of this medicinal can be avoided. I generally do not use amounts over 15g; furthermore, untreated Aconiti Radix lateralis *(fù zi)* is not to be used.

Historically and in modern times as well, there have been many old doctors with considerable experience in the use of Aconiti Radix lateralis preparata *(zhì fù zi)* who not only prescribed it for many different types of disease, but at rather large dosages; they quickly obtained clinical results. For example, the modern Shanghai physician Zhu Wei-Ju was so skilled at using Aconiti Radix lateralis preparata *(zhì fù zi)* that he was given the nickname 'Aconite Zhu' (祝 附子 *Zhù Fù-zi*).

The humidity in the southwestern Chinese provinces of Sichuan, Yunnan, and Guizhou is rather high, and the food and drink in these locales tends to be acrid and spicy. The people who live in these places view Aconiti Radix lateralis preparata *(zhì fù zi)* as a tonic and will use it when stewing meat to make a medicinal food. In summary, Aconiti Radix lateralis preparata *(zhì fù zi)* is an excellent herb, and the key to its effective use is to grasp its natural capacities and applicable clinical presentations. The primary clinical indications of Aconiti Radix lateralis preparata *(zhì fù zi)* are:

1. Profuse sweating, frigid extremities, chills, a sinking pulse, diminished heart sounds, and low blood pressure

2. Vomiting and diarrhea accompanied by cold hands and feet, abdominal pain and distention, a sinking and weak pulse, and a white, slippery tongue coating

3. Severe joint pain, localized swelling and distention, muscle and sinew spasms, reduced range of motion, and frigid extremities

4. Chronically ill, debilitated, or elderly patients with coldness in the lower half of the body, weakness and aching of lower back and knees; or cold pain, edema of the dorsal aspect of the foot, nighttime or frequent urination, an aversion to cold, and a sinking and feeble pulse

5. Chronic nephritis or cardiac insufficiency accompanied by symptoms of systemic weakness in physiological function along with edema

Aconite Presentation (附子證 *fù zǐ zhèng*)

These are the key indications for clinical use of Aconiti Radix lateralis preparata (*zhì fù zi*). Already described above are five types of illnesses that may, to a greater or lesser degree, be indicative of an aconite presentation. The following list also includes three other signs that indicate the use of Aconiti Radix lateralis preparata (*zhì fù zi*):

1. Listless and dispirited, exhausted with a desire to lie down, curl up, and sleep
2. Aversion to cold, frigid extremities, especially of the lower body, where from the knees down it feels icy cold
3. 'Aconite pulses': a pulse that is faint and weak (an extremely thin pulse that, when pressed, feels at times as if it is there and at times as if it is absent), sinking and hidden (only felt when using heavy pressure almost all the way to the bone), thin and weak (a pulse that is thin as a thread and forceless), or suddenly floating and large, but empty, soft, and without force

The first item in the list is accessed through observation. Although these patients' mental facilities are clear, they are extremely fatigued. They usually want to sleep, but do not sleep deeply, and when they are awoken, it is as if they are still half asleep. There are also some patients in the clinic who just appear quite fatigued, speak in a lackluster way about their condition, or whose mental processes are somewhat slow.

The second item concerns the patient's subjective sense of their symptoms. They feel cold, regardless of any objective measurements. The body temperature of these patients may be normal, or slightly lower than normal, or they may be frankly hypothermic.

The third item is what I call the 'aconite pulses.' The pulse is the most important part of the palpatory exam in Chinese medicine. The pulsations of the blood vessels have a subtle relationship with various elements, including cardiac output, the shape and quality of the vessel walls, the character of the blood itself and its rate of flow, the function of vasomotor nerves, and the patient's psychological state and external environment. By feeling the pulse, Chinese doctors can determine the abundance or lack of yang qi throughout the entire body, whether or not the patient is in good health, and especially the condition of the cardiovascular system. Pulse descriptions found in *Discussion of Cold Damage* (傷寒論 *Shāng hán lùn*) of "sinking," "minute," "so faint as to be on the point of being impalpable," "minute and thin," "sinking and minute," "collapsed without a pulse," "impalpable pulse after cessation of diarrhea," and "a pulse that suddenly bursts out" are all reflections of yang qi weakness, with the body's energy being in a state of decline and compromised heart function. Of course, if the blood pressure were to be checked, it would be low or lower than its usual pressure. On auscultation, the heart sounds would be low and soft. Descriptively, the aconite pulses are like a balloon that has leaked air: there is significant lack of force, and it is shriveled, thin, and soft.

The character of the aconite presentation is exactly the opposite of the gypsum, coptis, and rhubarb presentations discussed above. The gypsum presentation (feverishness, profuse sweating, irritability, thirst, and dry tongue), the coptis presentation (feverishness, irritability and irascibility, insomnia, and red tongue with a yellow, greasy tongue coating), and the rhubarb presentation (hot body with signs of constipation and a dry, burnt tongue) are all excessive heat presentations. Instead, with the aconite presentation, the body both feels cold and there is an aversion to cold. The patient is dispirited and listless, with a desire to lie down and sleep, the pulse is sinking, thin, or feeble, accompanied by a pale tongue with a white, slippery coating; all of these are deficiency-cold presentations. Excess heat presentations are yang presentations (陽證 *yáng zhèng*), while presentations of deficiency and cold are yin presentations (陰證 *yīn zhèng*); the character of these two are completely opposite of each other.

9.1 **Frigid Extremities Decoction** (四逆湯 *sì nì tāng*)

SOURCE: *Discussion of Cold Damage*

Aconiti Radix lateralis preparata (*zhì fù zǐ*) 3-10g
Zingiberis Rhizoma (*gān jiāng*) 3-6g
Glycyrrhizae Radix (*gān cǎo*) 3-6g

The words 'four reversals' (四逆 *sì nì*) in the name of this formula refer to frigid extremities and are indicative of severe coldness of the four limbs. Chinese medicine has two formulas in particular with the words Frigid Extremities, one being the bupleurum family formula Frigid Extremities Powder (*sì nì sǎn*) and the other being this formula. Although some of the symptoms are the same, the etiologies of the illnesses are quite different. The Frigid Extremities Powder presentation is a condition of interior heat, while the Frigid Extremities Decoction presentation is one of interior cold; the former falls into the category of excess, while the later is one of deficiency. Even though the names Frigid

Extremities Powder *(sì nì sǎn)* and Frigid Extremities Decoction *(sì nì tāng)* differ by only a single word, they have completely opposite presentations. The reader must not confuse them.

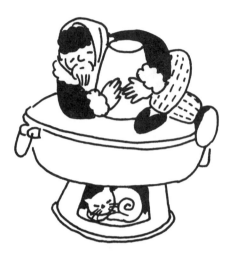

Frigid Extremities Decoction *(sì nì tāng)* is the representative prescription of the aconite formula family. Its yang-warming function is further strengthened by the pairing of Aconiti Radix lateralis preparata *(zhì fù zǐ)* and Zingiberis Rhizoma *(gān jiāng)*. This prescription has always been used for illnesses in that stage where yang turns into yin and the presentation goes from one of excess to one of deficiency. In practice, when this occurs, symptoms of yang deficiency with overabundant cold, such as frigid extremities, chills, being listless and dispirited, and a sinking, minute, and weak pulse, will manifest. The following passages in *Discussion of Cold Damage* refer to Frigid Extremities Decoction *(sì nì tāng)*:

- Paragraph 323: "*Shào yīn* diseases with a sinking pulse should be urgently warmed; Frigid Extremities Decoction *(sì nì tāng)* is appropriate."
- Paragraph 388: "When there is vomiting, diarrhea, and sweating with fever and chills, cramping of the limbs, and frigid hands and feet, Frigid Extremities Decoction *(sì nì tāng)* masters it."
- Paragraph 389: "When vomiting is followed by diarrhea, and then urination returns to normal along with profuse sweating, and diarrhea containing undigested food particles, this is interior cold with exterior heat. Where the pulse is minute and on the verge of being impalpable, Frigid Extremities Decoction *(sì nì tāng)* masters it."

- Paragraph 353: "If, after profuse sweating, the fever does not abate and there is internal tightness and contractions, pain in the extremities, along with diarrhea, frigid extremities, and chills, Frigid Extremities Decoction (*sì nì tāng*) masters it."

- Paragraph 225: "For those with a pulse that is floating and slow, the exterior is hot, and the interior is cold; if there is diarrhea with undigested food particles, Frigid Extremities Decoction (*sì nì tāng*) masters it."

- Paragraph 377, "For vomiting and a weak pulse when urination has returned to being smooth, the body is slightly hot, and inversion is observed, Frigid Extremities Decoction (*sì nì tāng*) masters it."

A glance at the above passages from the original text of *Discussion of Cold Damage* shows that Frigid Extremities Decoction (*sì nì tāng*) is primarily used to treat the aftermath of profuse sweating, severe episodes of vomiting, or diarrhea when the patient manifests the following three types of symptoms:

1. Minute and weak, or sinking and slow 'aconite pulse'
2. Frigid, stiff, and painful extremities
3. Chills, or a low-grade fever, or abdominal rigidity and spasms

Current clinical use of Frigid Extremities Decoction (*sì nì tāng*) is not dependent on the patient having a history of sweating, vomiting, or diarrhea. Patients who are constitutionally weak, whose yang qi is basically deficient, who are advanced in years, stressed, and overworked, have got chilled, lost blood, or have fevers, can also have a Frigid Extremities Decoction presentation. Other than the above-indicated symptoms, the tongue is of important diagnostic value. The tongue body will be pale or dark and pale, and the coating can be white and greasy, dry and greasy, or white and slippery. The tongue for this formula is the same as that for the dried ginger presentation. Furthermore, when these patients extend their tongue, they do so without much force. The specific formula presentation is as follows:

1. Pulse is either minute and weak, sinking and hidden, thin and soft, or suddenly becomes floating and large, but soft and empty with deep pressure, and without force (an aconite pulse)
2. Aversion to cold, frigid extremities; the lower half of the body (especially from the knees down) is icy cold and cannot be warmed up

3. Listless and dispirited with a desire to curl up and go to sleep
4. Pale, pale red, or dark pale tongue that usually is puffy and tender, with a white and greasy, grey and greasy, dry and greasy, or slippery and white coating ('dried ginger tongue')

From looking at the above list of symptoms, the most important points of the Frigid Extremities Decoction presentation are: an aconite pulse, frigid extremities, and 'dried ginger tongue.' Comparing and contrasting the presentation for this formula and that for Frigid Extremities Powder (*sì nì sǎn*) and Major Order the Qi Decoction (*dà chéng qì tāng*) will allow us to understand them better.

Sometimes the Major Order the Qi Decoction presentation can present with frigid extremities and a minute, weak pulse. If one just pays attention to these symptoms, it is easy to mix up these two presentations. However, the abdominal symptoms that are part of the Major Order the Qi Decoction presentation are rather obvious; furthermore, the tongue is dry and red with a burnt yellow coating. Frigid extremities is the symptom shared in common between Frigid Extremities Powder (*sì nì sǎn*) and Frigid Extremities Decoction (*sì nì tāng*). However, the cold versus heat and deficiency versus excess nature of these formula presentations are different. The important points of differentiation include the following:

- *The psycho-emotional states are different.* The overall body condition of patients with a Frigid Extremities Powder presentation is relatively good. They are in good spirits and their mental processes are clear. However, in Frigid Extremities Decoction presentations, the psycho-emotional situation is quite different as the patients are listless and dispirited, and it seems as if they are half asleep.

- *The pulses are different.* Although the pulse in a Frigid Extremities Powder presentation pulse is thin, it is also wiry, excessive, and forceful. The pulse in the presentation for Frigid Extremities Decoction, on the other hand, is totally deficient.

- *The tongues are also different.* The Frigid Extremities Powder (*sì nì sǎn*) tongue is red or dark red as well as often being tough and firm with a dry, yellow coating. By contrast, the Frigid Extremities Decoction (*sì nì tāng*) tongue is pale, pale red, or dark pale; it is often flabby or tender, and usually has a white, slippery, or greasy coating.

The frigid extremities and minute, almost impalpable, pulse that are core aspects of this formula's presentation can be seen in all types of shock. Chinese medicine refers to this condition as one of 'devastated yang' (亡陽 *wáng yáng*), where the yang qi within the body has collapsed. Frigid Extremities Decoction (*sì nì tāng*) is the prescription that effectively revives the yang and rescues from counterflow. There are reports of clinical success in using this formula to save the lives of those suffering from both septicemic and cardiogenic shock. One report details use of this formula, both unmodified and with the addition of Ginseng Radix (*rén shēn*), to treat 23 cases of cardiogenic shock. Among these cases, 10 underwent treatment by a combination of Western and Chinese medicine, and there were no fatalities.[1] There is another report concerning 20 patients suffering from cardiogenic shock. Among these, 17 were treated with injections of either Frigid Extremities Decoction (*sì nì tāng*) or Generate the Pulse Powder (*shēng mài sǎn*), with six of the patients using a combination of Chinese and Western medicine. One patient died while the blood pressure of the other 16 returned to normal. Of the three patients who were treated only with Western medicine, there was one fatality.

As observed in clinical practice, 10 to 20 minutes after giving injections of Frigid Extremities Decoction (*sì nì tāng*) or Generate the Pulse Powder (*shēng mài sǎn*) there are increases in blood pressure, but not significantly higher than normal, that can be maintained at normal levels. Furthermore, while these formulas did not have a significant effect on the heart rate in the above study, they did strengthen the heart sounds. In addition, the pulse changed from being thin and weak to having force, and there was an obvious improvement in the coldness of the arms and legs, ashen complexion, and cyanotic lips, thus pointing to an increase in the contractive force of the heart and improvement in microcirculation.[2] Experimental research also indicates that this formula has a significant protective effect in cases of shock from loss of blood, septic shock, cardiogenic shock, and shock secondary to intestinal ischemia. Anesthetized rabbits were used to model a condition of low blood pressure in order to investigate the effect of the complete formula and of each of the individual herbs of this formula; it was found that the complete formula's ability to protect against shock was superior to the use of the individual herbs by themselves. The formula had a more powerful impact with longer-lasting effects, and it was also capable of slowing down sinus rhythms as well as nonspecific arrthymias, thus showing that the formula's effect comes from the synergistic interaction of its constituent herbs.[3]

The relevant passages in *Discussion of Cold Damage* contain many references to vomiting and diarrhea, and clinically, digestive system disorders often are part of the presentation for this formula. There are clinical reports of this formula being effective in the treatment of diarrhea, especially for diarrhea in children. Wang used Frigid Extremities Decoction (sì nì tāng) with the addition of Coptidis Rhizoma (huáng lián) to treat 70 cases of pediatric diarrhea. Of these, 33 had taken Western medicine for three days without effect. Another 18 had taken at least three packets of another Chinese medicine prescription that was also ineffective. Two cases had been ineffectively treated by a combination of Western and Chinese medicine for over three weeks. The remaining 17 children had not been treated with any kind of medication. Treatment resulted in 58 cases obtaining a full recovery, eight recovering a short time after treatment, and four having no effect. From Wang's experience, he thinks it is appropriate to use this formula with children who have symptoms of loose stools, a temperature that is not significantly elevated, frigid extremities, a minute and weak pulse, and a white coated tongue.

Should there be an abundance of heat or dysentery, or if after taking the medicine the condition transforms into one with heat, then this formula is not appropriate.[4] Doctors at the Beijing College of Chinese Medicine observed six children with chronic diarrhea, all of whom had been unsuccessfully treated with the usual kinds of medicinals that warm the middle and build up the Spleen. Simply adding Aconiti Radix lateralis preparata (zhì fù zǐ) brought forth a significant result.[5] There are also reports of this formula being used to treat cor pulmonale leading to heart failure, stomach prolapse, severe hepatitis, sore throat, septicemia with persistent high fever, hypersomnia, schizophrenia, rheumatoid arthritis, nosebleeds, dysfunctional uterine bleeding, and prostatitis.

The clinical applications of Frigid Extremities Decoction (sì nì tāng) are quite extensive, but having a firm grasp of the pathodynamic of yang deficiency with overabundant yin is the key to using it well. In contemporary times, there have been many veteran doctors who have a wealth of experience in treating these types of problems; their work is worth studying. One example is the famous doctor from Yunnan, Wu Pei-Heng, who is quite skilled in the clinical use of Aconiti Radix lateralis preparata (zhì fù zǐ). He believes that Frigid Extremities Decoction (sì nì tāng) not only has the ability to revive the yang and rescue from counterflow, it can be used as well for every illness due to yang deficiency with an overabundance of yin-cold. Based on this, he used Frigid Extremities Decoction (sì nì tāng) to treat all types of internal medicine, gynecological, and pediatric illnesses. Additionally, he used Frigid Extremities Decoction (sì nì tāng) combined with a variety of herbs or other formulas to treat problems that have an aspect of cold or deficiency, some examples of which include:

- With Ephedrae Herba (*má huáng*), Asari Herba (*xì xīn*), and Two-Aged [Herb] Decoction (*èr chén tāng*) for coughs
- With Ephedrae Herba (*má huáng*), Asari Herba (*xì xīn*), and Cinnamomi Ramulus (*guì zhī*) for yang deficiency tooth pain
- With Cinnamomi Ramulus (*guì zhī*), Asari Herba (*xì xīn*), Atractylodis Rhizoma (*cāng zhú*), and Coicis Semen (*yì yǐ rén*) for rheumatic joint pain
- With the formula Licorice, Ginger, Poria, and White Atractrylodes Decoction (*gān cǎo gān jiāng fù líng bái zhú tāng*) for cold-damp back pain
- With Artemisiae scopariae Herba (*yīn chén*), Cinnamomi Cortex (*ròu guì*), and Five-Ingredient Powder with Poria (*wǔ líng sǎn*) for cirrhosis with ascites
- With Trichosanthes Fruit, Chinese Chive, and Wine Decoction (*gūa lǒu xìe bái bái jiǔ tāng*) for angina
- With Cinnamomi Cortex (*ròu guì*), Aucklandiae Radix (*mù xiāng*), Evodiae Fructus (*wú zhū yú*), Caryophylli Flos (*dīng xiāng*), and Poria (*fú líng*) for stomach ache
- With Astragali Radix (*huáng qí*), Angelicae sinensis Radix (*dāng guī*), and Gastrodiae Rhizoma (*tiān má*) for low blood pressure
- With Cinnamomi Cortex (*ròu guì*) and Actinolitum (*yáng qǐ shí*) for impotence and premature ejaculation
- With Ephedrae Herba (*má huáng*), Asari Herba (*xì xīn*), Cinnamomi Ramulus (*guì zhī*), and Zingiberis Rhizoma recens (*shēng jiāng*) for the early stages of mastitis
- With Artemisiae argyi Folium (*ài yè*), Astragali Radix (*huáng qí*), and Asini Corii Colla (*ē jiāo*) for dysfunctional uterine bleeding

Wu's experience in differential diagnosis comprises two mnemonic lists, each of which is only 16 characters in Chinese: "Yin presentations: a heavy body with chills, closed eyes, and a desire for sleep, soft voice with shortness of breath, not enough qi with laconic speech." At the same time, the mouth is moist and with a lack of thirst, or there is a desire for warm fluids but without an ability to drink much, and the breath of these patients does not warm one's hand. "Yang presentation: the patient is fidgety, manic or easily excitable with an aversion to heat, eyes that are open and insomnia; the voice is full and bright, along with bad breath and raspy breathing." At the same time, there is irritability and thirst with a desire for cold beverages, and the patient's breath feels hot. The use of

Frigid Extremities Decoction (sì nì tāng) is limited to the yin presentations.

Another example is the famous Sichuan doctor, Fan Zhong-Lin, who was also an expert in the clinical use of this formula. From a look at his case histories, we can see that he used Frigid Extremities Decoction (sì nì tāng) for diseases such as myasthenia gravis, dysfunctional uterine bleeding, thyroid enlargement, chronic pharyntitis, typhoid fever with high fever, pyelonephritis, and prostatitis, as well as for such symptoms as nosebleeds, dizziness, headaches, and asthma. In his differential diagnosis, he placed significant importance on the tongue, which is usually pale, pale red, or dark pale, and the tongue body itself being flabby or with teeth marks, and with a white and greasy, grey and greasy, or white and slippery coating.[6]

The toxicity of Aconiti Radix lateralis preparata (zhì fù zǐ) is relatively strong and comes primarily from the aconoitine. Aconoitine is not heat tolerant; decocting for a lengthy period of time breaks it down into aconine, thereby reducing its toxicity. Its active constituents, however, are not destroyed. Therefore, as a safety precaution, it is best to decoct Frigid Extremities Decoction (sì nì tāng) for an hour or more. Should the amount of Aconiti Radix lateralis preparata (zhì fù zǐ) in a prescription exceed 30g, it should be decocted even longer. According to other reports, decocting Aconiti Radix lateralis preparata (zhì fù zǐ) with Zingiberis Rhizoma (gān jiāng) and Glycyrrhizae Radix (gān cǎo) greatly reduces its toxicity. The Yunnan doctor noted above, Wu Pei-Heng, usually employs this method of detoxification by adding Zingiberis Rhizoma (gān jiāng) and Glycyrrhizae Radix (gān cǎo) when prescribing Aconiti Radix lateralis preparata (zhì fù zǐ). In addition, when decocting the herbs, patients are advised to first boil a pot of water, then add the herbs and cook for a longer period of time. Drawing from the expertise of others is helpful when considering ways to reduce the level of toxicity and improve clinical results when prescribing Aconiti Radix lateralis preparata (zhì fù zǐ).

It would be prudent to point out that both the Aconiti Radix lateralis preparata (zhì fù zǐ) and Zingiberis Rhizoma (gān jiāng) in Frigid Extremities Decoction (sì nì tāng) are acrid and hot medicinals. Pure yang prescriptions such as this one may only be used to treat yin-cold presentations. If this formula is used to treat a yang-heat presentation, it will result in symptoms of chest stuffiness, irritability and irascibility, and a dry tongue and mouth. Additionally, there will be a more pronounced reaction to the toxin in Aconiti Radix lateralis preparata (zhì fù zǐ). Therefore, distinguishing cold from heat and deficiency from excess is extremely important when using this prescription.

I have found that if there is a situation in my practice where deficiency and excess are difficult to differentiate and where there are syndromes of cold and heat being mixed together, then relying on constitutional diagnosis is the method to use. The presentation for Frigid Extremities Decoction (*sì nì tāng*) and other aconite family formulas is commonly seen in those with a yin-cold constitution; this body type is the complete opposite of the yang-heat constitution introduced in the Coptis Decoction to Resolve Toxicity (*huáng lián jiě dú tāng*) section. The yin-cold constitution consists of:

- *External distinguishing characteristics.* Tendency toward being overweight with loose musculature, dry skin, a dark or dark yellow complexion that lacks luster or appears edematous, eyes that lack spirit, feelings of being listless and dispirited, appears fatigued, pale, dark, withered, and dry lips, pale and flabby but dark tongue with a moist, white coating, soft and slack abdominal muscles, which feel weak when palpated
- *Predispositions.* Generally having an aversion to cold and being attracted to warmth, usually with frigid extremities (especially of the lower half of the body), easily fatigued, likes to be still and dislikes activity, stools that are watery and unformed, mouth is not dry and there is no thirst, or mild thirst with a desire for warm drinks, and copious, clear urination

9.2 Frigid Extremities Decoction plus Ginseng

(四逆加人參湯 *sì nì jiā rén shēn tāng*)

SOURCE: *Discussion of Cold Damage*

Aconiti Radix lateralis preparata (*zhì fù zǐ*) 3-10g
Glycyrrhizae Radix (*gān cǎo*) 3-6g
Zingiberis Rhizoma (*gān jiāng*) 3-5g
Ginseng Radix (*rén shēn*) 5-10

This formula is simply Frigid Extremities Decoction (*sì nì tāng*) plus Ginseng Radix (*rén shēn*). In *Discussion of Cold Damage*, it is used to treat those with "aversion to cold, a minute pulse, and diarrhea." Aversion to cold with a minute pulse are the typical signs of the Frigid Extremities Decoction presentation; these indicate the patient has suffered a loss of fluids from profuse sweating or severe diarrhea, which in turn leads to an extreme deficiency of yang qi. Continued diarrhea while the body is already in this weakened state advances the already severe fluid depletion and further injures the yang qi. This formula's presentation is a more advanced stage of the Frigid Extremities Decoction presentation. The Frigid Extremities Decoction presentation is one of yang deficiency with overabundant yin, while this formula's presentation, due to the depletion of internal body fluids, is one in which the yin and yang are both severely deficient.

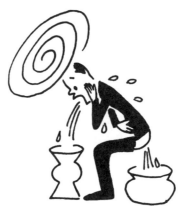

This formula's presentation then is simply that of the Frigid Extremities Decoction presentation combined with the ginseng presentation. Other than this formula, there are two others in *Discussion of Cold Damage* where the only addition is Ginseng Radix *(rén shēn)*. One is the cinnamon twig family formula Newly Augmented Decoction *(xīn jiā tāng)*, which is Cinnamon Twig Decoction *(guì zhī tāng)* plus Ginseng Radix *(rén shēn)* and larger amounts of both Paeoniae Radix *(sháo yào)* and Zingiberis Rhizoma recens *(shēng jiāng)*; it treats those who "after sweating, have body aches along with a sinking or slow pulse" (paragraph 62). The other is the gypsum family formula White Tiger plus Ginseng Decoction *(bái hǔ jiā rén shēn tāng)*; it treats "irritability and unquenchable thirst after profuse sweating" (paragraph 26), and "occasional aversion to wind, intense thirst, a dry and parched upper surface of the tongue, irritability, and a desire to drink large amounts of fluids" (paragraph 168). Additionally, a passage in *Discussion of Cold Damage* concerning Unblock the Pulse Decoction for Frigid Extremities *(tōng mài sì nì tāng)**** states that adding Ginseng Radix *(rén shēn)* treats "impalpable pulse after diarrhea has ceased." As seen in *Discussion of Cold Damage*, Ginseng Radix *(rén shēn)* is always added after profuse sweating or a serious bout of diarrhea when a patient will manifest

---

* This is the same as Frigid Extremities Decoction *(sì nì tāng)* except the amount of Zingiberis Rhizoma *(gān jiāng)* is increased.

with symptoms of a sinking, slow, minute, or weak pulse, body aches, dryness on the top of the tongue, and a significant degree of thirst. Furthermore, Ginseng Radix (rén shēn) combined with Aconiti Radix lateralis preparata (zhì fù zǐ) and Zingiberis Rhizoma (gān jiāng) is primarily used to treat those with diarrhea and a sinking, minute, or weak pulse.

The Frigid Extremities Decoction plus Ginseng presentation is as follows:

1. Aversion to cold, frigid limbs, being listless and dispirited
2. Diarrhea or watery stools, abdominal distention or epigastric focal distention with firmness, and poor appetite
3. A pulse that is minute, weak, sinking or slow; a dry tongue that lacks moisture

This formula's presentation is commonly seen in cases of diarrhea in children and the elderly. Additionally, it can be seen in cases of shock due to loss of blood, cardiogenic shock, myocardial infarction, or heart failure where a minute, sinking, or weak pulse is the primary manifestation.

If there are no symptoms of diarrhea or abdominal fullness, and the tongue is red and tender, then the Zingiberis Rhizoma (gān jiāng) and Glycyrrhizae Radix (gān cǎo) can be removed. The resulting formula is called Ginseng and Aconite Accessory Root Decoction (shēn fù tāng); it is primarily used in the treatment of all types of shock as well as a wide a variety of cardiovascular and cerebrovascular diseases.

9.3 **True Warrior Decoction** (真武湯 zhēn wǔ tāng)

SOURCE: *Discussion of Cold Damage*

Aconiti Radix lateralis preparata (zhì fù zǐ)	10g
Poria (fú líng)	10g
Atractylodis macrocephalae Rhizoma (bái zhú)	6g
Zingiberis Rhizoma recens (shēng jiāng)	10g
Paeoniae Radix (sháo yào)	10g

True Warrior Decoction (zhēn wǔ tāng) can be broken down into two parts: (1) Aconiti Radix lateralis preparata (zhì fù zǐ) with Poria (fú líng) and Atractylodis macrocephalae Rhizoma (bái zhú) and (2) Aconiti Radix lateralis preparata (zhì fù zǐ) with Paeoniae Radix alba (bái sháo). Poria (fú líng) and Atractylodis macrocephalae Rhizoma (bái zhú) are the essential medicinals used in Discus-

sion of Cold Damage for the treatment of urinary difficulty and edema. Aconiti Radix lateralis preparata *(zhì fù zǐ)* is added to this combination when there are aconite presentation signs of aversion to cold, listlessness and dispiritedness, and a minute, weak pulse. Paeoniae Radix alba *(bái sháo)* is the medicinal used in *Discussion of Cold Damage* to treat abdominal pain and leg cramps, and it is commonly combined with Glycyrrhizae Radix *(gān cǎo)*; this two-herb formula is called Peony and Licorice Decoction *(sháo yào gān cǎo tāng)*. The addition of Aconiti Radix lateralis preparata *(zhì fù zǐ)* results in the formula Peony, Licorice, and Aconite Accessory Root Decoction *(sháo yào gān cǎo fù zǐ tāng)*, which, according to paragraph 68 of *Discussion of Cold Damage*, is used "if, after inducing sweating, the disease is not released and instead there are chills." In True Warrior Decoction *(zhēn wǔ tāng)*, Aconiti Radix lateralis preparata *(zhì fù zǐ)* and Paeoniae Radix alba *(bái sháo)* are used together to treat the symptoms of abdominal pain, sweating, and aversion to cold. Glycyrrhizae Radix *(gān cǎo)* is not used in this formula, as there are symptoms of abdominal fullness and edema.

The True Warrior Decoction presentation is seen as the aconite presentation accompanied by the additional signs of urinary difficulty, edema, or abdominal fullness and pain. From the viewpoint of Chinese medicine, this type of disease is a yang deficiency thin mucus presentation.

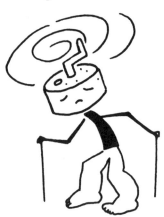

Chinese medicine recognizes thin mucus as a pathology of the fluid metabolism. In normal circumstances, the body's internal fluids are maintained in a certain state of equilibrium. If the yang qi is deficient, large amounts of internal body fluids, instead of circulating properly, are retained, thus themselves becoming a cause of disease. *Discussion of Cold Damage* (paragraph 82) uses this formula to treat greater yang diseases where "sweating that does not resolve the illness, these people have a persistent fever, palpitations in the epigastrium, dizziness, muscle twitches, or severe vertigo that makes it difficult to stand or easy for them to lose [their] balance and fall down" and "abdominal pain, urinary difficulty, a deep and heavy pain in the limbs, and diarrhea." All of these are signs of yang deficiency with thin mucus. The first set of symptoms—epigastric palpitations, dizziness, muscle twitches, and vertigo that makes standing up difficult—can be seen as rather severe manifestations of dizziness and palpitations. The latter set of symptoms—abdominal pain, urinary difficulty, a deep and heavy pain in the limbs, and diarrhea—is indicative of scanty urination that is neither smooth nor prompt, muscle cramping, edema, and coldness with pain, resulting in deep, heavy pain of the limbs, and spontaneous diarrhea that occurs even without the use of purgative herbs. All of these symptoms are actually the result of yang deficiency leading to thin mucus stagnating within the body. Other than the above-mentioned symptoms, there is a high probability of there being other associated symptoms, as noted in *Discussion of Cold Damage*: "These patients may have coughing, or urinary difficulty, or diarrhea, or vomiting." Some commonly seen signs of yang deficiency thin mucus presentations are as follows:

1. Dizziness, to the point where patients are unsteady on their feet
2. Palpitations, shortness of breath, muscle twitches
3. The body feels heavy and tired, penchant for sleep, deep, heavy limb pain, lower back pain, stiff joints
4. Scanty urine, watery stools, abdominal distention or pain, or nausea and vomiting
5. Edema of the lower extremities, or facial edema around the eyes
6. Coughing or wheezing, with clear, thin phlegm
7. Yellowish or dark complexion, pale and flabby tongue with a slippery and white or black and moist coating

In practice, as long as two or three items from the above list of symptoms are seen along with the following signs, True Warrior Decoction (*zhēn wǔ tāng*) can be used:

1. Listless and dispirited, desire to curl up and sleep, aversion to cold, frigid extremities, especially in the lower half of the body, with the area from the knees on down being icy cold

2. A minute and weak, sinking and hidden, or thin and weak
pulse

....

- The True Warrior Decoction presentation is often seen in cases of heart failure due to a wide variety of causes. There is a report of a modification of this formula being used to treat 15 patients with congestive heart failure. Among these patients were three with rheumatic mitral valve disease, one suffering from chronic cor pumonale, two with primary congestive cardiomyopathy, nine patients with acute right-sided heart failure, six with complete heart failure, seven with class IV heart function, another seven with class II, one with class I function, and three with accompanying arrhythmia. These cases of heart failure are all illnesses that develop relatively slowly over a long period of time. Furthermore, these cases did not respond well to treatment with the Western pharmaceutical digitalis or various diuretics; all were diagnosed with yang deficiency. A course of treatment consisted of one packet of herbs taken every day for five to seven days. If there was no improvement after the first course, treatment was considered ineffective for that patient. For those who showed improvement, another one to two courses of herbs were given. Treatment resulted in one case being cured, significant improvement for six cases, five experienced some improvement, and three experienced no effect. This treatment proved to be more effective for right ventricle failure than for complete heart failure. After the treatment, there were only two cases with class IV heart function, four cases with class III function, eight with class II functionality, and one for whom the situation was corrected. From the observations, it is believed that this treatment worked better for those with fewer instances of heart failure and where the disease process had been of shorter duration.[7]

- The True Warrior Decoction presentation is often seen with all types of cardiac and vascular disease. Use of True Warrior Decoction (zhēn wǔ tāng) is often effective for symptoms of dizziness and edema, which are commonly seen in cases of both high and low blood pressure. Japanese practitioners of Kampō use this formula to treat hypertension, and there are also reports from China that this formula reduces blood pressure in those with hypertension-induced heart disease with heart failure.[8] This formula is effective in the treatment of recurrent preventricular contractions, heart failure accompanied by atrial fibrillation, or from conduction delays.

- Cases of chronic nephritis and uremia, where edema is the primary symptom, are often seen with this formula's presentation. There is a report of using

True Warrior Decoction (*zhēn wǔ tāng*) with a small amount of prednisone to treat 12 cases of chronic nephritis. Treatment resulted in complete alleviation of symptoms for nine cases and partial relief for the other three. Among these cases, three were taking 20mg of prednisone per day, five were taking 30mg, three were taking 40mg, and one pediatric patient was taking 10mg. True Warrior Decoction (*zhēn wǔ tāng*) can increase the effectiveness of the ability of the prednisone to eliminate proteinuria and can reduce prednisone's side effects of immune suppression, metabolic disruption, and adrenal insufficiency.[9]

- Ménière's disease with dizziness as the primary symptom is commonly seen with the True Warrior Decoction presentation. There is a report of this formula, modified with the addition of Cinnamomi Ramulus (*guì zhī*), Asari Herba (*xì xīn*), Schisandrae Fructus (*wǔ wèi zǐ*), and Chuanxiong Rhizoma (*chuān xiōng*), being used to treat 41 cases of vertigo, resulting in 35 being completely cured. Among these, 18 cases were cured within two days, 13 recovered within four days, and four were cured within six days.[10]

- Frigid extremities are commonly seen in cases of thromboangitis obliterans along with symptoms of minute and weak arterial pulsation, a sinking and hidden pulse, or joint discomfort and edema; these symptoms are similar to those of the True Warrior Decoction presentation. There is reported use of this formula with the addition of Zingiberis Rhizoma (*gān jiāng*), Cinnamomi Ramulus (*guì zhī*), Codonopsis Radix (*dǎng shēn*), and Astragali Radix (*huáng qí*) being used to treat six cases of yin-type gangrene marked by the traditional findings of coldness, pain, hardness, swelling, and maceration. Among those six cases, four had accompanying nonpustulating, weeping ulcerations. Other than one case requiring amputation, all the remaining cases had their dorsal pedal pulse return to normal and their ulcers were healed. Generally, some results were seen after taking 10 to 20 packets of herbs. The least amount of herbs required was 22 packets, and the most was 60.[11]

- This formula can be considered for patients with digestive illnesses marked by abdominal fullness and distention, abdominal pain, a yellow or dark complexion with a pale, puffy tongue and a white and slippery, or black and moist coating. Cases of stomach prolapse, gastritis, peptic ulcers, constipation, diarrhea, and dumping syndromes seen after gastric surgery can be treated with this formula if they match its presentation.

- The True Warrior Decoction presentation is also seen in a wide variety of illnesses such as cases of neurosis, extrapyramidal diseases due to taking large amounts of chlorpromazine, recurrent neuralgia, sciatica, facial tics, essential tremor, profuse sweating, night sweats, vaginal discharge, amenorrhea, and fever in debilitated patients.

One needs to differentiate between the presentations for True Warrior Decoction (*zhēn wǔ tāng*) and Poria, Cinnamon Twig, Atractylodes, and Licorice Decoction (*líng guì zhú gān tāng*), as both formulas treat thin mucus. The Poria, Cinnamon Twig, Atractylodes, and Licorice Decoction presentation is the cinnamon twig presentation accompanied by signs of thin mucus, which results in symptoms of dizziness, palpitations with simultaneous sensation of something rushing upward on the chest, and counterflow with fullness in the epigastrium. These problems come on very quickly, and emotional stress is often the precipitant. However, once they calm down, it is as if nothing had happened. By contrast, the True Warrior Decoction presentation is the aconite presentation accompanied by signs of thin mucus with symptoms of dizziness, palpitations with simultaneous chills, being listless and dispirited, with a sinking, minute, or weak pulse, abdominal fullness and pain, or heavy and painful limbs.

9.4 Aconite Accessory Root Decoction to Drain the Epigastrium (附子瀉心湯 *fù zǐ xiè xīn tāng*)

SOURCE: *Discussion of Cold Damage*

Aconiti Radix lateralis preparata (*zhì fù zǐ*) 6-10g
Rhei Radix et Rhizoma (*dà huáng*) 6-10g
Coptidis Rhizoma (*huáng lián*) 3-6g
Scutellariae Radix (*huáng qín*) 3-10g

Aconite Accessory Root Decoction to Drain the Epigastrium (*fù zǐ xiè xīn tāng*) is the aconite family's prescription for clearing heat and purging downward. In clinical practice, aconite presentations, of course, occur in pure deficiency patterns; there are also aconite presentations in mixed patterns of cold/heat and deficiency/excess. One example would be when people with constitutional yang deficiency or a debilitated elderly person develops food damage (傷食 *shāng shí*) from an improper diet; another would be the result of the overuse of cold medicines in the treatment of what originally was an excess heat presentation. One aspect of this presentation are the rhubarb and coptis signs of abdominal fullness, upper abdominal focal distention, fullness, and pain, constipation or temesus, extreme irritability and agitation, and a greasy, yellow tongue coating.

The other aspect includes the aconite signs of chills, frigid extremities, cold sweats, and a sinking, minute, or weak pulse. Treatment must take into account both aspects of this presentation.

Discussion of Cold Damage (paragraph 155) states: "With epigastric focal distention, if there is also chills and sweating, Aconite Accessory Root Decoction to Drain the Epigastrium *(fù zǐ xiè xīn tāng)* masters it." Epigastric focal distention is the definitive sign for use of the herbal pair Coptidis Rhizoma *(huáng lián)* and Scutellariae Radix *(huáng qín)*; this presentation falls into the category of heat. Aversion to cold with sweating is an indication for the use of Aconiti Radix lateralis preparata *(zhì fù zǐ)*; it falls into the category of cold. Patients who commonly have the exterior deficiency symptoms of aversion to wind and cold with spontaneous sweating can, due to pathological changes in their condition, manifest with the interior heat presentation of epigastric focal distention. At the onset of the illness, the commonly seen symptoms of chills with sweating briefly manifest and then disappear. However, chills and sweating will return later at a more severe level and will be accompanied by the yang deficiency signs of frigid extremities, feeling listless and dispirited, along with a sinking, minute, or weak pulse. This is the presentation for which Aconite Accessory Root Decoction to Drain the Epigastrium *(fù zǐ xiè xīn tāng)* should be used. The Aconite Accessory Root Decoction to Drain the Epigastrium presentation is as follows:

1. Epigastric focal distention, or upper abdominal distention and pain, constipation or tememsus, extreme irritability and agitation, or a muddled consciousness, and a yellow, greasy tongue coating

2. Chills with sweating, or cold sweating from the forehead, frigid extremities, a sinking, minute, or weak pulse, or low blood pressure

The Aconite Accessory Root Decoction to Drain the Epigastrium presentation is often seen in cases of dysentery, chronic colitis, biliary tract disease, gastritis, or digestive illnesses in the elderly such as pancreatitis, cholecystitis, or cholelithitis.

While the traditional method of preparation, as outlined in *Discussion of Cold Damage*, is to infuse the 'three yellows,' in modern clinical practice, because formulas are often cooked at the pharmacy, this method is rarely used.

Discussion of Cold Damage has a unique method of decocting and administering this formula. First, the three herbs Rhei Radix et Rhizoma (*dà huáng*), Coptidis Rhizoma (*huáng lián*), and Scutellariae Radix (*huáng qín*) are steeped for five minutes in boiling water, the dregs are then removed, and the fluid saved for use. Next, Aconiti Radix lateralis preparata (*zhì fù zǐ*) is separately decocted, and the two fluids are then combined, divided into portions, and served warm. Traditionally, it is believed that this method of preparation can prevent possible side effects from the above-mentioned 'three yellows' overstimulating the intestines. Furthermore, combining that fluid with Aconiti Radix lateralis preparata (*zhì fù zǐ*) potentiates this formula's therapeutic effect. Modern pharmacological research on this has yet to be done.

In *Discussion of Cold Damage* are five prescriptions containing the phrase 'drain the epigastrium.' Pinellia Decoction to Drain the Epigastrium (*bàn xià xiè xīn tāng*), Fresh Ginger Decoction to Drain the Epigastrium (*shēng jiāng xiè xīn tāng*), Licorice Decoction to Drain the Epigastrium (*gān cǎo xiè xīn tāng*), Rhubarb and Coptis Decoction to Drain the Epigastrium (*dà huáng huáng lián xiè xīn tāng*), and this section's formula, Aconite Accessory Root Decoction to Drain the Epigastrium (*fù zǐ xiè xīn tāng*). Examination of the herbs used in these formulas shows that all contain both Coptidis Rhizoma (*huáng lián*) and Scutellariae Radix (*huáng qín*); analysis of the symptoms treated shows that all the 'drain the epigastrium' presentations include focal distention. Aconite Accessory Root Decoction to Drain the Epigastrium (*fù zǐ xiè xīn tāng*) uses Coptidis Rhizoma (*huáng lián*) and Scutellariae Radix (*huáng qín*) combined with Aconiti Radix lateralis preparata (*zhì fù zǐ*); its distinctive formula presentation is focal distention accompanied by the aconite presentation. In practice, it is not a difficult differentiation.

CHAPTER 10

PINELLIA FORMULA FAMILY

....

半夏類方 bàn xià lèi fāng

Every year in early summer in the shadowy damp places on hillsides, the sides of streams, and mulberry plantations, there is found a commonly seen small plant with long, thin petiole, tender green leaves, and an especially long calyx that produces small white flowers. It is the rhizome of this small plant that is used as Pinelliae Rhizoma preparatum (*zhì bàn xià*). Pinelliae Rhizoma preparatum (*zhì bàn xià*) has an acrid, spicy flavor. When chewed, it becomes pasty, numbs the tongue, and can irritate the throat. While toxic in its fresh state, treating it by frying with Zingiberis Rhizoma recens (*shēng jiāng*) or Alumen (*míng fán*) eliminates its toxicity. In the clinic, this is the form that is almost always used, which is why the term 'prepared' appears in Pinelliae Rhizoma preparatum (*zhì bàn xià*).

The scope of appropriate clinical uses for Pinelliae Rhizoma preparatum (*zhì bàn xià*) is quite extensive. *Discussion of Cold Damage* (傷寒論 *Shāng hán lùn*) includes 18 formulas that use Pinelliae Rhizoma preparatum (*zhì bàn xià*), and there are some 30-odd prescriptions in *Essentials from the Golden Cabinet* (金匱要略 *Jīn guì yào lüè*) that also include this herb. Formulas containing Pinelliae Rhizoma preparatum (*zhì bàn xià*) from later dynasties are even more numerous, to the point of being practically uncountable. Here is a simple introduction to some of the common uses of Pinelliae Rhizoma preparatum (*zhì bàn xià*):

- With Zingiberis Rhizoma (*gān jiāng*), it treats nausea and vomiting.
- With Poria (*fú líng*), it treats palpitations and insomnia.
- With Gastrodiae Rhizoma (*tiān má*) and Atractylodis macrocephalae Rhizoma (*bái zhú*), it treats headaches with dizziness.
- With Coptidis Rhizoma (*huáng lián*) and Trichosanthis Fructus (*guā lóu*), it treats chest fullness with coughing.

- With Coptidis Rhizoma (*huáng lián*) and Scutellariae Radix (*huáng qín*), it treats epigastric focal distention with irritability and restlessness.
- With Magnoliae officinalis Cortex (*hòu pò*), Perillae Folium (*zǐ sū yè*), and Poria (*fú líng*), it treats the sensation of something being stuck in the throat.
- With Aurantii Fructus immaturus (*zhǐ shí*), Poria (*fú líng*), Glycyrrhizae Radix (*gān cǎo*), Bambusae Caulis in taeniam (*zhú rú*), and Citri reticulatae Pericarpium (*chén pí*), it treats panic and being easily startled, nausea and vomiting, dizziness, and insomnia.
- With Zingiberis Rhizoma recens (*shēng jiāng*), Asari Herba (*xì xīn*), and Schisandrae Fructus (*wǔ wèi zǐ*), it treats coughing with profuse sputum.
- With Ephedrae Herba (*má huáng*), it treats those with whole body edema and a sallow complexion.
- With Magnoliae officinalis Cortex (*hòu pò*), Zingiberis Rhizoma recens (*shēng jiāng*), and Ginseng Radix (*rén shēn*), it reduces abdominal fullness.
- With Ginseng Radix (*rén shēn*) and Mel (*fēng mì*), it treats acid regurgitation and epigastric focal distention with firmness.
- With Trichosanthis Fructus (*guā lóu*) and Allii macrostemi Bulbus (*xiè bái*), it treats chest painful obstruction or chest pain.

Chinese medicine regards Pinelliae Rhizoma preparatum (*zhì bàn xià*) as a phlegm-transforming medicinal. It treats all types of phlegm, not only sputum that can be coughed up, but also phlegm retained in the body and formless phlegm that cannot be seen by the naked eye. In the Chinese medicine way of thinking, phlegm gets stuck in different places, which in turn generates different types of symptoms in those places. Here are some examples:

- 'Phlegm misting the orifices of the heart,' leading to mental derangement, epilepsy, irritability with an inability to calm down, and insomnia
- 'Phlegm in the Lungs,' generating coughing with chest stuffiness and profuse sputum that is difficult to expectorate
- 'Phlegm obstructing the qi of the diaphragm,' resulting in nausea, vomiting, or a sensation of something being caught in the throat
- 'Wind-phlegm harassing upward,' leading to dizziness, headache, numbness of the limbs, or spasms
- 'Phlegm-heat lodged in the Heart,' leading to chest stuffiness, profuse sputum, palpitations, and nausea

- 'Phlegm stagnation congealing in the channels and collaterals,' causing hemiplegia and numbness of the limbs

- 'Phlegm lodging in the joints,' causing joint swelling, pain, and deformity

- 'Phlegm nodules,' manifesting as lumps or swollen lymph nodes that are neither painful nor itchy nor red nor hot

- 'Phlegm obstructing the Womb,' resulting in obesity, infertility, amenorrhea, or profuse vaginal discharge

- 'Phlegm-fire,' with a phlegm presentation accompanied by symptoms of a red complexion with irritability and restlessness, dry mouth, constipation, and a red tongue

- 'Phlegm-dampness,' giving rise to a body that feels heavy and tired, with a sallow complexion, abdominal distention, watery stools, and a white, greasy tongue coating

Because in clinical practice there are numerous patients with phlegm-induced illnesses, Chinese doctors have coined the expression, "The hundred illnesses are due mostly to mischief caused by phlegm" (百病多由痰作祟 *bǎi bìng duō yóu tán zuò suì*). Pinelliae Rhizoma preparatum *(zhì bàn xià)* can be used to treat just about all of the above phlegm-induced illnesses. There are many opportunities to use this herb, particularly for diseases of the digestive, respiratory, or neuro-endocrine systems. How can one grasp the set of signs and symptoms that constitute the pinellia presentation? Apart from the above-mentioned symptoms, the following are the definitive signs that confirm the pinellia presentation:

1. Nausea or occasional nausea, which when severe results in vomiting
2. Slippery or greasy tongue coating
3. Sallow or dull, ashen complexion

Patients with phlegm disorders often have nausea with vomiting, tend to feel nauseous, and often respond with nausea to things that disgust them; constitutionally, they tend to be psycho-emotionally sensitive. Tongues with a white, slippery, and moist or greasy coating are frequently seen in the visual observation part of the clinical examination, and these coatings are relatively thick. Should the tongue be shiny, red, and without a coating, or the tongue surface dry, these are contraindications for the use of Pinelliae Rhizoma preparatum (*zhì bàn xià*); if the tongue coating is dry and burnt, Pinelliae Rhizoma preparatum (*zhì bàn xià*) also cannot be used. In short, the pinellia tongue must be moist and slippery. The complexion of patients with phlegm types of illness usually lack a normal amount of luster or is yellow-black, ashen and dark, or has a puffy appearance.

There are some important differences between the pinellia and dried ginger presentations. The dried ginger presentation often has abdominal fullness, watery stools, an aversion to cold, and a thick, white, greasy tongue coating, while the pinellia presentation usually includes nausea and vomiting, often accompanied by constipation, and no aversion to cold; the tongue has a white, greasy coating, but is not thick. The functions of the two medicinals are different: Pinelliae Rhizoma preparatum (*zhì bàn xià*) directs counterflow downward, stops vomiting, and disperses clumps, while Zingiberis Rhizoma (*gān jiāng*) warms the middle, stops diarrhea, and disperses cold.

Modern pharmacological experimentation has shown that Pinelliae Rhizoma preparatum (*zhì bàn xià*) functions to dilate the bronchioles and alleviate bronchospasms. It also functions to promote the urinary excretion of morphine and digitalis and stops vomiting caused by ingestion of copper sulfate. It functions as an antihypertensive, detoxifies, and has glucocorticoid-like effects.

10.1 Minor Pinellia Decoction (小半夏湯 *xiǎo bàn xià tāng*)

SOURCE: *Essentials from the Golden Cabinet*

Pinelliae Rhizoma preparatum (*zhì bàn xià*) 6-12g
Zingiberis Rhizoma recens (*shēng jiāng*).......................... 5-10g

This formula is the pinellia family prescription to stop vomiting. Apart from the anti-emetic effect of Pinelliae Rhizoma preparatum (*zhì bàn xià*), there is also the anti-emetic and stomachic function of Zingiberis Rhizoma recens (*shēng jiāng*). A common and effective Chinese folk remedy for unremitting vomiting is to drip ginger juice onto the tongue. Using the right amount of fresh ginger in cooking increases the flavor of the food and promotes the appetite. Modern pharmacological research has shown that a decoction of Zingiberis Rhizoma recens (*shēng jiāng*) stimulates secretions of the digestive glands and functions to protect the cells of the stomach mucosa. Therefore, both *Discussion of Cold Damage* and *Essentials from the Golden Cabinet* include many prescriptions that use this pairing of Pinelliae Rhizoma preparatum *(zhì bàn xià)* and Zingiberis Rhizoma recens *(shēng jiāng).*

Nausea and vomiting may be due to a variety of factors; the nausea and vomiting treated by Minor Pinellia Decoction *(xiǎo bàn xià tāng)* is seen in presentations of phlegm and dampness. Therefore, the tongue in these cases must have a white and slippery or white and greasy coating; there is a lack of thirst or an abundance of clear saliva; or there is coughing with profuse, thin sputum or watery sounds in the epigastrium. *Essentials from the Golden Cabinet* observes: "Those suffering from vomiting should have thirst, as the thirst is an indication that the condition will resolve. If, however, there is a lack of thirst, it is indicative of prodding thin mucus (支飲 *zhī yǐn*) in the epigastrium, and Minor Pinellia Decoction *(xiǎo bàn xià tāng)* masters it." What is called "prodding thin mucus in the epigastrium" is simply either watery sounds in the epigastrium or coughing with profuse, clear, thin sputum accompanied by chest and diaphragm fullness and distention. This formula's presentation is as follows:

1. Nausea and vomiting
2. No thirst or aversion to drinking, or abundant saliva in the mouth, or coughing with profuse, thin sputum, or watery sounds in the epigastrium, and chest and diaphragm fullness and distention
3. Relatively thick, white, and slippery or white and greasy tongue coating

If, apart from nausea and vomiting, there are also symptoms of headache, constipation, fever, abdominal or chest pain, one must then compare and differentiate with other formula presentations. In practice, it is not rare to see vomiting in rhubarb, gypsum, aconite, and coptis presentations.

• Minor Pinellia Decoction presentation is often seen in cases of neurogenic vomiting, morning sickness, gastrectomy, or drug-induced vomiting. There is a report of this formula having a significant effect in the treatment of vomiting from a variety of causes, including after a major gastrectomy.[1] Old Chinese medicine doctors in my hometown still use this formula with considerable success to treat vomiting of clear, watery fluids when accompanied by Ménière's disease.

• Those with bronchitis, asthma, and other respiratory tract disorders with coughing of profuse sputum or chest fullness and nausea can also use this formula. There is a reported use of ginger-treated Pinelliae Rhizoma prepara-tum (*jiāng bàn xià*) being administered, either by intramuscular injection or as an insufflation, to 144 subjects with silicosis. Patients' subjective sense of symptoms had varying degrees of improvement.[2]

MODIFICATIONS

In practice, a pure Minor Pinellia Decoction presentation is rarely seen; mixed patterns are more commonly encountered. For example, in the case of patients also having dizziness, palpitations, and epigastric focal distention, Poria (*fú líng*) can be added; this formula is called Minor Pinellia plus Poria Decoction (*xiǎo bàn xià jiā fú líng tāng*). In *Essentials from the Golden Cabinet* it is used to treat "sudden vomiting, epigastric focal distention, [pathogenic] water in the diaphragm, dizziness, and palpitations." Its distinguishing characteristic is the Minor Pinellia Decoction presentation accompanied by signs of thin mucus, with urinary difficulty, dizziness, or palpitations and muscle twitches. There is a report of using Pinelliae Rhizoma preparatum (*zhì bàn xià*) 40g, first decocted by itself for 30 minutes, then adding Poria (*fú líng*) 30g and Zingiberis Rhizoma recens (*shēng jiāng*) 30g, to treat a case of stomachache and hiccups brought about by eating too much cold and raw food. After taking four packets of herbs, all the symptoms disappeared. This patient presented with symptoms of vomiting clear, watery sputum mixed with saliva, having an aversion to cold, a desire for warmth and pressure on the abdomen during periods of pain, as well as abdominal distention, a poor appetite, no particular thirst but a desire for warm fluids, a white tongue coating, and a minute, sinking, and tight pulse.[3] Minor Pinellia plus Poria Decoction (*xiǎo bàn xià jiā fú líng tāng*) with the addition of Citri reticulatae Pericarpium (*chén pí*) and Glycyrrhizae Radix (*gān cǎo*) is the famous prescription Two-Aged [Herb] Decoction (*èr chén tāng*), which is the primary formula for treating disorders of phlegm-thin mucus. Later generations of doctors when treating coughing induced by phlegm-thin mucus, vomiting, dizziness, palpitations, and epigastric focal distention presen-tations invariably used it as the base formula to transform and reduce phlegm and modified it as needed.

10.2 Warm Gallbladder Decoction (溫膽湯 *wēn dǎn tāng*)

SOURCE: *Discussion of Illnesses, Patterns, and Formulas Related to the Unification of the Three Etiologies* (三因極一病證方論 *Sān yīn jí yī bìng zhèng fāng lùn*)

Pinelliae Rhizoma preparatum (*zhì bàn xià*) 6-12g

Poria (*fú líng*) 6-12g

Citri reticulatae Pericarpium (*chén pí*) 6-10g

Glycyrrhizae Radix (*gān cǎo*) 3g

Aurantii Fructus immaturus (*zhǐ shí*) 6-12g

Bambusae Caulis in taeniam (*zhú rú*) 6g

Jujubae Fructus (*dà zǎo*) 5-10g

Zingiberis Rhizoma recens (*shēng jiāng*) 3-6g

While this formula's name is Warm Gallbladder Decoction (*wēn dǎn tāng*), in fact, the nature of the medicinals that comprise it are not at all warm or hot; actually, it has a rather good sedative effect. The original text records this prescription as primarily treating those who "are easily startled by events, have dream-disturbed sleep, shortness of breath, palpitations and fatigue, or spontaneous sweating." Presently, it is often used clinically in the treatment of neuroses, mental illness, autonomic dystonia, biliary disease, gastrointestinal illness, cardiovascular disease, or cerebrovascular disease.

The Warm Gallbladder Decoction presentation is as follows:

1 Nausea, vomiting, bitter taste and/or sticky feeling in the mouth
2 Emotional lability, being easily startled, panicky, insomnia or dream-disturbed sleep
3 Greasy or slippery tongue coating

Those with the Warm Gallbladder presentation often express with prominent psycho-emotional symptoms that include sleep disorders, insomnia with excessive dreaming, irritability and restlessness with an inability to calm down, being easily startled, and a stifling feeling in the chest. Furthermore, these patients frequently suffer from panic attacks secondary to receiving some kind of severe emotional shock. These situations are similar to what Chinese folk sayings describe as being timid (膽小 *dǎn xiǎo*, literally 'small Gallbladder'), cowardly (膽怯 *dǎn qiè*, literally 'timid Gallbladder'), and scared stiff (嚇破膽 *xià pò dǎn*, literally 'scared and broken Gallbladder'). Accordingly, Warm Gallbladder Decoction (*wēn dǎn tāng*) can be regarded as a Gallbladder-strengthening/Gallbladder-emboldening medicinal (壯膽藥 *zhuàng dǎn yào*).

The Warm Gallbladder Decoction presentation is commonly seen in the following illnesses:

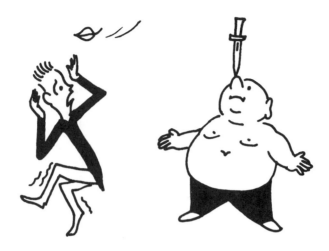

- *Mental illness.* There is a report of using a modification of Warm Gallbladder Decoction *(wēn dǎn tāng)* to treat 149 mentally ill patients with severe symptoms. Among these were 101 patients with schizophrenia, 13 with bipolar disorder, 13 with reactive psychosis, 10 with perimenopausal mental illness, and the remaining 12 had other psychological disorders. Of these patients, 64 were ill due to hereditary factors, and the remainder's illnesses were provoked by emotional factors. The length of illness for most patients ranged from three to five months. Treatment resulted in a complete cure for 117 patients, another two were significantly better, 24 showed some improvement, and six showed no effect. The most herbs administered were 34 packets, which was taken by one patient, but generally only three to 12 packets were required.[4] Another report used a modification of Warm Gallbladder Decoction *(wēn dǎn tāng)* to treat 30 schizophrenic patients. The herbs were administered from eight to 45 days, with most cases taking the herbs for 16 to 38 days. Treatment resulted in a complete recovery for 16 cases, improvement for another 12, and no effect for the remaining two cases.[5] Related reports are relatively numerous; most add in the medicinals Coptidis Rhizoma *(huáng lián)*, Acori tatarinowii Rhizoma *(shí chāng pǔ)*, Polygalae Radix *(yuǎn zhì)*, and Bambusae Concretio silicea *(tiān zhú huáng)*.

- *Insomnia.* Reports concerning insomnia are quite numerous. There is a report of this formula treating 50 subjects with Heart and Gallbladder deficiency type insomnia. All were cured, with the least amount of herbs required being three packets while the most was 20 packets.[6] There is another report of using Ten-Ingredient Decoction to Warm Gallbladder *(shí wèi wēn dǎn tāng)*[7] to treat 25 patients with yin deficiency phlegm-dampness type insomnia; excellent results were obtained.*

I once treated a young girl who, due to an automobile accident, would tremble with fear and suffered from insomnia where, every night, she would not be able to fall asleep until just before dawn and then slept for only a short time. Any little noise would wake her; it was as if although she slept, it was not real sleep. She spent her days as if in a trance, her appetite was poor, she was occasionally dizzy and/or nauseous, and her tongue had a white, greasy coating. Using Western pharmaceutical sedatives did not help much. Administering seven packets of Warm Gallbladder Decoction (*wēn dǎn tāng*) modified with Polygalae Radix (*yuǎn zhì*) and Acori tatarinowii Rhizoma (*shí chāng pú*) reduced her symptoms; continuing to take another 10 packets returned her to normal.

- *Neurosis.* According to one report, 77 patients with either menopausal syndrome or psycho-emotional changes after undergoing sterilization were treated, with 56 recovering completely and 21 showing improvement.[8] This formula with the addition of Bupleuri Radix (*chái hú*) and Scutellariae Radix (*huáng qín*) is also effective in treating neurosis and hysteria.[9]

- *Autonomic dystonia.* There is a report of using this formula to treat 165 cases, resulting in significant effect in 72 percent of the cases.[10]

- *Epilepsy.* This formula has been effective in treating epilepsy in children, primary epilepsy, and intracranial infections.

- *Head trauma.* There is a report concerning 15 head trauma cases where all had varying degrees of headache, nausea, constipation, irritability, and insomnia, and the tongue coating for the most part was either thick and greasy or thin and greasy. Treatment consisted of using Warm Gallbladder Decoction (*wēn dǎn tāng*) with the addition of Persicae Semen (*táo rén*), Carthami Flos (*hóng huā*), Salviae miltiorrhizae Radix (*dān shēn*), Cyperi Rhizoma (*xiāng fù*), and Polygalae Radix (*yuǎn zhì*). Five of the cases showed a significant improvement in their symptoms.[11]

- *Dizziness.* There is reported use of this formula with the addition of Puerariae Radix (*gé gēn*), Uncariae Ramulus cum Uncis (*gōu téng*), and Magnetitum (*cí shí*) as the primary treatment in 62 cases of Ménière's disease. Other than five cases, which, due to severe vomiting required the support of intravenous

---

* Warm Gallbladder Decoction (*wēn dǎn tāng*) with the additions of Ginseng Radix (*rén shēn*), Rehmanniae Radix preparata (*shú dì huáng*), Ziziphi spinosae Semen (*suān zǎo rén*), Polygalae Radix (*yuǎn zhì*), and Schisandrae Fructus (*wǔ wèi zǐ*).

fluids, all the rest only used the above medicinals. Generally, the symptoms were alleviated after the administration of one to three packets of herbs.[12]

• *Coronary heart disease and angina.* There are many reports of using this formula for these problems. This formula can reduce symptoms and improve electrocardiograms. Combined with Generate the Pulse Powder (*shēng mài sǎn*),* it treats coronary heart disease with preventricular contractions and cardiogenic shock; adding Ginseng Radix (*rén shēn*) and Astragali Radix (*huáng qí*) is effective for the treatment of coronary heart disease with atrial fibrillation.

• *Peptic ulcers, gastritis, and cholecystitis.* These digestive problems can be treated by using this formula with the addition of Coptidis Rhizoma (*huáng lián*) or combining it with Minor Decoction [for Pathogens] Stuck in the Chest (*xiǎo xiàn xiōng tāng*).

The key to using Warm Gallbladder Decoction (*wēn dǎn tāng*) well is first to master the pathomechinisms, complications, and various formula presentations that are seen in the above introduced neuropsychological, cardiovascular, and digestive system illnesses. Ordinarily, when using this formula, one needs to see nausea and vomiting, bitter taste and sticky feeling in the mouth, feelings of timidity and fright, insomnia with excessive dreaming, and a greasy or slippery tongue coating. The second key is to properly modify the formula in accordance with the patient's condition.

COMMONLY USED MODIFICATIONS

• Warm Gallbladder Decoction with Coptis (*huáng lián wēn dǎn tāng*) comes from *Warp and Woof of Warm-Heat Diseases* (溫熱經緯 *Wēn rè jīng wěi*), and, as the name suggests, is Warm Gallbladder Decoction (*wēn dǎn tāng*) with the addition of Coptidis Rhizoma (*huáng lián*). It is suitable to use when the Warm Gallbladder Decoction presentation is seen along with a red tongue, yellow and greasy tongue coating, epigastric focal distention, irritability and restless, insomnia, and a red complexion (coptis presentation). It is also commonly used to treat chronic gastritis, high blood pressure, mental disorders, hyperlipidemia, hypercholesterolemia, and dizziness.

• Guide Out Phlegm Decoction (*dǎo tán tāng*) comes from *Formulas to Aid the Living* (濟生方 *Jì shēng fāng*). It is Warm Gallbladder Decoction (*wēn dǎn tāng*) with the Bambusae Caulis in taeniam (*zhú rú*) and Zingiberis Rhizoma

---

* Ginseng Radix (*rén shēn*), Ophiopogonis Radix (*mài mén dōng*), and Schisandrae Fructus (*wǔ wèi zǐ*).

recens (*shēng jiāng*) removed, and Arisaema cum Bile (*dǎn nán xīng*) added. Arisaematis Rhizoma preparatum (*zhì tiān nán xīng*) functions to transform phlegm and calm spasms, treating dizziness, epilepsy, facial palsy, and paralysis from stroke. After being processed using bovine bile, Arisaematis Rhizoma (*tiān nán xīng*) is called Arisaema cum Bile (*dǎn nán xīng*); its nature is relatively even and harmonizing. Guide Out Phlegm Decoction (*dǎo tán tāng*) is primarily prescribed for those with dizziness, fainting, stroke, epilepsy, and facial palsy, when a stifling sensation in the chest and profusion of phlegm with a thick, greasy tongue coating are seen.

• Ten-Ingredient Decoction to Warm Gallbladder (*shí wèi wēn dǎn tāng*) comes from *Indispensable Tools for Pattern Treatment* (證治准繩 *Zhèng zhì zhǔn shéng*). It is Warm Gallbladder Decoction (*wēn dǎn tāng*) with the addition of Ginseng Radix (*rén shēn*), Rehmanniae Radix preparata (*shú dì huáng*), Ziziphi spinosae Semen (*suān zǎo rén*), and Polygalae Radix (*yuǎn zhì*). It is suitable for use with patients who have an emaciated physique and are dispirited and listless, or have been ill for a long time with a tongue body that is relatively thin and pale red, have a Warm Gallbladder Decoction presentation, and complain mainly of palpitations, insomnia, and forgetfulness. It is a formula that is often suitable for use in cases of heart disease and nervous exhaustion.

• Warm Gallbladder Decoction with Bamboo Shavings (*zhú rú wēn dǎn tāng*) is found in *Restoration of Health from the Myriad Diseases* (萬病回春 *Wàng bìng huí chūn*). It is comprised of Warm Gallbladder Decoction (*wēn dǎn tāng*) with the addition of Bupleuri Radix (*chái hú*), Ginseng Radix (*rén shēn*), Coptidis Rhizoma (*huáng lián*), Platycodi Radix (*jié gěng*), Ophiopogonis Radix (*mài mén dōng*), and Cyperi Rhizoma (*xiāng fù*). This formula is suitable for use in treating those with the Warm Gallbladder Decoction presentation when accompanied by chest and hypochondriac fullness and discomfort, a bitter taste in the mouth, coughing with yellow sputum, irritability, and insomnia.

10.3 **Major Pinellia Decoction** (大半夏湯 *dà bàn xià tāng*)

SOURCE: *Essentials from the Golden Cabinet*

Pinelliae Rhizoma preparatum (*zhì bàn xià*) 6-12g
Ginseng Radix (*rén shēn*) 6-10g
Mel (*fēng mì*) 10-15g

This formula, like Minor Pinellia Decoction (*xiǎo bàn xià tāng*), discussed above, is an anti-emetic, but their usages are quite different. *Essentials from the Golden Cabinet* states: "For regurgitation and vomiting, Major Pinellia Decoction (*dà bàn xià tāng*) masters it." Regurgitation (胃反 *wèi fǎn*) is a type of vomiting where a patient vomits at dusk what he ate at dawn. The course of this illness has already been rather long or has become chronic. The degree of vomiting is not severe, so food stays in the stomach for a relatively long period of time. Zhang Zhong-Jing used Ginseng Radix (*rén shēn*) to treat symptoms of epigastric distention with firmness, poor appetite, and vomiting; based on the medicinals used in this formula, the expected symptoms for this prescription would include epigastric focal distention with firmness and dry stools. Mel (*fēng mì*) is used to treat abdominal pain with a sense of urgency. From a clinical perspective, these patients for the most part present as dispirited and listless, have a thin physique, a withered, sallow complexion, poor appetite, occasional abdominal pain, dry stools that are difficult to pass, regurgitation, and vomiting of saliva. These types of symptoms are often diagnosed by Chinese doctors as Spleen and Stomach deficiency presentations, so medicinals that tonify the Spleen and Stomach, such as Ginseng Radix (*rén shēn*) and Mel (*fēng mì*), are used. The Major Pinellia Decoction presentation is as follows:

1. Regurgitation, vomiting in the evening of food eaten in the morning, vomitus that mostly contains saliva
2. Epigastric focal distention with firmness, dry stools, and a withered appearance
3. Pale red tongue, with a greasy coating that may be either thick or thin

The difference between the presentation of this formula and the Minor Pinellia Decoction presentation is that the signs of phlegm-thin mucus, such as a lack of thirst, vomiting of clear, watery fluids, water sounds in the epigastrium, dizziness, and palpitations, are more obvious in the Minor Pinellia Decoction presentation. On the other hand, the Major Pinellia Decoction presentation has more significant signs of fluid deficiency, such as a withered appearance and dry stools. The Major Pinellia Decoction presentation can be seen in cases of esophageal spasms, esophageal cancer, functional gastrointestinal disorders, and pyloric obstruction, especially in the debilitated or the elderly with chronic diseases.

10.4 **Pinellia and Magnolia Bark Decoction**
(半夏厚朴湯 *bàn xià hòu pò tāng*)

SOURCE: *Essentials from the Golden Cabinet*

Pinelliae Rhizoma preparatum (*zhì bàn xià*) 6-15g
Magnoliae officinalis Cortex (*hòu pò*) 6-10g
Poria (*fú líng*) 10-15g
Perillae Folium (*zǐ sū yè*) 6-10g
Zingiberis Rhizoma recens (*shēng jiāng*) 6-12g

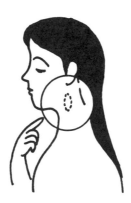

This formula specifically treats the feeling that there is something caught
in the throat (咽喉異物感 *yān hóu yì wù gǎn*). It comes from *Essentials from
Golden Cabinet* and treats "women who feel as if there is a piece of roasted meat
caught in the throat." *Important Formulas Worth a Thousand Gold Pieces* (千金
要方 *Qiān jīn yào fāng*) says that this formula treats "chest fullness, epigastric
firmness, the throat feels sticky as if there is a piece of meat lodged there that
can neither be spit out nor swallowed." *Formulary of the Pharmacy Service for
Benefiting the People in the Taiping Era* (太平惠民和劑局方 *Tài píng huì
mín hé jì jú fāng*) records in minute detail that it "treats the qi of joy, anger,
sadness, thinking, worry, fear, and fright knotting together to form phlegm and
thin mucus. It is as if there is a piece of cotton wadding or a plum pit caught
in the throat, which neither can be coughed out nor swallowed. It is from the
seven qi that this condition comes about. Or there may be focal distention
and fullness in the upper abdomen with the qi not feeling comfortable; or
phlegm blocking and overflowing with rising qi leading to urgent wheezing; or
phlegm-thin mucus that accumulates in the middle with vomiting and nausea."

In accord with the above historically recorded uses, the Pinellia and Magnolia Bark Decoction presentation is as follows:

1. Feeling of something being caught in the throat or chest stuffiness with a feeling of congestion as a result of some type of emotional factor
2. Coughing and wheezing with profuse phlegm and chest stuffiness, or abdominal distention, vomiting and nausea, and poor appetite
3. A tongue coating that is usually thick and greasy, or white and greasy, with the mouth having a sticky, greasy sensation

This formula's presentation is often seen in cases of neurosis and hysteria. There is a reported use of this formula in the treatment of 11 patients whose main complaint was a feeling of something odd in the area around the throat or esophagus. Patients were diagnosed with either anxiety neurosis, hypochondria, neurotic depression, or depression from chemical imbalances. Other than for the two patients who refused treatment after taking the herbs one time, the treatment had some effect. Five patients felt their symptoms had completely disappeared, and the other four only occasionally experienced symptoms. Furthermore, other psycho-emotional issues also improved. The time for the treatment to take effect was between two days and three weeks.[13]

The Japanese practitioner Okuda reports using this formula to treat seven cases of hypersensitivity of the vertebral spinous process, resulting in significant results in four cases, some effect in one, and no improvement in the remaining two. This illness manifests as intensely painful tenderness and pain on percussion of the vertebral spinal process; X-rays, however, do not show any abnormalities. These patients are often nervous and usually have epigastric focal distention. Furthermore, for those without this epigastric focal distention, this formula is not effective.[14]

I often use Pinellia and Magnolia Bark Decoction (*bàn xià hòu pò tāng*) to treat children who are picky eaters. Picky eaters, apart from having poor appetites, are often timid and tend to be introverted, and have sallow complexions and dry stools. After using this formula, their appetite increases significantly, bowel movements become regular, sleep improves, and personalities become more lively.

Other than being used to treat chronic illnesses, later generations of physicians modified this formula to treat some febrile and digestive system illnesses that have a damp presentation. For example, Patchouli/Agastache Powder to Rectify the Qi *(huò xiāng zhèng qì sǎn)** can be used to treat those contracting colds in the summer or fall with fever, diarrhea, poor appetite, nausea and vomiting, headaches, heavy lethargy, and productive coughs. It can also be used to treat those with chronic gastritis, chronic hepatitis, chronic colitis, and neuroses when seen with nausea and vomiting, headache with heavy lethargy, and a greasy tongue coating. Also, Patchouli/Agastache, Magnolia Bark, Pinellia, and Poria Decoction *(huò pò xià líng tāng)†* treats the Pinellia and Magnolia Bark Decoction presentation in those with urinary difficulty, a tendency toward edema, a stuffy feeling in the epigastrium, abdominal distention, or diarrhea, with a greasy tongue coating. It is also common to use this formula to treat febrile diseases in the summer and fall.

10.5 **Pinellia, White Atractylodes, and Gastrodia Decoction**
(半夏白朮天麻湯 *bàn xià bái zhú tiān má tāng*)

SOURCE: *Awakening of the Mind in Medical Studies*
(醫學心悟 *Yī xué xīn wù*)

Pinelliae Rhizoma preparatum *(zhì bàn xià)* 6g
Atractylodis macrocephalae Rhizoma *(bái zhú)* 10g
Gastrodiae Rhizoma *(tiān má)* 5g
Citri reticulatae Pericarpium *(chén pí)* 5g
Poria *(fú líng)* 5g
Glycyrrhizae Radix *(gān cǎo)* 3g
Jujubae Fructus *(dà zǎo)* 12g

This formula is effective for treating phlegm inversion headache with dizziness. The famous Jin-dynasty physician Li Dong-Yuan observed: "Without Pinelliae Rhizoma preparatum *(zhì bàn xià)*, phlegm inversion headaches cannot be treated; without Gastrodiae Rhizoma *(tiān má)*, blurry vision with dizziness or internal stirring of deficiency wind cannot be treated." Pinelliae Rhizoma

---

* *Formulary of the Pharmacy Service for Benefiting the People in the Taiping Era:* Pogostemonis/Agastaches Herba *(huò xiāng)*, Perillae Folium *(zǐ sū yè)*, Pinelliae Rhizoma preparatum *(zhì bàn xià)*, Magnoliae officinalis Cortex *(hòu pò)*, Poria *(fú líng)*, Angelicae dahuricae Radix *(bái zhǐ)*, Atractylodis macrocephalae Rhizoma *(bái zhú)*, Platycodi Radix *(jié gěng)*, Arecae Pericarpium *(dà fù pí)*, Glycyrrhizae Radix *(gān cǎo)*, Citri reticulatae Pericarpium *(chén pí)*, Zingiberis Rhizoma recens *(shēng jiāng)*, and Jujubae Fructus *(dà zǎo)*.

† *Bases of Medicine* (醫原 *Yī yuán*): Pogostemonis/Agastaches Herba *(huò xiāng)*, Pinelliae Rhizoma preparatum *(zhì bàn xià)*, Magnoliae officinalis Cortex *(hòu pò)*, Poria *(fú líng)*, Polyporus *(zhū líng)*, Alismatis Rhizoma *(zé xiè)*, Armeniacae Semen *(xìng rén)*, Coicis Semen *(yì yǐ rén)*, Amomi Fructus rotundus *(bái dòu kòu)*, and Sojae Semen preparatum *(dàn dòu chǐ)*.

preparatum *(zhì bàn xià)* and Gastrodiae Rhizoma *(tiān má)* are the essential herbs historically used by doctors to treat dizziness and headache. Obviously, this type of dizziness with headache is related to the influence of phlegm. In practice, it is not difficult to diagnose because the pinellia presentation is frequently seen. The range of action of the primary herbs in this formula, Pinelliae Rhizoma preparatum *(zhì bàn xià)* and Gastrodiae Rhizoma *(tiān má)*, becomes even broader when combined with Atractylodis macrocephalae Rhizoma *(bái zhú)* and Poria *(fú líng)*. Not only can they relieve pain and stop dizziness, they also regulate the Stomach and Intestines and promote urination. Therefore, they are especially suitable for those who are overweight, are prone to edema, or have headaches and dizziness along with weak digestive function. One should pay attention to the presence of the following principal signs and symptoms in order to make a clinical diagnosis:

1. Headache, dizziness, with a feeling of pressure in the head
2. Abdominal distention, borborygmus, loose stools or stool that starts off formed and later becomes loose
3. Soft and loose musculature, subjective feeling of water retention, or frequently has edema, or easily sweats
4. Red or pale red tongue body, the tongue itself is relatively large, and with a greasy or slightly yellow, greasy coating

This formula's presentation is often seen in cases of arteriosclerosis, hypertension, hyperlipidemia, Ménière's disease, nervous exhaustion, and anemia.

Because there are similarities, the presentation for this formula and that of True Warrior Decoction *(zhēn wǔ tāng)* should be differentiated. Both of these prescriptions can be used to treat dizziness and edema; however, they

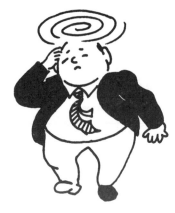

differ in the degree of severity. Generally speaking, illnesses seen with the True Warrior Decoction presentation are more severe than those with this formula's presentation, those differences being:

- The appearance of cold in the True Warrior Decoction presentation is more severe, with symptoms such as chills, body pain, cold limbs and a very pale tongue, whereas in the Pinellia, White Atractylodes, and Gastrodia Decoction presentation, these are not present.

- Patients with a True Warrior Decoction presentation are less fit, are listless and dispirited, and are unstable when standing. The psycho-emotional condition of patients with this formula's presentation is more solid.

- There is a more significant amount of edema in the True Warrior Decoction presentation, while digestive tract symptoms are more prevalent in the Pinellia, White Atractylodes, and Gastrodia Decoction presentation.

10.6 **Pinellia Decoction to Drain the Epigastrium**
(半夏瀉心湯 *bàn xià xiè xīn tāng*)

SOURCE: *Discussion of Cold Damage*

Pinelliae Rhizoma preparatum (*zhì bàn xià*) 6-15g
Coptidis Rhizoma (*huáng lián*) 3-5g
Scutellariae Radix (*huáng qín*) 5-10g
Zingiberis Rhizoma (*gān jiāng*) 3-6
Glycyrrhizae Radix (*gān cǎo*) 3-6g
Ginseng Radix (*rén shēn*) 6-10g
Jujubae Fructus (*dà zǎo*) 12g

Pinellia Decoction to Drain the Epigastrium (*bàn xià xiè xīn tāng*) originally appears in *Discussion of Cold Damage* where it is used to treat a particular type of symptom called 'focal distention' (痞 *pǐ*). The typical expression of a focal distention presentation is one of a full and stifling sensation in the area of the upper abdomen, but with a lack of intense pain. The formula contains neither Rhei Radix et Rhizoma (*dà huáng*), with its purgative actions, nor Bupleuri Radix (*chái hú*), which treats chest and hypochondriac fullness and distention and alternating fever and chills. As the ingredients of a formula determine its use, it can be seen that the presentation treated by this formula neither includes the constipation with abdominal pain and dislike of pressure of the rhubarb presentation, nor the distinctive signs of the bupleurum presentation.

Simply stated, fullness, stuffiness, and discomfort in the upper abdomen are the characteristic signs of this formula's presentation. Epigastric focal distention is a subjective feeling on the part of the patient where there is a feeling of discomfort or pain in the upper abdominal region; epigastric focal distention with firmness includes the aforementioned subjective feelings on the part of the patient plus a palpable feeling of firmness on the part of the practitioner. The Pinellia Decoction to Drain the Epigastrium presentation is as follows:

1. Upper abdominal fullness, stuffiness and discomfort, a slight degree of distention and pain, but little resistance when palpated; can be accompanied by digestive tract symptoms of nausea, vomiting, diarrhea, and borborygmus
2. Irritability and restlessness, a feeling of internal heat in the body, excessive dreaming, or insomnia
3. Thin and greasy, or yellow and greasy tongue coating

In practice, items number one and three are more commonly seen. While some patients don't have significant signs of item number two, the practitioner should still inquire about the state of their sleep and emotions. In my experience, generally speaking, patients with digestive illnesses often have accompanying problems with sleep, anxiety, depression, and other such psycho-emotional symptoms.

A passage in chapter 34 of *Basic Questions* (素問 *Sù wèn*) states: "When the Stomach is not in harmony, sleep will be uneasy." Especially for Pinellia Decoction to Drain the Epigastrium presentation patients, this type of situation is even more apparent. So, for patients with epigastric focal distention, or insomnia, or nervous exhaustion with a yellow, greasy tongue coating, I often treat using Pinellia Decoction to Drain the Epigastrium (*bàn xià xiè xīn tāng*) and get excellent results.

From the viewpoint of clinical application, Pinellia Decoction to Drain the Epigastrium (*bàn xià xiè xīn tāng*) is principally used in the treatment of digestive system illness. There are reports of this formula being effective in the treatment of acute gastroenteritis, chronic enteritis, dysentery, chronic atrophic gastritis, hypertrophic gastritis, peptic ulcers, gastrointestinal neurosis, pyloric obstruction, chronic cholecystitis, drunkenness, ulcers of the oral mucosa, autonomic dystonia, plum pit qi, and morning sickness.

The simultaneous coexistence of cold and heat presentations is the definitive characteristic of this formula's presentation. It is not easy to explain these clinical manifestations solely in terms of either a heat or cold presentation. These mixed cold-heat patterns can manifest as epigastric focal distention, abdominal fullness and distention that is aggravated when encountering cold, thirst with a lack of desire to drink, dry lips, and a red tongue with a yellow coating. It also can be seen as epigastric focal distention with pain where encountering either cold or heat both increase the patient's discomfort. The bowels can be either constipated or loose, and the urine can be either yellow or clear. When using this formula, some people will remove the Zingiberis Rhizoma (*gān jiāng*), Ginseng Radix (*rén shēn*), Glycyrrhizae Radix (*gān cǎo*), and Jujubae Fructus (*dà zǎo*) as these medicinals do not function to clear heat; they say that since they are counter to the nature of Coptidis Rhizoma (*huáng lián*) and Scutellariae Radix (*huáng qín*), they can be left out. Actually, this shows a lack of insight into the reason that Pinellia Decoction to Drain the Epigastrium (*bàn xià xiè xīn tāng*) should be used. One of the most profound aspects of how Chinese medicine formulas are composed is the combination of medicinals that have opposite effects: those that clear heat can be combined with those that tonify; those that cool with those that warm; and those that disperse with those that bind. This way of combining herbs is considered both opposite and complementary (相 反相成 *xiāng fǎn xiāng chéng*). Pinellia Decoction to Drain the Epigastrium (*bàn xià xiè xīn tāng*) is just such a mixture of cold, hot, tonifying, and purging medicinals. The Coptidis Rhizoma (*huáng lián*) and Scutellariae Radix (*huáng qín*) within this formula are cold heat-clearing herbs. Even though they are the principal herbs in the formula, were it not for the synergistic actions that come from combining them with Zingiberis Rhizoma (*gān jiāng*), Ginseng Radix (*rén shēn*), Glycyrrhizae Radix (*gān cǎo*), and Jujubae Fructus (*dà zǎo*), there would be no way for this prescription to bring out its particular curative effects. This is because all the warm, tonifying medicinals have the ability to preserve and harmonize the functioning of the Stomach and Intestines, promote the secretion of gastric juices, and improve the body's resistance to disease.

There is not much modern day pharmacological research material concerning Pinellia Decoction to Drain the Epigastrium (*bàn xià xiè xīn tāng*), however, the pharmacology of the individual herbs suggests that this formula possesses stomachic, anti-emetic, antibacterial, and anti-inflammatory effects, and that it promotes the immune function and has antispasmodic, analgesic, and gastro-intestinal-regulating functions. Of course, more penetrating research needs to be done.

Pinellia Decoction to Drain the Epigastrium (*bàn xià xiè xīn tāng*) and Warm Gallbladder Decoction with Coptis (*huáng lián wēn dǎn tāng*) have similar functions, the differences being that with this formula there are more significant digestive tract symptoms, such as epigastric focal distention, pain, and discomfort. In the Warm Gallbladder Decoction with Coptis presentation, psychoneurological symptoms such as insomnia, palpitations, being easily startled, and excessive dreaming are more prominent.

Pinellia Decoction to Drain the Epigastrium (*bàn xià xiè xīn tāng*) and the coptis family formula Coptis Decoction to Resolve Toxicity (*huáng lián jiě dú tāng*) both contain Coptidis Rhizoma (*huáng lián*) and Scutellariae Radix (*huáng qín*); their formula presentations also share the common points of epigastric focal distention and a restless spirit. The differences are that psychoneurologic symptoms are primary in the Coptis Decoction to Resolve Toxicity presentation, while for the Pinellia Decoction to Drain the Epigastrium presentation, it is the digestive symptoms that are primary.

Pinellia Decoction to Drain the Epigastrium (*bàn xià xiè xīn tāng*) is made by removing the Bupleuri Radix (*chái hú*) from Minor Bupleurum Decoction (*xiǎo chái hú tāng*), then adding Coptidis Rhizoma (*huáng lián*), increasing the doseage of Pinelliae Rhizoma preparatum (*zhì bàn xià*), and substituting Zingiberis Rhizoma recens (*shēng jiāng*) for Zingiberis Rhizoma (*gān jiāng*). It stands to reason that the presentations for both this formula and Minor Bupleurum Decoction (*xiǎo chái hú tāng*) would include significant digestive symptoms. The differences between them are that Pinellia Decoction to Drain the Epigastrium (*bàn xià xiè xīn tāng*) does not have the chest and hypochondriac fullness and discomfort, or alternating fever and chills, of the bupleurum presentation, while it does have the coptis presentation's epigastric focal distention, irritability, and restless spirit.

The composition of Pinellia Decoction to Drain the Epigastrium (*bàn xià xiè xīn tāng*) and Coptis Decoction (*huáng lián tāng*) are very similar, the only differences being whether or not there is Scutellariae Radix (*huáng qín*) or Cinnamomi Ramulus (*guì zhī*). As a result, the conditions they primarily treat are also quite similar. The main difference is that the Coptis Decoction presentation has the sweating and palpitations of the cinnamon twig presentation, while the Pinellia Decoction to Drain the Epigastrium presentation does not. Although the digestive symptoms are in large part the same, with the Coptis Decoction presentation there is more abdominal pain, while for the Pinellia Decoction to Drain the Epigastrium presentation, the primary symptom is epigastric focal distention. Of course, if the Pinellia Decoction to Drain the Epigastrium presentation is seen together with the cinnamon twig presentation, then Cinnamomi Ramulus (*guì zhī*) can be added, which would actually be a combination of the two formulas.

....

Formulas Arranged by Disease Names

THE FOLLOWING is a list of biomedically-defined diseases that often show with the presentations of the formulas in the table. This is not to say that for certain serious diseases these formulas would be the treatment of choice, nor that all the formulas within a category can be used to treat that illness, nor that even Chinese medicine is the best approach in a given patient. Rather, it is to say that certain disease processes through the course of an illness will exhibit certain presentations for which these formulas have proven useful.

1. Infectious Diseases

COMMON COLD

Ephedra Decoction (*má huáng tāng*), Cinnamon Twig Decoction (*guì zhī tāng*), Ephedra, Asarum, and Aconite Accessory Root Decoction (*má huáng xì xīn fù zǐ tāng*), Minor Bupleurum Decoction (*xiǎo chái hú tāng*), Pogostemon /Agastache Powder to Rectify the Qi (*huò xiāng zhèng qì sǎn*)

DYSENTERY, BACTERIAL

Coptis Decoction to Resolve Toxicity (*huáng lián jiě dú tāng*), Major Order the Qi Decoction (*dà chéng qì tāng*), Drain the Epigastrium Decoction (*xiè xīn tāng*), Cinnamon Twig plus Rhubarb Decoction (*guì zhī jiā dà huáng tāng*), Warm the Spleen Decoction (*wēn pí tāng*), Peach Pit Decoction to Order the Qi (*táo hé chéng qì tāng*), Frigid Extremities Powder (*sì nì sǎn*), Pinellia Decoction to Drain the Epigastrium (*bàn xià xiè xīn tāng*), Aconite Accessory Root Decoction to Drain the Epigastrium (*fù zǐ xiè xīn tāng*), Regulate the Middle Pill (*lǐ zhōng wán*), Aucklandia and Coptis Pill (*xiāng lián wán*), Coptis and Ass-Hide Gelatin Decoction (*huáng lián ē jiāo tāng*), Tonify the Middle to Augment the Qi Decoction (*bǔ zhōng yì qì tāng*)

ENCEPHALITIS B

Coptis Decoction to Resolve Toxicity (*huáng lián jiě dú tāng*), Major Order the Qi Decoction (*dà chéng qì tāng*), White Tiger Decoction (*bái hǔ tāng*)

EPIDEMIC HEMORRHAGIC FEVER

White Tiger Decoction (*bái hǔ tāng*), Peach Pit Decoction to Order the Qi (*táo hé chéng qì tāng*), Major Order the Qi Decoction (*dà chéng qì tāng*), Frigid Extremities Powder (*sì nì sǎn*)

HEPATITIS, SERIOUS

Virgate Wormwood Decoction (*yīn chén hāo tāng*), Major Order the Qi Decoction (*dà chéng qì tāng*), Frigid Extremities Decoction (*sì nì tāng*)

HEPATITIS, VIRAL

Virgate Wormwood Decoction (*yīn chén hāo tāng*), Coptis Decoction to Resolve Toxicity (*huáng lián jiě dú tāng*)

INFLUENZA

Ephedra Decoction (*má huáng tāng*), Ephedra, Asarum, and Aconite Accessory Root Decoction (*má huáng xì xīn fù zǐ tāng*), White Tiger Decoction (*bái hǔ tāng*)

LEPTOSPIROSIS

Coptis Decoction to Resolve Toxicity (*huáng lián jiě dú tāng*)

MEASLES

Ephedra, Apricot Kernel, Gypsum, and Licorice Decoction (*má xìng shí gān tāng*)

MENINGITIS

Coptis Decoction to Resolve Toxicity (*huáng lián jiě dú tāng*)

PERTUSSIS

Ephedra, Apricot Kernel, Gypsum, and Licorice Decoction (*má xìng shí gān tāng*)

RABIES

Purge Static Blood Decoction (*xià yū xuè tāng*)

TYPHOID FEVER

Coptis and Ass-Hide Gelatin Decoction (*huáng lián ē jiāo tāng*), Aucklandia and Coptis Pill (*xiāng lián wán*)

2. Digestive System Diseases

BILIARY ASCARIASIS

Frigid Extremities Powder *(sì nì sǎn)*, Regulate the Middle Pill *(lǐ zhōng wán)*, Minor Decoction [for Pathogens] Stuck in the Chest *(xiǎo xiàn xiōng tāng)*, Minor Construct the Middle Decoction *(xiǎo jiàn zhōng tāng)*

BLEEDING, UPPER DIGESTIVE TRACT

Regulate the Middle Pill *(lǐ zhōng wán)*, Drain the Epigastrium Decoction *(xiè xīn tāng)*

CHOLECYSTITIS, CHOLELITHIASIS

Aconite Accessory Root Decoction to Drain the Epigastrium *(fù zǐ xiè xīn tāng)*, Virgate Wormwood Decoction *(yīn chén hāo tāng)*, Major Order the Qi Decoction *(dà chéng qì tāng)*, Major Bupleurum Decoction *(dà chái hú tāng)*, Bupleurum and Cinnamon Twig Decoction *(chái hú guì zhī tāng)*, Pinellia Decoction to Drain the Epigastrium *(bàn xià xiè xīn tāng)*, Warm Gallbladder Decoction *(wēn dǎn tāng)*, Rhubarb and Aconite Accessory Root Decoction *(dà huáng fù zǐ tāng)*, Left Metal Pill *(zuǒ jīn wán)*, Minor Decoction [for Pathogens] Stuck in the Chest *(xiǎo xiàn xiōng tāng)*, Frigid Extremities Powder *(sì nì sǎn)*, Peony and Licorice Decoction *(sháo yào gān cǎo tāng)*

COLITIS, CHRONIC

Regulate the Middle Pill *(lǐ zhōng wán)*, Jade Windscreen Powder *(yù píng fēng sǎn)*, Pogostemon/Agastache Powder to Rectify the Qi *(huò xiāng zhèng qì sǎn)*, Cinnamon Twig and Ginseng Decoction *(guì zhī rén shēn tāng)*, Regulating Decoction with Coptis *(lián lǐ tāng)*, Aucklandia and Coptis Pill *(xiāng lián wán)*, Tonify the Middle to Augment the Qi Decoction *(bǔ zhōng yì qì tāng)*, Astragalus Decoction to Construct the Middle *(huáng qí jiàn zhōng tāng)*

ESOPHAGEAL SPASMS

Major Pinellia Decoction *(dà bàn xià tāng)*

GASTRITIS, ALLERGIC

Frigid Extremities Powder *(sì nì sǎn)*, Bupleurum and Cinnamon Twig Decoction *(chái hú guì zhī tāng)*, Minor Construct the Middle Decoction *(xiǎo jiàn zhōng tāng)*, Cinnamon Twig and Ginseng Decoction *(guì zhī rén shēn tāng)*, Regulate the Middle Pill *(lǐ zhōng wán)*

GASTRITIS, CHRONIC

Regulate the Middle Pill (lǐ zhōng wán), Regulating Decoction with
Coptis (lián lǐ tāng), Major Construct the Middle Decoction (dà jiàn
zhōng tāng), Left Metal Pill (zuǒ jīn wán), Coptis and Ass-Hide Gelatin
Decoction (huáng lián ē jiāo tāng), Drain the Epigastrium Decoction
(xiè xīn tāng), Minor Decoction [for Pathogens] Stuck in the Chest
(xiǎo xiàn xiōng tāng), Astragalus Decoction to Construct the Middle
(huáng qí jiàn zhōng tāng), Minor Construct the Middle Decoction (xiǎo
jiàn zhōng tāng), Poria, Cinnamon Twig, Atractylodes, and Licorice
Decoction (líng guì zhú gān tāng)

GASTRO-ENTERITIS, ACUTE

Coptis Decoction (huáng lián tāng), Aucklandia and Coptis Pill (xiāng
lián wán), Pinellia Decoction to Drain the Epigastrium (bàn xià xiè
xīn tāng), Frigid Extremities Powder (sì nì sǎn), Aconite Accessory
Root Decoction to Drain the Epigastrium (fù zǐ xiè xīn tāng), Coptis
Decoction to Resolve Toxicity (huáng lián jiě dú tāng)

HEPATITIS, CHRONIC

Rhubarb and Ground Beetle Pill (dà huáng zhè chóng wán), Frigid
Extremities Powder (sì nì sǎn), Pogostemon/Agastache Powder to
Rectify the Qi (huò xiāng zhèng qì sǎn), Regulate the Middle Pill (lǐ zhōng
wán), Tonify the Middle to Augment the Qi Decoction (bǔ zhōng yì
qì tāng), Astragalus Decoction to Construct the Middle (huáng qí jiàn
zhōng tāng), Drive Out Stasis from the Mansion of Blood Decoction
(xuè fǔ zhú yū tāng)

ILEUS

Rhubarb and Aconite Accessory Root Decoction (dà huáng fù zǐ tāng),
Regulate the Stomach and Order the Qi Decoction (tiáo wèi chéng
qì tāng), Major Order the Qi Decoction (dà chéng qì tāng), Frigid
Extremities Powder (sì nì sǎn), Major Construct the Middle Decoction
(dà jiàn zhōng tāng), Drive Out Stasis from the Mansion of Blood
Decoction (xuè fǔ zhú yū tāng)

INDIGESTION

Regulate the Middle Pill (lǐ zhōng wán)

PANCREATITIS, ACUTE

Major Order the Qi Decoction (dà chéng qì tāng), Major Bupleurum

Decoction *(dà chái hú tāng)*, Frigid Extremities Powder *(sì nì sǎn)*, Bupleurum and Cinnamon Twig Decoction *(chái hú guì zhī tāng)*

PSEUDO-ILEUS

Peach Pit Decoction to Order the Qi *(táo hé chéng qì tāng)*, Major Order the Qi Decoction *(dà chéng qì tāng)*

PYLORIC OBSTRUCTION

Pinellia Decoction to Drain the Epigastrium *(bàn xià xiè xīn tāng)*, Major Pinellia Decoction *(dà bàn xià tāng)*, Regulate the Middle Pill *(lǐ zhōng wán)*

STOMACH CANCER

Minor Construct the Middle Decoction *(xiǎo jiàn zhōng tāng)*

STOMACH DISORDERS, FUNCTIONAL

Frigid Extremities Powder *(sì nì sǎn)*, Major Pinellia Decoction *(dà bàn xià tāng)*, Major Construct the Middle Decoction *(dà jiàn zhōng tāng)*, Astragalus Decoction to Construct the Middle *(huáng qí jiàn zhōng tāng)*

STOMACH PAINS, SPASMODIC

Peony and Licorice Decoction *(sháo yào gān cǎo tāng)*

STOMACH PROLAPSE

Tonify the Middle to Augment the Qi Decoction *(bǔ zhōng yì qì tāng)*

STOMACH PROLAPSE

Frigid Extremities Powder *(sì nì sǎn)*, True Warrior Decoction *(zhēn wǔ tāng)*, Tonify the Middle to Augment the Qi Decoction *(bǔ zhōng yì qì tāng)*, Poria, Cinnamon Twig, Atractylodes, and Licorice Decoction *(líng guì zhú gān tāng)*

ULCERS, PEPTIC

Frigid Extremities Powder *(sì nì sǎn)*, Bupleurum and Cinnamon Twig Decoction *(chái hú guì zhī tāng)*, Warm Gallbladder Decoction *(wēn dǎn tāng)*, True Warrior Decoction *(zhēn wǔ tāng)*, Major Construct the Middle Decoction *(dà jiàn zhōng tāng)*, Cinnamon Twig and Ginseng Decoction *(guì zhī rén shēn tāng)*, Regulate the Middle Pill *(lǐ zhōng wán)*, Minor Construct the Middle Decoction *(xiǎo jiàn zhōng tāng)*, Astragalus Decoction to Construct the Middle *(huáng qí jiàn zhōng tāng)*, Cinnamon Twig Decoction plus Dragon Bone and Oyster Shell *(guì zhī jiā lóng gǔ mǔ lì tāng)*, Peony and Licorice Decoction *(sháo yào gān cǎo tāng)*, Poria, Cinnamon Twig, Atractylodes, and Licorice Decoction *(líng guì zhú gān tāng)*, Major Bupleurum Decoction *(dà chái hú tāng)*

Vomiting, neurogenic

Minor Pinellia Decoction *(xiǎo bàn xià tāng)*, Poria, Cinnamon Twig, Atractylodes, and Licorice Decoction *(líng guì zhú gān tāng)*, Drive Out Stasis from the Mansion of Blood Decoction *(xuè fǔ zhú yū tāng)*

3. Respiratory System Diseases

Asthma

Minor Bluegreen Dragon Decoction *(xiǎo qīng lóng tāng)*, Minor Pinellia Decoction *(xiǎo bàn xià tāng)*, Bupleurum and Magnolia Bark Decoction *(chái pò tāng)*, Ephedra, Apricot Kernel, Gypsum, and Licorice Decoction *(má xìng shí gān tāng)*, Frigid Extremities Powder *(sì nì sǎn)*, Three-Unbinding Decoction *(sān ǎo tāng)*, Balmy Yang Decoction *(yáng hé tāng)*

Bronchitis

Cinnamon Twig Decoction *(guì zhī tāng)*, *Bupleurum and Magnolia Bark Decoction (chái pò tāng)*, Minor Bluegreen Dragon Decoction *(xiǎo qīng lóng tāng)*, Ephedra, Asarum, and Aconite Accessory Root Decoction *(má huáng xì xīn fù zǐ tāng)*, Minor Pinellia Decoction *(xiǎo bàn xià tāng)*, Minor Decoction [for Pathogens] Stuck in the Chest *(xiǎo xiàn xiōng tāng)*, Minor Bupleurum Decoction *(xiǎo chái hú tāng)*, Three-Unbinding Decoction *(sān ǎo tāng)*, Lophatherum and Gypsum Decoction *(zhú yè shí gāo tāng)*, Poria, Cinnamon Twig, Atractylodes, and Licorice Decoction *(líng guì zhú gān tāng)*, Ephedra, Apricot Kernel, Gypsum, and Licorice Decoction *(má xìng shí gān tāng)*

Hemoptysis, acute

Drain the Epigastrium Decoction *(xiè xīn tāng)*

Pleurisy

Drive Out Stasis from the Mansion of Blood Decoction *(xuè fǔ zhú yū tāng)*, Drain the Epigastrium Decoction *(xiè xīn tāng)*, Minor Decoction [for Pathogens] Stuck in the Chest *(xiǎo xiàn xiōng tāng)*, Minor Bupleurum Decoction *(xiǎo chái hú tāng)*

PNEUMONIA, ACUTE

Major Order the Qi Decoction (*dà chéng qì tāng*), Minor Decoction [for Pathogens] Stuck in the Chest (*xiǎo xiàn xiōng tāng*), Ephedra, Apricot Kernel, Gypsum, and Licorice Decoction (*má xìng shí gān tāng*), White Tiger plus Ginseng Decoction (*bái hǔ jiā rén shēn tāng*), Cinnamon Twig Decoction (*guì zhī tāng*)

PULMONARY TUBERCULOSIS

Minor Bupleurum Decoction (*xiǎo chái hú tāng*)

SILICOSIS

Drive Out Stasis from the Mansion of Blood Decoction (*xuè fǔ zhú yū tāng*)

4. Cardiovascular and Cerebrovascular Diseases

ANGINA PECTORIS

Minor Decoction [for Pathogens] Stuck in the Chest (*xiǎo xiàn xiōng tāng*), Unripe Bitter Orange, Chinese Garlic, and Cinnamon Twig Decoction (*zhǐ shí xiè bái guì zhī tāng*), Tonify the Yang to Restore Five-Tenths Decoction (*bǔ yáng huán wǔ tāng*), Drive Out Stasis from the Mansion of Blood Decoction (*xuè fǔ zhú yū tāng*), Warm Gallbladder Decoction (*wēn dǎn tāng*)

ARRHYTHMIA

Drive Out Stasis from the Mansion of Blood Decoction (*xuè fǔ zhú yū tāng*), Prepared Licorice Decoction (*zhì gān cǎo tāng*)

ARTERITIS

Drive Out Stasis from the Mansion of Blood Decoction (*xuè fǔ zhú yū tāng*)

ATHEROSCLEROSIS

Pinellia, White Atractylodes, and Gastrodia Decoction (*bàn xià bái zhú tiān má tāng*), Tonify the Yang to Restore Five-Tenths Decoction (*bǔ yáng huán wǔ tāng*), Peach Pit Decoction to Order the Qi (*táo hé chéng qì tāng*), Drive Out Stasis from the Mansion of Blood Decoction (*xuè fǔ zhú yū tāng*), Drain the Epigastrium Decoction (*xiè xīn tāng*), Tonify the Middle to Augment the Qi Decoction (*bǔ zhōng yì qì tāng*)

CARDIAC FAILURE

True Warrior Decoction (*zhēn wǔ tāng*), Frigid Extremities Decoction plus Ginseng (*sì nì jiā rén shēn tāng*)

HEART DISEASE, CORONARY

Tonify the Yang to Restore Five-Tenths Decoction (*bǔ yáng huán wǔ tāng*), Frigid Extremities Powder (*sì nì sǎn*), Drive Out Stasis from the Mansion of Blood Decoction (*xuè fǔ zhú yū tāng*), Warm Gallbladder Decoction (*wēn dǎn tāng*), Prepared Licorice (*zhì gān cǎo tāng*), Minor Decoction [for Pathogens] Stuck in the Chest (*xiǎo xiàn xiōng tāng*)

HEART DISEASE, PULMONARY

Drive Out Stasis from the Mansion of Blood Decoction (*xuè fǔ zhú yū tāng*), Frigid Extremities Powder (*sì nì sǎn*)

HEART DISEASE, RHEUMATIC

Poria, Cinnamon Twig, Atractylodes, and Licorice Decoction (*líng guì zhú gān tāng*), Drive Out Stasis from the Mansion of Blood Decoction (*xuè fǔ zhú yū tāng*)

HYPERTENSION

Peach Pit Decoction to Order the Qi (*táo hé chéng qì tāng*), Drive Out Stasis from the Mansion of Blood Decoction (*xuè fǔ zhú yū tāng*), Bupleurum plus Dragon Bone and Oyster Shell Decoction (*chái hú jiā lóng gǔ mǔ lì tāng*), Major Bupleurum Decoction (*dà chái hú tāng*), Warm Gallbladder Decoction with Coptis (*huáng lián wēn dǎn tāng*), Coptis Decoction to Resolve Toxicity (*huáng lián jiě dú tāng*), Drain the Epigastrium Decoction (*xiè xīn tāng*), Poria, Cinnamon Twig, Atractylodes, and Licorice Decoction (*líng guì zhú gān tāng*)

HYPOTENSION

Tonify the Middle to Augment the Qi Decoction (*bǔ zhōng yì qì tāng*)

KESHAN DISEASE

Ephedra, Asarum, and Aconite Accessory Root Decoction (*má huáng xì xīn fù zǐ tāng*)

MYOCARDIAL INFARCTION

Tonify the Yang to Restore Five-Tenths Decoction (*bǔ yáng huán wǔ tāng*)

MYOCARDITIS

Prepared Licorice *(zhì gān cǎo tāng)*, Coptis Decoction *(huáng lián tāng)*

PULSELESS DISEASE

Tonify the Yang to Restore Five-Tenths Decoction *(bǔ yáng huán wǔ tāng)*, Cinnamon Twig Decoction *(guì zhī tāng)*

RAYNAUD'S DISEASE

Astragalus and Cinnamon Twig Five-Substance Decoction *(huáng qí guì zhī wǔ wù tāng)*, Tangkuei Decoction for Frigid Extremities *(dāng guī sì nì tāng)*

SICK SINUS SYNDROME

Ephedra, Asarum, and Aconite Accessory Root Decoction *(má huáng xì xīn fù zǐ tāng)*, Balmy Yang Decoction *(yáng hé tāng)*, Prepared Licorice *(zhì gān cǎo tāng)*

TACHYCARDIA

Coptis and Ass-Hide Gelatin Decoction *(huáng lián ē jiāo tāng)*, Coptis Decoction *(huáng lián tāng)*, Cinnamon Twig Decoction *(guì zhī tāng)*

5. Urogenital System Diseases

CHYLURIA

Tonify the Middle to Augment the Qi Decoction *(bǔ zhōng yì qì tāng)*

CYSTITIS, URINARY TRACT INFECTION

Drain the Epigastrium Decoction *(xiè xīn tāng)*, Frigid Extremities Powder *(sì nì sǎn)*, Coptis Decoction to Resolve Toxicity *(huáng lián jiě dú tāng)*

IMPOTENCE AND SEMINAL EMISSIONS

Frigid Extremities Powder *(sì nì sǎn)*, Cinnamon Twig Decoction plus Dragon Bone and Oyster Shell *(guì zhī jiā lóng gǔ mǔ lì tāng)*

LOW SPERM COUNT

Tonify the Middle to Augment the Qi Decoction *(bǔ zhōng yì qì tāng)*

Nephritis, acute

Bupleurum and Poria Decoction *(chái líng tāng)*, Ephedra Decoction plus Atractylodes *(má huáng jiā zhú tāng)*, Eliminate Wind Powder *(xiāo fēng sǎn)*, Maidservant from Yue's Decoction plus Atractylodes *(Yuè bì jiā zhú tāng)*, Minor Bupleurum Decoction *(xiǎo chái hú tāng)*

Nephritis, chronic

Jade Windscreen Powder *(yù píng fēng sǎn)*, Tonify the Yang to Restore Five-Tenths Decoction *(bǔ yáng huán wǔ tāng)*, Stephania and Astragalus Decoction *(fáng jǐ huáng qí tāng)*, True Warrior Decoction *(zhēn wǔ tāng)*

Nephrotic syndrome

Tonify the Yang to Restore Five-Tenths Decoction *(bǔ yáng huán wǔ tāng)*

Prostate hypertrophy, benign

Cinnamon Twig and Poria Pill *(guì zhī fú líng wán)*

Prostatitis

Frigid Extremities Powder *(sì nì sǎn)*

Uremia

True Warrior Decoction *(zhēn wǔ tāng)*

Urinary tract stones

Rhubarb and Aconite Accessory Root Decoction *(dà huáng fù zǐ tāng)*, Peach Pit Decoction to Order the Qi *(táo hé chéng qì tāng)*, Frigid Extremities Powder *(sì nì sǎn)*, Peony and Licorice Decoction *(sháo yào gān cǎo tāng)*

6. Blood System Diseases

Anemia

Astragalus Decoction to Construct the Middle *(huáng qí jiàn zhōng tāng)*

Favism

Virgate Wormwood Decoction *(yīn chén hāo tāng)*, Coptis Decoction to Resolve Toxicity *(huáng lián jiě dú tāng)*

Jaundice, hemolytic

Astragalus Decoction to Construct the Middle *(huáng qí jiàn zhōng tāng)*

Leukopenia

Tonify the Middle to Augment the Qi Decoction *(bǔ zhōng yì qì tāng)*

Purpura, allergic

Jade Windscreen Powder *(yù píng fēng sǎn)*, Regulate the Middle Pill *(lǐ zhōng wán)*, Coptis Decoction to Resolve Toxicity *(huáng lián jiě dú tāng)*, Bupleurum and Cinnamon Twig Decoction *(chái hú guì zhī tāng)*, Drive Out Stasis from the Mansion of Blood Decoction *(xuè fǔ zhú yū tāng)*

Purpura, thrombocytopenic

Regulate the Middle Pill *(lǐ zhōng wán)*

7. Metabolic Diseases

Diabetes

White Tiger plus Ginseng Decoction *(bái hǔ jiā rén shēn tāng)*, Lophatherum and Gypsum Decoction *(zhú yè shí gāo tāng)*, Major Bupleurum Decoction *(dà chái hú tāng)*

Gout

Major Bupleurum Decoction *(dà chái hú tāng)*, Cinnamon Twig, Peony, and Anemarrhena Decoction *(guì zhī sháo yào zhī mǔ tāng)*

Hypercholesterolemia

Drain the Epigastrium Decoction *(xiè xīn tāng)*, Saposhnikovia Powder that Sagely Unblocks *(fáng fēng tōng shèng sǎn)*

Hyperlipidemia

Saposhnikovia Powder that Sagely Unblocks *(fáng fēng tōng shèng sǎn)*, Warm Gallbladder Decoction with Coptis *(huáng lián wēn dǎn tāng)*, Pinellia, White Atractylodes, and Gastrodia Decoction *(bàn xià bái zhú tiān má tāng)*, Drain the Epigastrium Decoction *(xiè xīn tāng)*

Obesity

Stephania and Astragalus Decoction *(fáng jǐ huáng qí tāng)*

Porphyria

Astragalus Decoction to Construct the Middle *(huáng qí jiàn zhōng tāng)*

8. Connective Tissue Diseases

ARTHRITIS, RHEUMATOID

White Tiger plus Ginseng Decoction (*bái hǔ jiā rén shēn tāng*), Cinnamon Twig, Peony, and Anemarrhena Decoction (*guì zhī sháo yào zhī mǔ tāng*), Tangkuei Decoction for Frigid Extremities (*dāng guī sì nì tāng*), Maidservant from Yue's Decoction plus Atractylodes (*Yuè bì jiā zhú tāng*), Stephania and Astragalus Decoction (*fáng jǐ huáng qí tāng*)

BEHCET'S DISEASE

Coptis Decoction to Resolve Toxicity (*huáng lián jiě dú tāng*)

FEVER, RHEUMATIC

White Tiger Decoction (*bái hǔ tāng*), White Tiger plus Ginseng Decoction (*bái hǔ jiā rén shēn tāng*), White Tiger plus Cinnamon Twig Decoction (*bái hǔ jiā guì zhī tāng*)

LUPUS ERYTHEMATOSUS, SYSTEMIC

Tonify the Yang to Restore Five-Tenths Decoction (*bǔ yáng huán wǔ tāng*)

9. Neuropsychological Diseases

AUTONOMIC DYSTONIA

Drive Out Stasis from the Mansion of Blood Decoction (*xuè fǔ zhú yū tāng*), Bupleurum and Cinnamon Twig Decoction (*chái hú guì zhī tāng*), Pinellia Decoction to Drain the Epigastrium (*bàn xià xiè xīn tāng*), Warm Gallbladder Decoction (*wēn dǎn tāng*), Astragalus and Cinnamon Twig Five-Substance Decoction (*huáng qí guì zhī wǔ wù tāng*), Frigid Extremities Powder (*sì nì sǎn*), Ephedra, Asarum, and Aconite Accessory Root Decoction (*má huáng xì xīn fù zǐ tāng*), Cinnamon Twig plus Aconite Accessory Root Decoction (*guì zhī jiā fù zǐ tāng*), Cinnamon Twig Decoction (*guì zhī tāng*)

CEREBRAL INFARCTION

Coptis Decoction to Resolve Toxicity (*huáng lián jiě dú tāng*)

CEREBRAL THROMBOSIS

Rhubarb and Ground Beetle Pill (*dà huáng zhè chóng wán*), Tonify the Yang to Restore Five-Tenths Decoction (*bǔ yáng huán wǔ tāng*)

CEREBRAL VASCULAR ACCIDENT

Major Order the Qi Decoction (*dà chéng qì tāng*), Drain the Epigastrium Decoction (*xiè xīn tāng*)

DEMENTIA, CEREBROVASCULAR

Coptis Decoction to Resolve Toxicity (*huáng lián jiě dú tāng*)

DEMENTIA, SENILE

Bupleurum plus Dragon Bone and Oyster Shell Decoction (*chái hú jiā lóng gǔ mǔ lì tāng*)

EPILEPSY

Drive Out Stasis from the Mansion of Blood Decoction (*xuè fǔ zhú yū tāng*), Bupleurum plus Dragon Bone and Oyster Shell Decoction (*chái hú jiā lóng gǔ mǔ lì tāng*), Bupleurum and Cinnamon Twig Decoction (*chái hú guì zhī tāng*), Guide Out Phlegm Decoction (*dǎo tán tāng*), Warm Gallbladder Decoction (*wēn dǎn tāng*), Frigid Extremities Powder (*sì nì sǎn*)

FACIAL PALSY

Guide Out Phlegm Decoction (*dǎo tán tāng*)

FACIAL TICS

Peony and Licorice Decoction (*sháo yào gān cǎo tāng*)

HEADACHE, MIGRAINE

Tangkuei Decoction for Frigid Extremities (*dāng guī sì nì tāng*)

HEADACHE, NEUROGENIC

Drive Out Stasis from the Mansion of Blood Decoction (*xuè fǔ zhú yū tāng*)

ISCHEMIA, CEREBROVASCULAR

Tonify the Yang to Restore Five-Tenths Decoction (*bǔ yáng huán wǔ tāng*)

MYASTHENIA GRAVIS

Frigid Extremities Decoction (*sì nì tāng*), Tonify the Middle to Augment the Qi Decoction (*bǔ zhōng yì qì tāng*)

Nervous exhaustion

Bupleurum, Cinnamon Twig, and Ginger Decoction (*chái hú guì jiāng tāng*), Bupleurum and Cinnamon Twig Decoction (*chái hú guì zhī tāng*), Ten-Ingredient Warm Gallbladder Decoction (*shí wèi wēn dǎn tāng*), Tonify the Middle to Augment the Qi Decoction (*bǔ zhōng yì qì tāng*), Astragalus Decoction to Construct the Middle (*huáng qí jiàn zhōng tāng*), Ephedra, Asarum, and Aconite Accessory Root Decoction (*má huáng xì xīn fù zǐ tāng*), Cinnamon Twig Decoction plus Dragon Bone and Oyster Shell (*guì zhī jiā lóng gǔ mǔ lì tāng*), Lophatherum and Gypsum Decoction (*zhú yè shí gāo tāng*), Poria, Cinnamon Twig, Atractylodes, and Licorice Decoction (*líng guì zhú gān tāng*), Drive Out Stasis from the Mansion of Blood Decoction (*xuè fǔ zhú yū tāng*), Cinnamon Twig Decoction (*guì zhī tāng*)

Neuralgia, intercostal

Drive Out Stasis from the Mansion of Blood Decoction (*xuè fǔ zhú yū tāng*), Frigid Extremities Powder (*sì nì sǎn*)

Neuralgia, trigeminal

Drive Out Stasis from the Mansion of Blood Decoction (*xuè fǔ zhú yū tāng*), Drain the Epigastrium Decoction (*xiè xīn tāng*), Frigid Extremities Powder (*sì nì sǎn*), Ephedra, Asarum, and Aconite Accessory Root Decoction (*má huáng xì xīn fù zǐ tāng*), Coptis Decoction to Resolve Toxicity (*huáng lián jiě dú tāng*), Peony and Licorice Decoction (*sháo yào gān cǎo tāng*)

Neuritis

Tonify the Yang to Restore Five-Tenths Decoction (*bǔ yáng huán wǔ tāng*)

Neuritis, recurrent

True Warrior Decoction (*zhēn wǔ tāng*)

Neuropathy, diabetic

Astragalus and Cinnamon Twig Five-Substance Decoction (*huáng qí guì zhī wǔ wù tāng*)

Neuropathy, peripheral

Astragalus and Cinnamon Twig Five-Substance Decoction (*huáng qí guì zhī wǔ wù tāng*), Balmy Yang Decoction (*yáng hé tāng*)

NEUROSIS

Drive Out Stasis from the Mansion of Blood Decoction (*xuè fǔ zhú yū tāng*), Rambling Powder (*xiāo yáo sǎn*), Bupleurum, Cinnamon Twig, and Ginger Decoction (*chái hú guì jiāng tāng*), Bupleurum and Cinnamon Twig Decoction (*chái hú guì zhī tāng*), Bupleurum and Magnolia Bark Decoction (*chái pò tāng*), Pinellia Decoction to Drain the Epigastrium (*bàn xià xiè xīn tāng*), Pinellia and Magnolia Bark Decoction (*bàn xià hòu pò tāng*), Warm Gallbladder Decoction (*wēn dǎn tāng*), True Warrior Decoction (*zhēn wǔ tāng*), Poria, Cinnamon Twig, Jujubae, and Licorice Decoction (*líng guì zǎo tāng*)

PARKINSON'S DISEASE

Bupleurum plus Dragon Bone and Oyster Shell Decoction (*chái hú jiā lóng gǔ mǔ lì tāng*), True Warrior Decoction (*zhēn wǔ tāng*)

POISONING, CARBON MONOXIDE

Tonify the Yang to Restore Five-Tenths Decoction (*bǔ yáng huán wǔ tāng*)

SCHIZOPHRENIA

Peach Pit Decoction to Order the Qi (*táo hé chéng qì tāng*), Bupleurum plus Dragon Bone and Oyster Shell Decoction (*chái hú jiā lóng gǔ mǔ lì tāng*), Warm Gallbladder Decoction (*wēn dǎn tāng*), Frigid Extremities Decoction (*sì nì tāng*), Warm Gallbladder Decoction with Coptis (*huáng lián wēn dǎn tāng*), Drain the Epigastrium Decoction (*xiè xīn tāng*)

SCIATICA

True Warrior Decoction (*zhēn wǔ tāng*), Astragalus and Cinnamon Twig Five-Substance Decoction (*huáng qí guì zhī wǔ wù tāng*), Ephedra, Asarum, and Aconite Accessory Root Decoction (*má huáng xì xīn fù zǐ tāng*), Tangkuei Decoction for Frigid Extremities (*dāng guī sì nì tāng*), Peony and Licorice Decoction (*sháo yào gān cǎo tāng*), Balmy Yang Decoction (*yáng hé tāng*)

SLEEP WALKING

Drive Out Stasis from the Mansion of Blood Decoction (*xuè fǔ zhú yū tāng*)

Stroke, sequelae of

Tonify the Yang to Restore Five-Tenths Decoction *(bǔ yáng huán wǔ tāng)*, Rhubarb and Ground Beetle Pill *(dà huáng zhè chóng wán)*, Astragalus and Cinnamon Twig Five-Substance Decoction *(huáng qí guì zhī wǔ wù tāng)*, Coptis Decoction to Resolve Toxicity *(huáng lián jiě dú tāng)*

Throat, odd sensations in

Pinellia and Magnolia Bark Decoction *(bàn xià hòu pò tāng)*, Bupleurum and Magnolia Bark Decoction *(chái pò tāng)*, Rambling Powder *(xiāo yáo sǎn)*, Frigid Extremities Powder *(sì nì sǎn)*

Vertebral spinous process, hypersensitivity of

Pinellia and Magnolia Bark Decoction *(bàn xià hòu pò tāng)*

10. Endocrine System Diseases

Hypertrophic thyroid

Frigid Extremities Decoction *(sì nì tāng)*

Hyperthyroidism

Bupleurum plus Dragon Bone and Oyster Shell Decoction *(chái hú jiā lóng gǔ mǔ lì tāng)*

11. Surgical Diseases and Infectious Disorders Affecting the Musculoskeletal System

Abscess, acute

Drain the Epigastrium Decoction *(xiè xīn tāng)*

Abscess, deep

Balmy Yang Decoction *(yáng hé tāng)*

Appendicitis, acute

Drain the Epigastrium Decoction *(xiè xīn tāng)*, Major Order the Qi Decoction *(dà chéng qì tāng)*

Appendicitis, chronic

Cinnamon Twig and Poria Pill *(guì zhī fú líng wán)*

APPENDIX, ABSCESSED

Frigid Extremities Powder *(sì nì sǎn)*, Rhubarb and Aconite Accessory Root Decoction *(dà huáng fù zǐ tāng)*

ARTHRITIS, DEGENERATIVE

Ephedra, Asarum, and Aconite Accessory Root Decoction *(má huáng xì xīn fù zǐ tāng)*

ARTHRITIS, RHEUMATOID

Cinnamon Twig, Peony, and Anemarrhena Decoction *(guì zhī sháo yào zhī mǔ tāng)*, Astragalus and Cinnamon Twig Five-Substance Decoction *(huáng qí guì zhī wǔ wù tāng)*, Maidservant from Yue's Decoction plus Atractylodes *(Yuè bì jiā zhú tāng)*, Tangkuei Decoction for Frigid Extremities *(dāng guī sì nì tāng)*

BONE AND JOINT TUBERCULOSIS

Balmy Yang Decoction *(yáng hé tāng)*

CERVICAL SPINE PAIN

Astragalus and Cinnamon Twig Five-Substance Decoction *(huáng qí guì zhī wǔ wù tāng)*

CHEST TRAUMA

Drive Out Stasis from the Mansion of Blood Decoction *(xuè fǔ zhú yū tāng)*

CHILBLAINS

Tangkuei Decoction for Frigid Extremities *(dāng guī sì nì tāng)*, Balmy Yang Decoction *(yáng hé tāng)*, Cinnamon Twig Decoction *(guì zhī tāng)*

CONCUSSION, SEQUELAE OF

Drive Out Stasis from the Mansion of Blood Decoction *(xuè fǔ zhú yū tāng)*

COSTOCHONDRITIS

Drive Out Stasis from the Mansion of Blood Decoction *(xuè fǔ zhú yū tāng)*, Frigid Extremities Powder *(sì nì sǎn)*

CRUSH SYNDROME

Peach Pit Decoction to Order the Qi *(táo hé chéng qì tāng)*, Major Order the Qi Decoction *(dà chéng qì tāng)*

HERNIA

> Tonify the Middle to Augment the Qi Decoction (*bǔ zhōng yì qì tāng*), Minor Construct the Middle Decoction (*xiǎo jiàn zhōng tāng*)

LOWER LEG, ULCERS OF

> Cinnamon Twig and Poria Pill (*guì zhī fú líng wán*)

LUMBER DISC DISEASE

> Balmy Yang Decoction (*yáng hé tāng*)

LYMPHADENITIS, CHRONIC

> Balmy Yang Decoction (*yáng hé tāng*)

MASTITIS, ACUTE

> Drain the Epigastrium Decoction (*xiè xīn tāng*), Frigid Extremities Powder (*sì nì sǎn*)

OSTEOMYELITIS, CHRONIC

> Balmy Yang Decoction (*yáng hé tāng*)

PHLEBITIS

> Drive Out Stasis from the Mansion of Blood Decoction (*xuè fǔ zhú yū tāng*)

SHOULDER, FROZEN

> Astragalus and Cinnamon Twig Five-Substance Decoction (*huáng qí guì zhī wǔ wù tāng*), Tangkuei Decoction for Frigid Extremities (*dāng guī sì nì tāng*)

THROMBOANGIITIS OBLITERANS

> Tonify the Yang to Restore Five-Tenths Decoction (*bǔ yáng huán wǔ tāng*), True Warrior Decoction (*zhēn wǔ tāng*), Ephedra, Asarum, and Aconite Accessory Root Decoction (*má huáng xì xīn fù zǐ tāng*), Tangkuei Decoction for Frigid Extremities (*dāng guī sì nì tāng*), Peony and Licorice Decoction (*sháo yào gān cǎo tāng*), Balmy Yang Decoction (*yáng hé tāng*)

THROMBOSIS, VENOUS

> Cinnamon Twig and Poria Pill (*guì zhī fú líng wán*)

TRAUMA LEADING TO PAIN IN BACK AND LOWER LEGS

> Rhubarb and Ground Beetle Pill (*dà huáng zhè chóng wán*)

TRAUMA TO FOREHEAD

Drive Out Stasis from the Mansion of Blood Decoction (*xuè fǔ zhú yū tāng*), Warm Gallbladder Decoction (*wēn dǎn tāng*)

TRAUMATIC HEADACHES

Drive Out Stasis from the Mansion of Blood Decoction (*xuè fǔ zhú yū tāng*)

12. Obstetrical and Gynecological Diseases

ADNEXAL INFECTION

Cinnamon Twig and Poria Pill (*guì zhī fú líng wán*), Drain the Epigastrium Decoction (*xiè xīn tāng*)

AMENORRHEA

Rambling Powder (*xiāo yáo sǎn*), Rhubarb and Ground Beetle Pill (*dà huáng zhè chóng wán*), Peach Pit Decoction to Order the Qi (*táo hé chéng qì tāng*), Jade Candle Powder (*yù zhú sǎn*), Drive Out Stasis from the Mansion of Blood Decoction (*xuè fǔ zhú yū tāng*), Cinnamon Twig and Poria Pill (*guì zhī fú líng wán*)

BREAST SWELLING

Drive Out Stasis from the Mansion of Blood Decoction (*xuè fǔ zhú yū tāng*), Rambling Powder (*xiāo yáo sǎn*)

DYSMENORRHEA, PRIMARY

Balmy Yang Decoction (*yáng hé tāng*), Tangkuei Decoction to Construct the Middle (*dāng guī jiàn zhōng tāng*), Frigid Extremities Powder (*sì nì sǎn*), Peach Pit Decoction to Order the Qi (*táo hé chéng qì tāng*), Rambling Powder (*xiāo yáo sǎn*), Tangkuei Decoction for Frigid Extremities (*dāng guī sì nì tāng*), Drive Out Stasis from the Mansion of Blood Decoction (*xuè fǔ zhú yū tāng*)

ENDOMETRIOSIS

Rambling Powder (*xiāo yáo sǎn*)

FALLOPIAN TUBE OBSTRUCTION

Frigid Extremities Powder (*sì nì sǎn*), Drive Out Stasis from the Mansion of Blood Decoction (*xuè fǔ zhú yū tāng*)

FEVER, POSTPARTUM

Minor Bupleurum Decoction (*xiǎo chái hú tāng*)

GENERALIZED PAIN, POSTPARTUM

Tangkuei Decoction to Construct the Middle (*dāng guī jiàn zhōng tāng*)

INFERTILITY

Cinnamon Twig and Poria Pill (*guì zhī fú líng wán*), Rambling Powder (*xiāo yáo sǎn*), Drive Out Stasis from the Mansion of Blood Decoction (*xuè fǔ zhú yū tāng*)

LACTATION, PROBLEMATIC

Rambling Powder (*xiāo yáo sǎn*)

LIBIDO, LOW

Rambling Powder (*xiāo yáo sǎn*)

LOCHIA, PROLONGED

Peach Pit Decoction to Order the Qi (*táo hé chéng qì tāng*)

LOWER BACK PAIN, POSTPARTUM

Purge Static Blood Decoction (*xià yū xuè tāng*)

MENOPAUSAL SYNDROME

Bupleurum, Cinnamon Twig, and Ginger Decoction (*chái hú guì jiāng tāng*), Warm Gallbladder Decoction (*wēn dǎn tāng*), Frigid Extremities Powder (*sì nì sǎn*), Drive Out Stasis from the Mansion of Blood Decoction (*xuè fǔ zhú yū tāng*)

MENSTRUATION, IRREGULAR

Bupleurum, Cinnamon Twig, and Ginger Decoction (*chái hú guì jiāng tāng*), Cinnamon Twig and Poria Pill (*guì zhī fú líng wán*), Purge Static Blood Decoction (*xià yū xuè tāng*), Rambling Powder (*xiāo yáo sǎn*), Frigid Extremities Powder (*sì nì sǎn*), Tonify the Middle to Augment the Qi Decoction (*bǔ zhōng yì qì tāng*), Drive Out Stasis from the Mansion of Blood Decoction (*xuè fǔ zhú yū tāng*), Flow-Warming Decoction (*wēn jīng tāng*)

MENSTRUATION, MANIA DURING

Peach Pit Decoction to Order the Qi (*táo hé chéng qì tāng*)

MISCARRIAGE

Drive Out Stasis from the Mansion of Blood Decoction (*xuè fŭ zhú yū tāng*), Peach Pit Decoction to Order the Qi (*táo hé chéng qì tāng*), Tonify the Middle to Augment the Qi Decoction (*bŭ zhōng yì qì tāng*)

MISCARRIAGE, HABITUAL

Cinnamon Twig and Poria Pill (*guì zhī fú líng wán*)

MORNING SICKNESS

Cinnamon Twig Decoction (*guì zhī tāng*), Pinellia Decoction to Drain the Epigastrium (*bàn xià xiè xīn tāng*), Regulate the Middle Pill (*lĭ zhōng wán*), Minor Pinellia Decoction (*xiăo bàn xià tāng*)

PELVIC INFLAMMATORY DISEASE

Peach Pit Decoction to Order the Qi (*táo hé chéng qì tāng*), Rhubarb and Ground Beetle Pill (*dà huáng zhè chóng wán*), Drive Out Stasis from the Mansion of Blood Decoction (*xuè fŭ zhú yū tāng*)

PLACENTA, RETENTION OF

Peach Pit Decoction to Order the Qi (*táo hé chéng qì tāng*)

PREGNANCY, ECTOPIC

Peach Pit Decoction to Order the Qi (*táo hé chéng qì tāng*), Drive Out Stasis from the Mansion of Blood Decoction (*xuè fŭ zhú yū tāng*)

PREMENSTRUAL TENSION

Bupleurum and Cinnamon Twig Decoction (*chái hú guì zhī tāng*), Rambling Powder (*xiāo yáo săn*), Frigid Extremities Powder (*sì nì săn*)

URINARY RETENTION, POSTPARTUM

Tonify the Middle to Augment the Qi Decoction (*bŭ zhōng yì qì tāng*)

UTERINE BLEEDING

Rambling Powder (*xiāo yáo săn*), Frigid Extremities Powder (*sì nì săn*), Regulate the Middle Pill (*lĭ zhōng wán*), Coptis and Ass-Hide Gelatin Decoction (*huáng lián ē jiāo tāng*)

UTERINE LEIOMYOMA

Cinnamon Twig and Poria Pill (*guì zhī fú líng wán*), Rhubarb and Ground Beetle Pill (*dà huáng zhè chóng wán*), Rambling Powder (*xiāo yáo săn*)

UTERINE PROLAPSE

Tonify the Middle to Augment the Qi Decoction (*bŭ zhōng yì qì tāng*)

13. Pediatric Diseases

APPETITE, LACK OF (PEDIATRIC)

Pinellia and Magnolia Bark Decoction (*bàn xià hòu pò tāng*)

ASTHMA, PEDIATRIC

Ephedra, Apricot Kernel, Gypsum, and Licorice Decoction (*má xìng shí gān tāng*), Three-Unbinding Decoction (*sān ǎo tāng*)

BRONCHITIS, PEDIATRIC

Minor Decoction [for Pathogens] Stuck in the Chest (*xiǎo xiàn xiōng tāng*)

CANKER SORES, PEDIATRIC

Regulate the Middle Pill (*lǐ zhōng wán*), White Tiger Decoction (*bái hǔ tāng*)

CONVULSIONS, INFANTILE

Regulate the Middle Pill (*lǐ zhōng wán*)

DIARRHEA WITH ANAL PROLAPSE, PEDIATRIC

Tonify the Middle to Augment the Qi Decoction (*bǔ zhōng yì qì tāng*)

DIARRHEA, PEDIATRIC

Frigid Extremities Decoction (*sì nì tāng*), Regulate the Middle Pill (*lǐ zhōng wán*)

ENURESIS, PEDIATRIC

Cinnamon Twig Decoction plus Dragon Bone and Oyster Shell (*guì zhī jiā lóng gǔ mǔ lì tāng*), Minor Construct the Middle Decoction (*xiǎo jiàn zhōng tāng*)

INDIGESTION,

Regulate the Middle Pill (*lǐ zhōng wán*)

INTESTINAL SPASMS, PEDIATRIC

Regulate the Middle Pill (*lǐ zhōng wán*), Minor Construct the Middle Decoction (*xiǎo jiàn zhōng tāng*)

JAUNDICE, NEONATAL

Drain the Epigastrium Decoction (*xiè xīn tāng*), Virgate Wormwood Decoction (*yīn chén hāo tāng*)

NIGHT TERRORS

Cinnamon Twig Decoction plus Dragon Bone and Oyster Shell (*guì zhī jiā lóng gǔ mǔ lì tāng*)

OSTEOMALACIA, PEDIATRIC (RICKETS)

Cinnamon Twig Decoction plus Dragon Bone and Oyster Shell (*guì zhī jiā lóng gǔ mǔ lì tāng*)

PNEUMONIA, PEDIATRIC

Regulate the Middle Pill (*lǐ zhōng wán*), Cinnamon Twig Decoction plus Dragon Bone and Oyster Shell (*guì zhī jiā lóng gǔ mǔ lì tāng*), Minor Bluegreen Dragon Decoction (*xiǎo qīng lóng tāng*), Ephedra, Apricot Kernel, Gypsum, and Licorice Decoction (*má xìng shí gān tāng*)

SUMMERTIME FEVERS, PEDIATRIC

White Tiger plus Ginseng Decoction (*bái hǔ jiā rén shēn tāng*), Jade Windscreen Powder (*yù píng fēng sǎn*)

14. Dermatological Diseases

ACNE

Schizonepeta and Forsythia Decoction (*jīng jiè lián qiào tāng*)

DERMATITIS, ALLERGIC

Virgate Wormwood Decoction (*yīn chén hāo tāng*), Eliminate Wind Powder (*xiāo fēng sǎn*)

DERMATITIS, CHRONIC

Drive Out Stasis from the Mansion of Blood Decoction (*xuè fǔ zhú yū tāng*)

DERMATITIS, SUMMERTIME

White Tiger Decoction (*bái hǔ tāng*)

DERMATITIS, WINTER

Cinnamon Twig Decoction (*guì zhī tāng*)

ECZEMA

Drive Out Stasis from the Mansion of Blood Decoction (*xuè fǔ zhú yū tāng*), Eliminate Wind Powder (*xiāo fēng sǎn*), Cinnamon Twig Decoction (*guì zhī tāng*)

ERYTHEMA MULTIFORME

Cinnamon Twig Decoction (*guì zhī tāng*)

FOLLICULITIS

Schizonepeta and Forsythia Decoction (*jīng jiè lián qiào tāng*)

FURUNCLE, RECURRENT

Drain the Epigastrium Decoction (*xiè xīn tāng*), Saposhnikovia Powder that Sagely Unblocks (*fáng fēng tōng shèng sǎn*)

HAIR LOSS

Bupleurum plus Dragon Bone and Oyster Shell Decoction (*chái hú jiā lóng gǔ mǔ lì tāng*), Cinnamon Twig Decoction plus Dragon Bone and Oyster Shell (*guì zhī jiā lóng gǔ mǔ lì tāng*)

NEURODERMATITIS

Eliminate Wind Powder (*xiāo fēng sǎn*)

PIGMENTATION DISORDERS

Drive Out Stasis from the Mansion of Blood Decoction (*xuè fǔ zhú yū tāng*)

PRURITUS, SENILE

Eliminate Wind Powder (*xiāo fēng sǎn*)

PSORIASIS

Drain the Epigastrium Decoction (*xiè xīn tāng*), Virgate Wormwood Decoction (*yīn chén hāo tāng*)

SEBORRHEIC BALDNESS

Drain the Epigastrium Decoction (*xiè xīn tāng*)

STEATOCYSTOMA MULTIPLEX

Saposhnikovia Powder that Sagely Unblocks (*fáng fēng tōng shèng sǎn*), Coptis Decoction to Resolve Toxicity (*huáng lián jiě dú tāng*)

URTICARIA

Virgate Wormwood Decoction (*yīn chén hāo tāng*), Eliminate Wind Powder (*xiāo fēng sǎn*), Ephedra, Apricot Kernel, Gypsum, and Licorice Decoction (*má xìng shí gān tāng*), Cinnamon Twig Decoction (*guì zhī tāng*), Cinnamon Twig plus Rhubarb Decoction (*guì zhī jiā dà huáng tāng*)

URTICARIA, CHRONIC

Drive Out Stasis from the Mansion of Blood Decoction (*xuè fǔ zhú yū tāng*), Bupleurum and Cinnamon Twig Decoction (*chái hú guì zhī tāng*)

15. Diseases of the Eyes, Ears, Nose, and Throat

CATARACTS

Tonify the Middle to Augment the Qi Decoction (*bǔ zhōng yì qì tāng*)

CONJUNCTIVITIS

Coptis Decoction to Resolve Toxicity (*huáng lián jiě dú tāng*), Drain the Epigastrium Decoction (*xiè xīn tāng*), Saposhnikovia Powder that Sagely Unblocks (*fáng fēng tōng shèng sǎn*)

EAR FURUNCLE

Drain the Epigastrium Decoction (*xiè xīn tāng*)

EYES, DRY

Tonify the Middle to Augment the Qi Decoction (*bǔ zhōng yì qì tāng*)

FUNDAL BLEEDING

Drive Out Stasis from the Mansion of Blood Decoction (*xuè fǔ zhú yū tāng*)

HAY FEVER

Minor Bluegreen Dragon Decoction (*xiǎo qīng lóng tāng*)

KERATITIS

Major Order the Qi Decoction (*dà chéng qì tāng*)

LARYNGITIS

Ephedra, Asarum, and Aconite Accessory Root Decoction (*má huáng xì xīn fù zǐ tāng*)

NASAL BOILS

Drain the Epigastrium Decoction (*xiè xīn tāng*)

NASOSINUSITIS

Ephedra, Apricot Kernel, Gypsum, and Licorice Decoction (*má xìng shí gān tāng*)

NOSEBLEEDS

Drain the Epigastrium Decoction (*xiè xīn tāng*), White Tiger Decoction (*bái hǔ tāng*)

OPHTHALMIA, SYMPATHETIC

White Tiger Decoction (*bái hǔ tāng*)

OPTIC ATROPHY

Tonify the Middle to Augment the Qi Decoction (*bǔ zhōng yì qì tāng*)

OPTIC NERVE PHLEBITIS

Drive Out Stasis from the Mansion of Blood Decoction (*xuè fǔ zhú yū tāng*)

OPTIC NEURITIS

White Tiger Decoction (*bái hǔ tāng*)

ORAL MUCOSAL ULCERS

Pinellia Decoction to Drain the Epigastrium (*bàn xià xiè xīn tāng*), Regulating Decoction with Coptis (*lián lǐ tāng*), Tonify the Middle to Augment the Qi Decoction (*bǔ zhōng yì qì tāng*), Coptis and Ass-Hide Gelatin Decoction (*huáng lián ē jiāo tāng*)

OTITIS MEDIA

Schizonepeta and Forsythia Decoction (*jīng jiè lián qiào tāng*)

PAPILLEDEMA

Tonify the Middle to Augment the Qi Decoction (*bǔ zhōng yì qì tāng*)

PERIODONTITIS

White Tiger Decoction (*bái hǔ tāng*)

PHARYNGITIS

Ephedra, Asarum, and Aconite Accessory Root Decoction (*má huáng xì xīn fù zǐ tāng*)

RETINAL VEIN THROMBOSIS

Drive Out Stasis from the Mansion of Blood Decoction (*xuè fǔ zhú yū tāng*)

RETINITIS

Tonify the Middle to Augment the Qi Decoction (*bǔ zhōng yì qì tāng*)

RHINITIS

Major Order the Qi Decoction (*dà chéng qì tāng*)

RHINITIS, CHRONIC

Tonify the Middle to Augment the Qi Decoction (*bǔ zhōng yì qì tāng*)

RHINITIS, ALLERGIC

Jade Windscreen Powder (*yù píng fēng sǎn*), Bupleurum and Cinnamon Twig Decoction (*chái hú guì zhī tāng*), Minor Bluegreen Dragon Decoction (*xiǎo qīng lóng tāng*), Frigid Extremities Powder (*sì nì sǎn*), Ephedra, Asarum, and Aconite Accessory Root Decoction (*má huáng xì xīn fù zǐ tāng*), Cinnamon Twig plus Aconite Accessory Root Decoction (*guì zhī jiā fù zǐ tāng*), Cinnamon Twig Decoction (*guì zhī tāng*)

SORE THROAT, CHRONIC

Tonify the Middle to Augment the Qi Decoction (*bǔ zhōng yì qì tāng*)

STOMATITIS, ACUTE

Drain the Epigastrium Decoction (*xiè xīn tāng*), White Tiger Decoction (*bái hǔ tāng*), Lophatherum and Gypsum Decoction (*zhú yè shí gāo tāng*), Coptis Decoction (*huáng lián tāng*)

STRABISMUS, PARALYTIC

Tonify the Middle to Augment the Qi Decoction (*bǔ zhōng yì qì tāng*)

TINNITUS

Tonify the Middle to Augment the Qi Decoction (*bǔ zhōng yì qì tāng*)

TONSILLITIS, ACUTE

Major Order the Qi Decoction (*dà chéng qì tāng*), Schizonepeta and Forsythia Decoction (*jīng jiè lián qiào tāng*), Drain the Epigastrium Decoction (*xiè xīn tāng*)

TOOTH PAIN

Tangkuei Decoction for Frigid Extremities (*dāng guī sì nì tāng*), Saposhnikovia Powder that Sagely Unblocks (*fáng fēng tōng shèng sǎn*)

Tʏᴍᴘᴀɴɪᴄ ᴍᴇᴍʙʀᴀɴᴇ, ʀᴇᴛʀᴀᴄᴛᴇᴅ

Tonify the Middle to Augment the Qi Decoction (*bǔ zhōng yì qì tāng*)

Vᴇʀᴛɪɢᴏ, ɪɴɴᴇʀ ᴇᴀʀ ɪɴᴅᴜᴄᴇᴅ

Bupleurum plus Dragon Bone and Oyster Shell Decoction (*chái hú jiā lóng gǔ mǔ lì tāng*), Pinellia, White Atractylodes, and Gastrodia Decoction (*bàn xià bái zhú tiān má tāng*), Minor Pinellia Decoction (*xiǎo bàn xià tāng*), True Warrior Decoction (*zhēn wǔ tāng*), Poria, Cinnamon Twig, Atractylodes, and Licorice Decoction (*líng guì zhú gān tāng*)

Basic Formulary for Important Symptoms

Appetite, poor

Minor Bupleurum Decoction (*xiǎo chái hú tāng*), Bupleurum, Cinnamon Twig, and Ginger Decoction *(chái hú guì jiāng tāng)*, Bupleurum and Cinnamon Twig Decoction (*chái hú guì zhī tāng*), Regulate the Middle Pill *(lǐ zhōng wán)*, Four-Gentleman Decoction (*sì jūn zǐ tāng*), Newly Augmented Decoction (*xīn jiā tāng*), Rambling Powder (*xiāo yáo sǎn*)

Chest and hypochondriac fullness and discomfort

Minor Bupleurum Decoction (*xiǎo chái hú tāng*), Bupleurum and Cinnamon Twig Decoction (*chái hú guì zhī tāng*), Bupleurum, Cinnamon Twig, and Ginger Decoction *(chái hú guì jiāng tāng)*, Bupleurum plus Dragon Bone and Oyster Shell Decoction (*chái hú jiā lóng gǔ mǔ lì tāng*), Major Bupleurum Decoction (*dà chái hú tāng*), Tonify the Middle to Augment the Qi Decoction (*bǔ zhōng yì qì tāng*)

Chills and aversion to cold

Ephedra Decoction *(má huáng tāng)*, Ephedra, Asarum, and Aconite Accessory Root Decoction (*má huáng xì xīn fù zǐ tāng*), Minor Bluegreen Dragon Decoction (*xiǎo qīng lóng tāng*), Cinnamon Twig plus Aconite Accessory Root Decoction (*guì zhī jiā fù zǐ tāng*), Frigid Extremities Decoction (*sì nì tāng*), Aconite Accessory Root Decoction to Drain the Epigastrium (*fù zǐ xiè xīn tāng*), Rhubarb and Aconite Accessory Root Decoction (*dà huáng fù zǐ tāng*), Regulate the Middle Pill (*lǐ zhōng wán*), Aconite Accessory Root Decoction to Regulate the Middle (*fù zǐ lǐ zhōng tāng*)

Constipation

Major Order the Qi Decoction (*dà chéng qì tāng*), Regulate the Stomach and Order the Qi Decoction (*tiáo wèi chéng qì tāng*), Drain the Epigastrium Decoction (*xiè xīn tāng*), Cinnamon Twig plus Rhubarb Decoction (*guì zhī jiā dà huáng tāng*), Rhubarb and Aconite Accessory

Root Decoction (*dà huáng fù zǐ tāng*), Warm the Spleen Decoction
(*wēn pí tāng*), Saposhnikovia Powder that Sagely Unblocks (*fáng
fēng tōng shèng sǎn*), Major Bupleurum Decoction (*dà chái hú tāng*),
Tonify the Middle to Augment the Qi Decoction (*bǔ zhōng yì qì tāng*),
Minor Construct the Middle Decoction (*xiǎo jiàn zhōng tāng*), Frigid
Extremities Powder (*sì nì sǎn*)

Cough

Minor Bupleurum Decoction (*xiǎo chái hú tāng*), Bupleurum Sinking
Decoction (*chái xiàn tāng*), Pinellia and Magnolia Bark Decoction (*bàn
xià hòu pò tāng*), Two-Aged [Herb] Decoction (*èr chén tāng*), Warm
Gallbladder Decoction with Bamboo Shavings (*zhú rú wēn dǎn tāng*),
Minor Pinellia Decoction (*xiǎo bàn xià tāng*), Minor Decoction [for
Pathogens] Stuck in the Chest (*xiǎo xiàn xiōng tāng*), Frigid Extremities
Powder (*sì nì sǎn*), Cinnamon Twig Decoction plus Magnolia Bark and
Apricot Kernels (*guì zhī jiā hòu pò xìng zǐ tāng*)

Diarrhea

Frigid Extremities Powder (*sì nì sǎn*), Regulate the Middle Pill (*lǐ zhōng
wán*), Aconite Accessory Root Decoction to Regulate the Middle (*fù
zǐ lǐ zhōng tāng*), Five-Ingredient Powder with Poria (*wǔ líng sǎn*),
Pogostemon/Agastache Powder to Rectify the Qi (*huò xiāng zhèng qì
sǎn*), Patchouli/Agastache, Magnolia Bark, Pinellia, and Poria Decoction
(*huò pò xià líng tāng*), Aucklandia and Coptis Pill (*xiāng lián wán*),
Pinellia Decoction to Drain the Epigastrium (*bàn xià xiè xīn tāng*),
Regulating Decoction with Coptis (*lián lǐ tāng*), Cinnamon Twig and
Ginseng Decoction (*guì zhī rén shēn tāng*)

Distention, abdominal

Minor Order the Qi Decoction (*xiǎo chéng qì tāng*), Pinellia and
Magnolia Bark Decoction (*bàn xià hòu pò tāng*), Regulate the Middle
Pill (*lǐ zhōng wán*), Unripe Bitter Orange, Chinese Garlic, and Cinnamon
Twig Decoction (*zhǐ shí xiè bái guì zhī tāng*)

Dizziness

Pinellia, White Atractylodes, and Gastrodia Decoction (*bàn xià bái
zhú tiān má tāng*), Poria, Cinnamon Twig, Atractylodes, and Licorice
Decoction (*líng guì zhú gān tāng*), True Warrior Decoction (*zhēn wǔ
tāng*), Minor Pinellia plus Poria Decoction (*xiǎo bàn xià jiā fù líng tāng*),
Warm Gallbladder Decoction with Coptis (*huáng lián wēn dǎn tāng*),
Guide Out Phlegm Decoction (*dǎo tán tāng*)

Edema

Stephania and Astragalus Decoction (*fáng jǐ huáng qí tāng*), Bupleurum and Poria Decoction (*chái líng tāng*), Ephedra Decoction plus Atractylodes (*má huáng jiā zhú tāng*), Maidservant from Yue's Decoction plus Atractylodes (*Yuè bì jiā zhú tāng*), Five-Ingredient Powder with Poria (*wǔ líng sǎn*), True Warrior Decoction (*zhēn wǔ tāng*)

Fever

Cinnamon Twig Decoction (*guì zhī tāng*), Ephedra Decoction (*má huáng tāng*), Ephedra, Apricot Kernel, Gypsum, and Licorice Decoction (*má xìng shí gān tāng*), Ephedra, Asarum, and Aconite Accessory Root Decoction (*má huáng xì xīn fù zǐ tāng*), Major Order the Qi Decoction (*dà chéng qì tāng*), Coptis Decoction to Resolve Toxicity (*huáng lián jiě dú tāng*), Saposhnikovia Powder that Sagely Unblocks (*fáng fēng tōng shèng sǎn*), Bupleurum and Cinnamon Twig Decoction (*chái hú guì zhī tāng*), Tonify the Middle to Augment the Qi Decoction (*bǔ zhōng yì qì tāng*), Frigid Extremities Powder (*sì nì sǎn*), White Tiger Decoction (*bái hǔ tāng*), White Tiger plus Cinnamon Twig Decoction (*bái hǔ jiā guì zhī tāng*), White Tiger plus Atractylodes Decoction (*bái hǔ jiā cāng zhú tāng*), Lophatherum and Gypsum Decoction (*zhú yè shí gāo tāng*), Coptis Decoction (*huáng lián tāng*), Coptis Decoction to Resolve Toxicity (*huáng lián jiě dú tāng*), Frigid Extremities Decoction (*sì nì tāng*)

Fever, low-grade

Astragalus Decoction to Construct the Middle (*huáng qí jiàn zhōng tāng*), Tonify the Middle to Augment the Qi Decoction (*bǔ zhōng yì qì tāng*), Cinnamon Twig Decoction plus Dragon Bone and Oyster Shell (*guì zhī jiā lóng gǔ mǔ lì tāng*), Lophatherum and Gypsum Decoction (*zhú yè shí gāo tāng*), Cinnamon Twig Decoction (*guì zhī tāng*)

Focal distention with firmness

Cinnamon Twig and Ginseng Decoction (*guì zhī rén shēn tāng*), Major Pinellia Decoction (*dà bàn xià tāng*), Four-Gentleman Decoction (*sì jūn zǐ tāng*), Regulate the Middle Pill (*lǐ zhōng wán*), Newly Augmented Decoction (*xīn jiā tāng*)

Focal distention with pain

Bupleurum Sinking Decoction (*chái xiàn tāng*), Pinellia Decoction to Drain the Epigastrium (*bàn xià xiè xīn tāng*), Drain the Epigastrium Decoction (*xiè xīn tāng*), Aconite Accessory Root Decoction to Drain the Epigastrium *(fù zǐ xiè xīn tāng)*, Coptis Decoction to Resolve Toxicity *(huáng lián jiě dú tāng)*

Hands and feet, cold

Frigid Extremities Powder *(sì nì sǎn)*, Frigid Extremities Decoction *(sì nì tāng)*, Tangkuei Decoction for Frigid Extremities *(dāng guī sì nì tāng)*, Cinnamon Twig plus Aconite Accessory Root Decoction *(guì zhī jiā fù zǐ tāng)*, Rhubarb and Aconite Accessory Root Decoction *(dà huáng fù zǐ tāng)*, Aconite Accessory Root Decoction to Drain the Epigastrium *(fù zǐ xiè xīn tāng)*, Tonify the Middle to Augment the Qi Decoction *(bǔ zhōng yì qì tāng)*, Aconite Accessory Root Decoction to Regulate the Middle *(fù zǐ lǐ zhōng tāng)*, Ephedra, Asarum, and Aconite Accessory Root Decoction *(má huáng xì xīn fù zǐ tāng)*

Headache

White Tiger Decoction *(bái hǔ tāng)*, Saposhnikovia Powder that Sagely Unblocks *(fáng fēng tōng shèng sǎn)*, Frigid Extremities Powder *(sì nì sǎn)*, Drive Out Stasis from the Mansion of Blood Decoction *(xuè fǔ zhú yū tāng)*, Bupleurum plus Dragon Bone and Oyster Shell Decoction *(chái hú jiā lóng gǔ mǔ lì tāng)*, Augmented Rambling Powder *(jiā wèi xiāo yáo sǎn)*, Tonify the Yang to Restore Five-Tenths Decoction *(bǔ yáng huán wǔ tāng)*, Tangkuei Decoction for Frigid Extremities *(dāng guī sì nì tāng)*, Tangkuei Decoction for Frigid Extremities plus Evodia and Fresh Ginger *(dāng guī sì nì jiā wú zhū yú shēng jiāng tāng)*

Hiccup

Peony and Licorice Decoction *(sháo yào gān cǎo tāng)*, Frigid Extremities Powder *(sì nì sǎn)*, Drive Out Stasis from the Mansion of Blood Decoction *(xuè fǔ zhú yū tāng)*

Insomnia

Drive Out Stasis from the Mansion of Blood Decoction *(xuè fǔ zhú yū tāng)*, Bupleurum plus Dragon Bone and Oyster Shell Decoction *(chái hú jiā lóng gǔ mǔ lì tāng)*, Pinellia Decoction to Drain the Epigastrium *(bàn xià xiè xīn tāng)*, Warm Gallbladder Decoction *(wēn dǎn tāng)*, Ten-Ingredient Warm Gallbladder Decoction *(shí wèi wēn dǎn tāng)*, Coptis and Ass-Hide Gelatin Decoction *(huáng lián ē jiāo tāng)*, Coptis Decoction *(huáng lián tāng)*, Drain the Epigastrium Decoction *(xiè xīn tāng)*, Tonify the Middle to Augment the Qi Decoction *(bǔ zhōng yì qì tāng)*, Cinnamon Twig Decoction plus Dragon Bone and Oyster Shell *(guì zhī jiā lóng gǔ mǔ lì tāng)*

Irritability

Coptis and Ass-Hide Gelatin Decoction *(huáng lián ē jiāo tāng)*, Coptis Decoction *(huáng lián tāng)*, Pinellia Decoction to Drain the Epigastrium *(bàn xià xiè xīn tāng)*, Coptis Decoction to Resolve Toxicity *(huáng lián jiě dú tāng)*, Drain the Epigastrium Decoction *(xiè xīn tāng)*

Jaundice

Virgate Wormwood Decoction *(yīn chén hāo tāng)*

Listless and dispirited

Ephedra, Asarum, and Aconite Accessory Root Decoction *(má huáng xì xīn fù zǐ tāng)*, Frigid Extremities Decoction *(sì nì tāng)*, Frigid Extremities Decoction plus Ginseng *(sì nì jiā rén shēn tāng)*, Ginseng and Aconite Accessory Root Decoction *(shēn fù tāng)*

Numbness

Astragalus and Cinnamon Twig Five-Substance Decoction *(huáng qí guì zhī wǔ wù tāng)*, Tonify the Yang to Restore Five-Tenths Decoction *(bǔ yáng huán wǔ tāng)*

Pain, abdominal

Minor Construct the Middle Decoction *(xiǎo jiàn zhōng tāng)*, Astragalus Decoction to Construct the Middle *(huáng qí jiàn zhōng tāng)*, Tangkuei Decoction to Construct the Middle *(dāng guī jiàn zhōng tāng)*, Warm the Spleen Decoction *(wēn pí tāng)*, Rhubarb and Aconite Accessory Root Decoction *(dà huáng fù zǐ tāng)*, Minor Order the Qi Decoction *(xiǎo chéng qì tāng)*, Bupleurum and Cinnamon Twig Decoction *(chái hú guì zhī tāng)*, Rambling Powder *(xiāo yáo sǎn)*, Frigid Extremities Powder *(sì nì sǎn)*, Coptis Decoction *(huáng lián tāng)*, Aconite Accessory Root Decoction to Drain the Epigastrium *(fù zǐ xiè xīn tāng)*, Major Construct the Middle Decoction *(dà jiàn zhōng tāng)*, Aucklandia and Coptis Pill *(xiāng lián wán)*, Coptis and Ass-Hide Gelatin Decoction *(huáng lián ē jiāo tāng)*, Tangkuei Decoction for Frigid Extremities *(dāng guī sì nì tāng)*, Tangkuei Decoction for Frigid Extremities plus Evodia and Fresh Ginger *(dāng guī sì nì jiā wú zhū yú shēng jiāng tāng)*, Cinnamon Twig Decoction plus Dragon Bone and Oyster Shell *(guì zhī jiā lóng gǔ mǔ lì tāng)*

Pain, joint

Cinnamon Twig Decoction *(guì zhī tāng)*, Bupleurum and Cinnamon Twig Decoction *(chái hú guì zhī tāng)*, Ephedra Decoction *(má huáng tāng)*, Ephedra Decoction plus Atractylodes *(má huáng jiā zhú tāng)*, Maidservant from Yue's Decoction plus Atractylodes *(Yuè bì jiā zhú tāng)*, Licorice, Ginger, Poria and Atractrylodes Macrocephala Decoction *(gān cǎo gān jiāng fú líng bái zhú tāng)*, Cinnamon Twig, Peony, and Anemarrhena Decoction *(guì zhī sháo yào zhī mǔ tāng)*, Tangkuei Decoction for Frigid Extremities *(dāng guī sì nì tāng)*, White Tiger plus Cinnamon Twig Decoction *(bái hǔ jiā guì zhī tāng)*, Cinnamon Twig plus Aconite Accessory Root Decoction *(guì zhī jiā fù zǐ tāng)*, Cinnamon Twig plus Atractylodes and Aconite Accessory Root Decoction *(guì zhī jiā zhú fù tāng)*, Tangkuei Decoction to Construct the Middle *(dāng guī jiàn zhōng tāng)*

Pain, lower abdominal

Peach Pit Decoction to Order the Qi *(táo hé chéng qì tāng)*, Rhubarb and Ground Beetle Pill *(dà huáng zhè chóng wán)*, Flow-Warming Decoction *(wēn jīng tāng)*, Cinnamon Twig and Poria Pill *(guì zhī fú líng wán)*

Pain, lower back

Licorice, Ginger, Poria and Atractrylodes Macrocephala Decoction *(gān cǎo gān jiāng fú líng bái zhú tāng)*, Ephedra, Asarum, and Aconite Accessory Root Decoction *(má huáng xì xīn fù zǐ tāng)*, Tangkuei Decoction for Frigid Extremities *(dāng guī sì nì tāng)*

Palpitations

Cinnamon Twig Decoction *(guì zhī tāng)*, Minor Construct the Middle Decoction *(xiǎo jiàn zhōng tāng)*, Cinnamon Twig Decoction plus Dragon Bone and Oyster Shell *(guì zhī jiā lóng gǔ mǔ lì tāng)*, Prepared Licorice *(zhì gān cǎo tāng)*, Bupleurum plus Dragon Bone and Oyster Shell Decoction *(chái hú jiā lóng gǔ mǔ lì tāng)*, Bupleurum, Cinnamon Twig, and Ginger Decoction *(chái hú guì jiāng tāng)*, Poria, Cinnamon Twig, Atractylodes, and Licorice Decoction *(líng guì zhú gān tāng)*, Poria, Cinnamon Twig, Jujubae, and Licorice Decoction *(líng guì zǎo tāng)*, True Warrior Decoction *(zhēn wǔ tāng)*, Minor Pinellia plus Poria Deoction *(xiǎo bàn xià jiā fù líng tāng)*, Ten-Ingredient Warm Gallbladder Decoction *(shí wèi wēn dǎn tāng)*

Palpitations

Prepared Licorice *(zhì gān cǎo tāng)*

Phlegm

Pinellia and Magnolia Bark Decoction *(bàn xià hòu pò tāng)*, Two-Aged

[Herb] Decoction (*èr chén tāng*), Guide Out Phlegm Decoction (*dǎo tán tāng*), Minor Bluegreen Dragon Decoction (*xiǎo qīng lóng tāng*) Minor Decoction [for Pathogens] Stuck in the Chest (*xiǎo xiàn xiōng tāng*), Poria, Cinnamon Twig, Atractylodes, and Licorice Decoction (*líng guì zhú gān tāng*)

Shock

Major Order the Qi Decoction (*dà chéng qì tāng*), Frigid Extremities Decoction (*sì nì tāng*), Frigid Extremities Decoction plus Ginseng (*sì nì jiā rén shēn tāng*), Ginseng and Aconite Accessory Root Decoction (*shēn fù tāng*), Regulate the Middle Pill (*lǐ zhōng wán*)

Spasms, muscle

Peony and Licorice Decoction (*sháo yào gān cǎo tāng*)

Stupor

White Tiger Decoction (*bái hǔ tāng*), Major Order the Qi Decoction (*dà chéng qì tāng*)

Sweating, abnormal

Cinnamon Twig Decoction (*guì zhī tāng*), Cinnamon Twig Decoction plus Dragon Bone and Oyster Shell (*guì zhī jiā lóng gǔ mǔ lì tāng*), Jade Windscreen Powder (*yù píng fēng sǎn*), Bupleurum and Cinnamon Twig Decoction (*chái hú guì zhī tāng*), True Warrior Decoction (*zhēn wǔ tāng*), Astragalus Decoction to Construct the Middle (*huáng qí jiàn zhōng tāng*), Stephania and Astragalus Decoction (*fáng jǐ huáng qí tāng*), Astragalus and Cinnamon Twig Five-Substance Decoction (*huáng qí guì zhī wǔ wù tāng*), White Tiger Decoction (*bái hǔ tāng*), Cinnamon Twig plus Aconite Accessory Root Decoction (*guì zhī jiā fù zǐ tāng*), Cinnamon Twig Decoction plus Astragalus (*guì zhī jiā huáng qí tāng*)

Thirst, severe

White Tiger Decoction (*bái hǔ tāng*), White Tiger plus Ginseng Decoction (*bái hǔ jiā rén shēn tāng*), Ephedra, Apricot Kernel, Gypsum, and Licorice Decoction (*má xìng shí gān tāng*)

Urinary difficulty

Ephedra Decoction plus Atractylodes (*má huáng jiā zhú tāng*), Maidservant from Yue's Decoction plus Atractylodes (*Yuè bì jiā zhú tāng*), Poria, Cinnamon Twig, Atractylodes, and Licorice Decoction (*líng guì zhú gān tāng*), Pinellia, White Atractylodes, and Gastrodia Decoction (*bàn xià bái zhú tiān má tāng*), Jade Windscreen Powder (*yù píng fēng sǎn*), True Warrior Decoction (*zhēn wǔ tāng*)

Vomiting

Pinellia Decoction to Drain the Epigastrium (*bàn xià xiè xīn tāng*), Minor Pinellia Decoction (*xiǎo bàn xià tāng*), Major Pinellia Decoction (*dà bàn xià tāng*), Pinellia and Magnolia Bark Decoction (*bàn xià hòu pò tāng*), Two-Aged [Herb] Decoction (*èr chén tāng*), Warm Gallbladder Decoction (*wēn dǎn tāng*), Minor Bupleurum Decoction (*xiǎo chái hú tāng*), Left Metal Pill (*zuǒ jīn wán*), Coptis Decoction (*huáng lián tāng*), Tangkuei Decoction for Frigid Extremities plus Evodia and Fresh Ginger (*dāng guī sì nì jiā wú zhū yú shēng jiāng tāng*)

Weariness and fatigue

Tonify the Middle to Augment the Qi Decoction (*bǔ zhōng yì qì tāng*), Ephedra, Asarum, and Aconite Accessory Root Decoction (*má huáng xì xīn fù zǐ tāng*), Frigid Extremities Decoction plus Ginseng (*sì nì jiā rén shēn tāng*)

Wheezing

Ephedra, Apricot Kernel, Gypsum, and Licorice Decoction (*má xìng shí gān tāng*), Ephedra Decoction (*má huáng tāng*), Three-Unbinding Decoction (*sān ǎo tāng*), Minor Bluegreen Dragon Decoction (*xiǎo qīng lóng tāng*), Unripe Bitter Orange, Chinese Garlic, and Cinnamon Twig Decoction (*zhǐ shí xiè bái guì zhī tāng*), Cinnamon Twig Decoction plus Dragon Bone and Oyster Shell (*guì zhī jiā lóng gǔ mǔ lì tāng*)

Wind, aversion to

Cinnamon Twig Decoction (*guì zhī tāng*), Bupleurum and Cinnamon Twig Decoction (*chái hú guì zhī tāng*), Tonify the Middle to Augment the Qi Decoction (*bǔ zhōng yì qì tāng*)

Notes

Chapter 1: **Cinnamon Twig Formula Family**

1 Chen Ke-Ji et al. 陳可冀 等. *New Chinese Medicine* 新中醫 4: 8, 1983.

2 Lin Zong-Guang 林宗廣. *Journal of Chinese Medicine* 中醫雜誌 4: 1, 1965.

3 Gu Bo-Quan 顧柏泉. *Zhejiang Chinese Medicine* 浙江中醫 5: 30, 1965.

4 Lai Chun-Mao 來春茂. *New Chinese Medicine* 新中醫 1: 4, 1978.

5 Wang Chun-Xian 王春賢. *Hunan Journal of Chinese Medicine* 湖南中醫雜誌 3: 17, 1988.

6 Shao Ji-Tang 邵繼棠. *Sichuan Chinese Medicine* 四川中醫 1: 34, 1986.

7 Guo Zi-Guang 郭子光. *New Compilation of Shang Han Lun Formula Patterns* 傷寒論湯證新編 Shanghai: Shanghai Science and Technology Publishing House, page 45, 1983.

8 Cai Yu-Quan 蔡漁琴. *Liaoning Journal of Chinese Medicine* 遼寧中醫雜誌 4: 29, 1984.

9 Ye Ju-Quan 葉橘泉. *Jiangsu Chinese Medicine* 江蘇中醫 1: 27, 1962.

10 Wang San-Hu [trans.] 王三虎. *Journal of the Nanjing College of Traditional Chinese Medicine* 南京中醫學院報 2: 55, 1986.

11 Gu Jie-Shan 顧介山. *Jiangsu Chinese Medicine* 江蘇中醫 2: 25, 1958.

12 Wang Ping-Fen 王萍芬. *Journal of Chinese Medicine* 中醫雜誌 10: 12, 1964.

13 You Guo-Xiong et al. 游國雄等. *Tianjin Chinese Medicine* 天津中醫 6: 25, 1985.

14 You Guo-Xiong et al. 游國雄等. *China Journal of Medicine* 中華醫學雜誌 1:57, 1981.

15 You Guo-Xiong et al. 游國雄等. *People's Army Medicine* 人民軍醫 8: 43, 1983.

16 Wu De-Xiu 吳德秀. *Hubei Journal of Chinese Medicine* 湖北中醫雜誌 2: 39, 1986.

17 Zhang Xin-Feng et al. 張心鳳等. *Journal of the Chengdu University of Chinese Medicine* 成都中醫學院學報 1: 26 1986.

18 Huang Mu-Jun 黃慕君. *Railway Medicine* 鐵道醫學 2: 50, 1976.

19 Beijing Jishui Tan Hospital 北京積水潭醫院. *Selected Readings in Coronary Heart Disease* 冠心病資料選編 page 25, 1975.

20 Tianjin Hospital of Chinese Medicine 天津中醫學院. *Selected Readings from Tianjin City Prevention of Coronary Heart Disease* 天津市冠心病防治資料選編 page 55, 1974.

21 Gao Er-Xin 高爾鑫. *Journal of Chinese Medicine* 中醫雜誌 10: 24, 254, 1983.

22 Xu De-Xian 徐德先. *Jiangsu Journal of Chinese Medicine* 江蘇中醫雜誌 1: 25, 1984.

23 Shandong Provincial Chinese Medicine Research Institute 山東省中醫研究所. *Selected Readings in Combining Chinese and Western Medicine* 中西醫結合研究資料選編 page 25, 1972.

24 Zhang Feng-Qiang 張豐強. *Practical Compendium of Famous Chinese Medicine Formulas* 中醫名方應用大全 China Medical and Technology Publishing House, 1992.

Chapter 2: **Ephedra Formula Family**

1 Zhang Yun-Peng 張雲鵬. *Shanghai Journal of Chinese Medicine* 上海中醫藥雜誌 8: 10, 1965.

2 Shang Village Coal Mine Public Health Clinic of the Fengcheng Mining Bureau 豐成礦務局尚莊煤礦衛生所. *Materials on the New Medicine and Pharamcology* 新醫藥資料 4: 32, 1975.

3 Li Feng-Lin et al. 李鳳林等. *New Chinese Medicine* 新中醫 9: 28, 1985.

4 Gong Ke-Chang 龔克昌. *Journal of Integrated Chinese and Western Medicine* 中西醫結合雜誌 11: 691, 1988.

5 Jing Jie 經捷. *Journal of the Nanjing College of Traditional Chinese Medicine* 南京中醫學院報 2: 11, 1987.

6 Fujihara Ken 藤平健. *Kampo Research Journal* 漢方の研究 6: 210, 1982.

7 Cao Guo-Xing 曹國星. *New Chinese Medicine* 新中醫 11: 43, 1984.

8 Chu Jie-Qiu 初結秋譯 (translator). *Overseas Medicine: Chinese Medicine and Pharmacology Fascicle* 國外醫學中醫中藥分冊 6: 15, 1984.

9 Hong Zhi-Lin 洪智林. *Zhejiang Journal of Chinese Medicine* 浙江中醫雜誌 6: 247, 1985.

10 Yu Yun-Zhong 余雲中. *Sichuan Chinese Medicine* 四川中醫 11: 38, 1985.

11 Liu Guan-Jun 劉冠軍. *Shanghai Journal of Chinese Medicine and Pharmacology* 上海中醫藥雜誌 6: 14, 1964.

12 Zhang Zhen-Dong 張振東. *Zhejiang Journal of Chinese Medicine* 浙江中醫雜誌 6: 254, 1988.

13 Nakamura 脹麗娟譯. *Overseas Medicine: Chinese Medicine and Pharmacology Fascicle* 國外醫學中醫中藥分冊 5: 19, 1990.

14 Morishima Akira 森島昭: *Diagnosis and Treatment in Pediatrics* 小兒科診療 41(2): 103, 1978.

15 Wang Hua-Ming et al. 王華明等. *Shanghai Journal of Chinese Medicine* 上海中醫雜誌 12: 15, 1981.

16 Wang Hua-Ming et al. 王華明等. *Fujian Chinese Medical Herbology* 福建中醫藥 5: 61 1983.

17 Okazaki 岡崎等. *Clinical Otolaryngology* 耳鼻咽喉科臨床 74(3): 367, 1981.

18 Imai Nao 今井直. *Research in Chinese Medical Formulas* 中醫方劑研究 5: 11, 1979.

19 Kuriyama 栗山一夫等. *Allergy* アレルギー 29(5): 227, 1980.

20 Miyata et al. 宮天隆夫等. *Pediatric Clinical Medicine* 小兒科臨床 39 (9): 2101, 1986.

21 Pediatric Department of the Tianjin College of Chinese Medicine 天津中醫學院附屬小兒科. *Chinese Journal of Pediatrics* 中華兒科雜誌 10(2): 101, 1959.

22 Pang Hua-Wei 龐華威. *Shanghai Journal of Chinese Traditional Chinese Medicine* 上海中醫藥雜誌 1: 26 1986.

23 Tianjin Donglou Public Health Clinic 天津東樓衛生院. *Tianjin Pharmacology* 天津醫藥 12: 626, 1975.

24 Dai An-Sheng 戴安生. *Hubei Journal of Chinese Medicine* 湖北中醫雜誌 6: 23, 1983.

25 Xu Wei-Lin 徐蔚霖. *Shanghai Journal of Chinese Traditional Chinese Medicine* 上海中醫藥雜誌 1: 14, 1960.

26 Hunan Yiyangou River Public Health Clinic 湖南益陽歐江岔公社衛生院. *Jiangxi Journal of Chinese Herbology* 江西中醫藥 10: 25, 1960.

27 Fujian Province People's Hospital Eye, Ear, Nose and Throat Department 福建省人民醫院五宮科. *Fujian Journal of Chinese Traditional Chinese Medicine* 福建中醫藥 3: 42, 1959.

28 Pan Wen-Kui 潘文奎. *New Chinese Medicine* 新中醫 1: 20, 1990.

29 Zhao Shou-Zhen 趙守真. *Recollections of Clinical Experience* 治驗回憶錄 Beijing: People's Medical Publishing House, 1962.

30 Zhang Zhen-Dong 張振東. *Liaoning Journal of Traditional Chinese Medicine* 遼寧中醫雜誌 10: 16, 1988.

31 Shang De-Jun 尚德俊. *Treatment of Thromboangiitis Obliterans with Chinese and Western Medicine* 中西醫結合治療血拴閉塞性脈管炎 Jinan: Shandong Science and Technology Press, 1983.

32 Dong Guo-Long 董國隆. *Shanxi Traditional Chinese Medicine* 陝西中醫 4: 160, 1991.

33 Dong Guo-Ban 董國半. *Hunan Journal of Traditional Chinese Medicine* 湖南中醫雜誌 3: 10, 1986.

Chapter 3: **Bupleurum Formula Family**

1 Honsono Shiro 細野史郎. *Ten Lectures on the Study of Kampo* 漢方醫學十講 Tokyo: Sogensha, page 104, 1982.

2 Traditional Chinese Medicine Teaching and Research Section of the First Teaching Hospital of the Harbin University of Medical Sciences 哈爾濱醫科大學附屬一院中醫教研室. *Journal of Traditional Chinese Medicine* 中醫雜誌 10: 24, 1965.

3 Shen Zhao-Xiong 沈兆熊. *Journal of the Nanjing TCM University* 南京中醫學院學報 1: 34, 1993.

4 Gu Yue-Ping 顧躍平. *Sichuan Traditional Chinese Medicine* 四川中醫 5: 36, 1986.

5 Wada Tadashi. et al. 和田正系. *Kampo and Chinese Medicine* 漢方と漢藥 3(10): 27, 1936.

6 Shen Heng-Fu 沈衡甫. *Shanghai Journal of Traditional Chinese Medicine* 上海中醫藥雜誌 10: 14, 1965.

7 Yashiki Michiaki 矢數道明. *Clinical Kampo* 漢方の臨床 22(9): 37, 1975.

8 Hasegawa Hisashi 長谷川久. *Kampo Research* 漢方研究 75(9): 29, 1975.

9 Ogawa Yukio et al. 小川辛男 等. *Journal of the Japanese Medical Society* 日本東洋醫學會志 4: 30, 1970.

10 Wada Tadashi et al. 和田正系. *Clinical Kampo* 漢方の臨床 10(8): 13, 1963.

11 Yashiki Michiaki 矢數道明. *Clinical Kampo* 漢方の臨床 11(2): 24, 1964.

12 Zhang Qin-Song et al. 張琴松等. *Fujian Traditional Chinese Medicine* 福建中醫藥 5: 3, 1963.

13 Yashiki Michiaki 矢數道明. *Clinical Kampo* 漢方の臨床 15(11-12): 133, 1968.

14 Soumi Ichiro 相見一郎. *Journal of Japanese Medicine* 日本東洋醫學志 19(11): 33, 1968.

15 Soumi Ichiro 相見一郎. *Kampo Research Journal* 漢方研究 6: 15, 1976.

16 Soumi Ichiro 相見一郎. *Clinical Kampo* 漢方の臨床 15(11-12): 189, 1968.

17 Soumi Ichiro 相見一郎. *Clinical Kampo* 漢方の臨床 5(6): 15, 1958.

18 Kubo Michinori 久保道德. *Study of Kampo* 漢方醫學 8(1): 11, 1984.

19 Marunoto Masahiko 丸本正彥等. *Overseas Medicine: Chinese Medicine and Pharmacology Fascicle* 國外醫學中醫藥分冊 6(2): 121, 1984.

20 Hayakawa Masanori 早川政兼等. *Overseas Medicine: Chinese Medicine and Pharmacology Fascicle* 國外醫學中醫藥分冊 6(5): 307, 1984.

21 Soumi Ichiro 相見一郎. *Kampo Research Journal* 漢方研究 6: 15, 1976.

22 Abe Hiroko 阿部博子等. *Journal of Pharmacology* 藥學雜誌 100(6): 602, 1980.

23 Abe Hiroko 阿部博子等. *Journal of Pharmacology* 藥學雜誌 100(6): 607, 1980.

24 Yue Mei-Zhong 岳美中. *New Chinese Medicine* 新中醫 1: 24, 1974.

25 Sakaguchi Hiroshi 阪口弘. *Sino-Japanese Medicines: Clinical Supplement* 臨床增刊號和漢藥 10(5): 702, 1973.

26 Ge Ping et al. 葛萍等. *Journal of Integrated Chinese and Western Medicine* 中西醫結合雜誌 6(12): 753, 1986.

27 Zhou Kang 周康. *Shanghai Journal of Chinese Medicine* 上海中醫藥雜誌 8: 33, 1962.

28 Yu Ji-Xian 喻繼先. *Journal of the Hunan TCM University* 湖南中醫學院報 2: 29, 1986.

29 Zhou Kang 周康. *Shanghai Journal of Traditional Chinese Medicine* 上海中醫藥雜誌 11: 30, 1958.

30 Kaneko Yoshihiko 金子善彥. *Clinical Research* 臨床と研究 57(10): 3379, 1980.

31 Muroka Akizon 室賀昭三. *Kampo Medicine* 漢方醫藥 2: 44, 1973.

32 Xie Huan-Rong 謝煥榮. *Inner Mongolian Chinese Medicine and Pharmacology* 內蒙古中醫藥 1: 20, 1989.

33 Fan Zhong-Lin Case Study Organization Group 范中林議案整理小組. *Fan Zhong-Lin's Selected Six Stage Diagnosis Case Studies* 范中林六經辨證議案選, Shenyang: Liaoning Science and Technology Publishing Company 遼寧科學技術出版社 page 50, 1984.

34 Wang Lie 王烈. *Zhejiang Journal of Traditional Chinese Medicine* 浙江中醫雜誌 9: 425, 1983.

35 Tian De-Yin 田德蔭. *Tianjin Traditional Medicine* 天津醫藥 2: 112, 1980.

36 Wu Qi-Fu 吳啓富. *China Journal of Traditional Medicine* 中國醫藥學報 4: 28, 1990.

37 Zhang Rui-Jin 張銳金. *Journal of Traditional Chinese Medicine* 中醫雜誌 6: 35, 1980.

38 Luo Yu-Hua 駱玉華. *Sichuan Traditional Chinese Medicine* 四川中醫 3: 22, 1987.

39 Sun You-Li 孫幼立. *Journal of Traditional Chinese Medicine* 中醫雜誌 7: 15, 1963.

40 Zhang Liang-Dong 張良棟. *Journal of Integrated Chinese and Western Medicine* 中西結合雜誌 4(8): 465, 1984.

41 Huang Yin-Fu 黃銀富. *Fujian Traditional Chinese Medicine and Pharmacology* 福建中醫藥 3: 4, 1961.

42 Wang Cheng-Xun 王承訓. *Journal of Traditional Chinese Medicine* 中醫雜誌 27(10): 44, 1986.

43 Zheng Xian-Li et al. 鄭顯理等. *Journal of Traditional Chinese Medicine* 中醫雜誌 7: 12, 1965.

Chapter 4: **Rhubarb Formula Family**

1 Hunan Province Intestinal Adhesion and Obstruction Prevention Association 湖南省防治腸粘連，粘連性腸梗阻協作組. *Hunan Journal of Traditional Chinese Medicine* 湖南醫藥雜誌 2: 11, 1978.

2 Gu Xuan-Wen顧選文. *Shanghai Journal of Traditional Chinese Medicine* 上海中醫藥雜誌 2: 15, 1980.

3 Shuguang Hospital Internal Medicine Department Ward 5 曙光醫院內科五病區. *Shanghai Journal of Traditional Chinese Medicine* 上海中醫藥雜誌 4: 14, 1979.

4 Wang Peng-Mei 汪朋梅等. *Jiangsu Journal of Traditional Chinese Medicine* 江蘇中醫雜誌 8: 342, 1985.

5 Wang Rong-Gen王榮根. *Zhejiang Journal of Traditional Chinese Medicine* 浙江中醫雜誌 3: 113, 1980.

6 Tan Zheng-Yu et al. 譚正宇等. *Midlevel Medicine* 中級醫刊 10: 629, 1985.

7 Tianjin First Central Hospital 天津第一中心醫院. *Zhejiang Journal of Traditional Medicine* 浙江中醫雜誌 10: 342, 1985.

8 Liu Tao et al. 劉濤等. *Proceedings of the Combined China Medical Association and Chinese Western Medicine Academic Conference on the Treatment of Serious Illness* 中華醫學會中國西醫結合研究會全國危重症急救醫學學術會議論文彙扁 (Hangzhou), page 209, November 1982.

9 Liaoning Hospital of Chinese Medicine 遼寧中醫學院. *China Journal of Traditional Chinese Medicine* 中華醫學雜誌 1: 57, 1978.

10 Tianjin City Guhan Hospital 天津市沽漢醫院. *Tianjin Medicine* 天津醫藥 29: 75, 1977.

11 Tang Zong-Ming 湯宗明. *Journal of Integrated Chinese and Western Medicine* 中西醫結合雜誌 3(1): 19, 1983.

12 Xue Fang 薛芳. *Tianjin Medicine* 天津醫藥 9: 566, 1980.

13 Xue Fang 薛芳. *Journal of Traditional Chinese Medicine* 中醫雜誌 22(9): 664, 1981.

14 Xue Fang 薛芳. *New Chinese Medicine* 新中醫 10: 21, 1983.

15 Liu Gui-Lian 劉桂蓮. *Journal of Traditional Chinese Medicine* 中醫雜誌 26(10): 766, 1985.

16 Shen Ji-Ze 沈繼澤. *Jiangsu Journal of Traditional Chinese Medicine* 江蘇中醫雜誌 1: 40, 1083.

17 Wang Yun-Feng 王雲峰. *Zhejiang Journal of Traditional Chinese Medicine* 浙江中醫雜誌 10: 472, 1982.

18 Higuchi Kazuko, et al. 樋和自等 (Zhuo Shu-Li, translator 濯書利節譯). *Overseas Medicine: Chinese Medicine and Pharmacology Fascicle* 國外醫學 (中醫中藥分冊) 6: 19, 1981.

19 Zhou Guan-Ying 趙冠英. *Selected Materials on Our Motherland's Medicine* 祖國醫學資料選編, Beijing: People's Liberation Army General Hospital 中國人民解放軍總醫院 page 201, 1978.

20 Niu Shu-Hua 牛淑華. *Medical Science Report* 醫藥科技簡報 4: 23, 1977.

21 Arichi Shigeshi 有地滋. *Medicine and Pharmacology* 醫學と藥學 9(3): 901, 1983.

22 Zheng Jin-Feng 鄭晉豐. *New Traditional Chinese Medicine* 新中醫 1: 37, 1979.

23 Chen Hou-Zhong 陳厚忠. *Hunan Journal of Traditional Chinese Medicine* 湖南醫藥雜誌 3: 44, 1984.

24 Zhao Shi-Kui 趙士魁. *Shanghai Journal of Traditional Chinese Medicine* 上海中醫藥雜誌 6: 20, 1984.

25 Gai Shi-Chang 蓋世昌. *Journal of Traditional Chinese Medicine* 中醫藥學報
    1: 34, 1987.

26 Yao Guang-Bi 姚光弼. *Medical Information Exchange* 醫學情報交流 4: 54,
    1977.

27 Chinese International Mother and Child Peace and Welfare Pediatric Conference
    中國福利會國際和平婦幼保健院兒科. *New Journal of Traditional Chinese
    Medicine* 新醫藥學雜誌 8: 21, 1973.

28 Ma Rong-Geng 馬榮庚. *Journal of Integrated Chinese and Western Medicine*
    中西結合雜誌 4(7): 402,1984.

29 *Compilation of the Experience from Modern Chinese Traditional Medicine Currents*
    近代中醫流派經驗選集. Shanghai: Shanghai Science and Technology
    Publishing House 上海科技出版社 page 136, 1962.

Chapter 5: **Astragalus Formula Family**

1   Yi Ning-Yu 易寧育. *Collected Abstracts from the Plenary Meeting of the First
    Congress of the Chinese Pharmacological Society* 全國藥理學會成立大會第一屆
    全國藥理會學術會議文摘要彙編 (Chengdu), page 88, 1977.

2   Chen Mei-Fang 陳梅芳. *Shanghai Journal of Traditional Chinese Medicine*
    上海中醫藥雜誌 6: 16, 1979.

3   Wu Bao-De 吳葆德. *New Medicine* 新醫學 6: 298, 1984.

4   Gu Zhi-Ping 谷志平. *Hebei Traditional Chinese Medicine* 河北中醫 6: 11,
    1987.

5   Li Liang-De 李量德. *Clinical Chinese Traditional Medicine and Health
    Preservation* 中醫臨床與保健 4: 14, 1990.

6   Jin Xue-Ren 金學仁. *Journal of Traditional Chinese Medicine* 中醫雜誌
    1: 72, 1982.

7   Fu Zhong-Fen付忠芬. *Jilin Traditional Chinese Medicine* 吉林中醫藥
    4: 29, 1982.

8   Liu Shan-Yuan 劉善元. *Journal of Traditional Chinese Medicine* 中醫雜誌
    3: 20, 1963.

9   Li Wei-Pu 李蔚普. *Jiangxi Traditional Chinese Medicine* 江西中醫藥
    6: 43, 1955.

10 Gan Can-Qi甘燦其. *Guangxi Traditional Chinese Medicine* 廣西中醫藥
    3: 9, 1979.

11   Li Guo-Zhi 李國治. *Hubei Journal of Traditional Chinese Medicine* 湖北中醫雜誌 5: 30, 1980.

12   Zou Zhi-Sheng 鄒志生. *Journal of New Medicine* 新醫藥學雜誌 11: 26, 1974.

13   Gu Xiao-Chi 顧小痴. *Tianjin Journal of Medicine* 天津醫藥雜誌 2(1): 4, 1960.

14   Chen Zhi-Gao 陳芝高. *Shanghai Journal of Traditional Chinese Medicine* 上海中醫藥雜誌 10: 28, 1983.

15   He Zhi-Jun 何志軍. *Hebei Traditional Chinese Medicine* 河北中醫 2: 33, 1984.

16   Cao Ming-Gao 曹鳴高. *Journal of Traditional Chinese Medicine* 中醫雜誌 6: 397, 1958.

17   Cao Ming-Gao 曹鳴高. *Journal of the Nanjing College of Traditional Chinese Medicine* 南京中醫學院報 1: 44, 1959.

18   Takada Shigeru 武田重之等. *Study of Kampo* 漢方醫學 8(12): 32, 1984.

19   Wang Xing-Jie et al. 王行潔等. *Journal of Traditional Chinese Medicine* 中醫雜誌 6: 434, 1984.

20   Zheng Yuan-Pang 鄭源龐. *Zhejiang Journal of Traditional Chinese Medicine* 浙江中醫雜誌 12: 547, 1986.

Chapter 6: **Gypsum Formula Family**

1   Guo Zi-Guang 郭子光. *New Edition of the Discussion of Cold Damage Decoction Presentations* 傷寒論湯證新編. Shanghai: Shanghai Science and Technology Press 上海科學技術出版社 page 162, 1983.

2   Qiu Fu-Xi 丘福喜. *China Journal of Medicine* 中醫學雜誌 7: 456, 1964.

3   Heilong River Production-Construction Corps Medical Team 黑龍江生產建設兵團衛生隊. *Heilong River Medicine* 黑龍江醫藥 1: 31, 1976.

4   Yao Hua 姚華. *Jiangsu Journal of Traditional Chinese Medicine* 江蘇中醫雜誌 1: 9, 1986.

5   Tao Jun-Ren 陶君仁. *Jiangsu Traditional Chinese Medicine* 江蘇中醫 39: 12, 1963.

6   Xia Yi-Jun 夏奕鈞. *Journal of the Nanjing University of Traditional Chinese Medicine* 南京中醫學院學報 3: 39, 1994.

7   Xiao Run-Hua 肖潤華. *Integrated Chinese and Western Ophthalmology* 中西結合眼科 1: 31, 1982.

8 Yao Fang-Wei 姚芳蔚. *Shanghai Journal of Traditional Chinese Medicine* 上海中醫雜誌 4: 23, 1964.

9 Cheng Rong-Zhao et al. 程榮昭等. *Sichuan Traditional Medical Study* 四川醫學 2: 100, 1982.

10 Xu Yi-Hou 徐宜厚. *Liaoning Journal of Traditional Chinese Medicine* 遼寧中醫雜誌 7: 29, 1982.

11 Yue Mei-Zhong 岳美中. *New Chinese Medicine* 新醫學 3: 32, 1973.

12 Kimura Masayasu 木村正康. *Proceedings of the First Sino-Japanese Medicine Symposium* 第一回和漢藥討論會記錄 page 14, 1967.

13 Dong Zhi-Zhong 董治中. *Jilin Traditional Chinese Medicine* 吉林中醫藥 1: 19, 1983.

14 Guo Zhen-Qiu 郭振球. *Shanghai Journal of Traditional Chinese Medicine* 上海中醫雜誌 7: 29, 1959.

15 Shanghai College of Traditional Chinese Medicine 上海中醫學院. *Chinese Medicine Almanac* 中醫年鑒, Beijing: People's Medical Publishing House 人民衛生出版社 page 88, 1983.

16 Cheng Zhen-Xiang 程珍祥. *Hebei Journal of Traditional Chinese Medicine* 河北中醫雜誌 2: 28, 1981.

17 Li Da-Xiang 李達祥. *Journal of Traditional Chinese Medicine* 中醫雜誌 8: 14, 1963.

18 Wang Yan-Bin 王彥彬. *People's Liberation Army Medicine* 人民軍醫 3: 69, 1981.

19 Li Xue-Sheng 李學聲. *Hubei Journal of Traditional Chinese Medicine* 湖北中醫雜誌 3: 20, 1985.

20 Xu Rong-Xi 徐榮喜. *Journal of Integrated Chinese and Western Medicine* 中西結合雜誌 12: 725, 1988.

Chapter 7: Coptis Formula Family

1 Araki Goro 荒木五郎. *Kampo for Sequela of Cerebral Vascular Accidents in the Elderly* 高齢者の脳血管障礙後遺證と漢方 Iyaku Journal Company, page 198, 1991.

2 Ibid., 124.

3 Ibid., 51.

4 Ma Xiao-Zhong 馬曉中. *Hubei Journal of Traditional Chinese Medicine* 湖北中醫雜誌 19: 33, 1984.

5　Guo Wen-rong 郭文榮. *Sichuan Traditional Chinese Medicine* 四川中醫 7: 38, 1986.

6　Xu Guang-Bin 徐光彬. *Journal of the Chengdu University of Traditional Chinese Medicine* 成都中醫學院報 10: 45, 1980.

7　Pang Hua-Wei 龐華威. *Shanghai Journal of Traditional Chinese Medicine and Pharmacology* 上海中醫藥雜誌 19: 26, 1986.

8　Zhou Wei-Xin 周維新. *Chinese Journal of Internal Medicine* 中華內科雜誌 59: 464, 1960.

9　Jinan City Number Three Hospital 濟南市立第三醫院. *Periodical of Shandong Medicine* 山東醫刊 8: 43, 1960.

10　Li Huan-Ruo 李煥若. *Sichuan Traditional Chinese Medicine* 四川中醫 7: 31, 1986.

11　Gao Feng-Cai 高鳳才. *Zhejiang Journal of Traditional Chinese Medicine* 浙江中醫雜誌 3: 105, 1987.

12　Zheng Chang-Xiong 鄭昌雄. *Shanghai Journal of Traditional Chinese Medicine and Pharmacology* 上海中醫藥雜誌 12: 21, 1963.

Chapter 8: **Dried Ginger Formula Family**

1　China Kongmou Hospital Department of Internal Medicine 中國空某醫院內科. *New Journal of Medicine and Pharmocology* 新醫藥雜誌 7: 30, 1977.

2　Diao Ben-Shu 刁本恕. *Sichuan Traditional Chinese Medicine* 四川中醫 3: 25, 1986.

3　Zhang Xiu-Yun 張岫雲. *Journal of Traditional Chinese Medicine* 中醫雜誌 2: 23, 1966.

4　Chen Qi-Wu 陳其五. *Journal of the Chengdu University of Traditional Chinese Medicine* 成都中醫學院報 2: 21, 1988.

5　Ma Shu-Sheng 馬蜀生. *Journal of New Medicine and Pharmacology* 新醫藥學雜誌 2: 39, 1976.

6　Nie Ji-Nan 聶季南. *Zhejiang Journal of Traditional Chinese Medicine* 浙江中醫雜誌 2: 77, 1980.

Chapter 9: **Aconite Formula Family**

1　Tianjin Nankai Hospital 天津南開醫院. *Tianjin Medicine Report* 天津醫藥通訊 11: 1, 1972.

2 Tianjin Nankai Hospital 天津南開醫院. *Journal of New Medicine* 新醫藥學雜誌 3: 117, 1974.

3 Han Xin et al. 韓新等. *Chinese Patent Medicine Research* 中成藥研究 2: 26, 1983.

4 Wang Wan-Qing 汪萬頃. *Zhejiang Journal of Traditional Chinese Medicine* 浙江中醫雜誌 8: 14, 1984.

5 Beijing College of Chinese Medicine 北京醫學院. *Journal of the Beijing College of Traditional Chinese Medicine* 北京醫學院報 3: 1974.

6 Editorial Committee for the Case Histories of Fan Zhong-Lin 范中林醫案整理小組編. *Fan Zhong-Lin's Selected Cases Using Six Stage Differentiation* 范中林六經辨證醫案選 Shenyang: Liaoning Science and Technology Publishing Press 遼寧科技出版社 1984.

7 Pei Liang-Huan et al. 裴良懷等. *Journal of Traditional Chinese Medicine* 中醫雜誌 21(3): 190, 1980.

8 Ke Xue-Fan 柯雪帆. *Shanghai Journal of Traditional Chinese Medicine and Pharmacology* 上海中醫藥雜誌 6: 7, 1964.

9 Ma Shu-Sheng 馬蜀生. *Anqing Medicine* 安慶醫學 1: 35, 1987.

10 Yao Tian-Yuan 姚天源. *Fujian Traditional Chinese Medicine* 福建醫藥 5: 20, 1981.

11 Zhou Lian-Shan, et al. 周連山等. *Journal of Traditional Chinese Medicine* 中醫雜誌 9: 20, 1965.

Chapter 10: **Pinellia Formula Family**

1 *Journal of the Xian College of Medicine* 西安醫學院報 5: 105, 1958.

2 Chinese Academy of Medical Sciences Information Group 中國醫學科學院情報組. *New Medicine* 新醫學 1: 25, 1974.

3 Wang Zi-De 王子德. *Sichuan Traditional Medicine* 西川中醫 2: 26, 1983.

4 Cai Hui-Qun 蔡惠群. *Zhejiang Journal of Traditional Chinese Medicine* 浙江用以雜誌 5: 5, 1958.

5 Wang Jun-Guo 王俊國. *Shanxi Traditional Chinese Medicine* 陝西中醫 3: 139, 1987.

6 Wang Ji-You 王吉友. *Liaoning Intermediate Medical Journal* 遼寧中級醫刊 6: 51, 1978.

7 Lin Jia-Kun 林家坤. *Jiangxi Traditional Chinese Medicine* 江西中醫藥 2: 20, 1986.

8   Yan Zong-Ling 閻宗玲. *Barefoot Doctor* 赤腳醫生 1: 15, 1979. (Shandong Changwei District Department of Health)

9   Wang Hai-Zhou 王海州. *Henan Traditional Chinese Medicine* 河南中醫 3: 24, 1985.

10 Chen Ke-Zhong et al. 陳克忠等. *Journal of the Shandong Medical College* 山東醫學院報 3: 61, 1978.

11 Guo Guo-Dong 郭國棟. *Zhejiang Journal of Traditional Chinese Medicine* 浙江中醫雜誌 11: 496, 1986.

12 Zhang Xiao-Ping 張笑平. *Journal of New Medicine* 新醫藥學雜誌 8(3): 19, 1984.

13 Sugimoto Kotaro 杉本浩郎. *Kampo Medicine* 漢方醫學 8 (3): 19, 1984.

14 Okuda Takashi 奧田隆司. *Japanese Journal of Traditional Japanese Medicine* 日本東洋醫學雜誌 4: 16, 1986.

Index